MW01000263

Geriatric Physical Therapy

A Case Study Approach

NOTICE

Medicine is an ever-changing science. As new research and clinical experience broaden our knowledge, changes in treatment and drug therapy are required. The authors and the publisher of this work have checked with sources believed to be reliable in their efforts to provide information that is complete and generally in accord with the standards accepted at the time of publication. However, in view of the possibility of human error or changes in medical sciences, neither the authors nor the publisher nor any other party who has been involved in the preparation or publication of this work warrants that the information contained herein is in every respect accurate or complete, and they disclaim all responsibility for any errors or omissions, or for the results obtained from use of the information contained in this work. Readers are encouraged to confirm the information contained herein with other sources. For example and in particular, readers are advised to check the product information sheet included in the package of each drug they plan to administer to be certain that the information contained in this work is accurate and that changes have not been made in the recommended dose or in the contraindications for administration. This recommendation is of particular importance in connection with new or infrequently used drugs.

Geriatric Physical Therapy
A Case Study Approach

Editor

William H. Staples, PT, DHSc, DPT, GCS, CEEAA

President, Academy of Geriatric Physical Therapy
Associate Professor of Physical Therapy
Krannert School of Physical Therapy
University of Indianapolis
Indianapolis, Indiana

Section Editors:

Jill Heitzman, PT, DPT, GCS, NCS, CWS, CEEAA, FACCWS
Associate Professor of Physical Therapy Program
College of Health Sciences
Alabama State University
Montgomery, Alabama

Meri Goehring, PT, PhD, GCS, CWS
Asssociate Professor of Physical Therapy
College of Health Professions
Grand Valley State University
Cook-DeVos Center
Grand Rapids, Michigan

Deborah A. Kegelmeyer, PT, DPT, MS, GCS
Associate Professor of Clinical Health and Rehabilitation Sciences
Physical Therapy Division
The Ohio State University
Columbus, Ohio

William H. Staples, PT, DHSc, DPT, GCS, CEEAA
President, Academy of Geriatric Physical Therapy
Associate Professor of Physical Therapy
Krannert School of Physical Therapy
University of Indianapolis
Indianapolis, Indiana

New York   Chicago   San Francisco   Athens   London   Madrid
Mexico City   Milan   New Delhi   Singapore   Sydney   Toronto

Geriatric Physical Therapy

Copyright © 2016 by McGraw-Hill Education. All rights reserved. Printed in China.
Except as permitted under the United States Copyright Act of 1976, no part of this
publication may be reproduced or distributed in any form or by any means, or stored
in a database or retrieval system, without the prior written permission of the publisher.

1 2 3 4 5 6 7 8 9 0 DSS/DSS 20 19 18 17 16

ISBN 978-0-07-182542-9
MHID 0-07-182542-8

This book was set in Minion Pro 9/11 by MPS Limited.
The editors were Michael Weitz and Brian Kearns.
The production supervisor was Richard Ruzycka.
Project management was provided by Charu Khanna, MPS Ltd.
The text designer was Alan Barnett.
The cover designer was Dreamit, Inc.
RR Donnelley/Shenzhen was printer and binder.

This book was printed on acid-free paper.

Library of Congress Cataloging-in-Publication Data
Names: Staples, William, 1956- , author. | Kegelmeyer, Deb, author. | Heitzman, Jill, author.
Title: Geriatric physical therapy / William Staples, Deb Kegelmeyer, Jill Heitzman.
Description: New York : McGraw-Hill, 2016. | Includes bibliographical references.
Identifiers: LCCN 2015046543 (print) | LCCN 2015047053 (ebook) | ISBN 9780071825429 |
  ISBN 0071825428 | ISBN 007182409X ()
Subjects: | MESH: Physical Therapy Modalities | Aged | Geriatric Assessment | Geriatrics—methods | Case Reports
Classification: LCC RC953.5 (print) | LCC RC953.5 (ebook) | NLM WB 460 | DDC
  615.5/47—dc23
LC record available at http://lccn.loc.gov/2015046543

McGraw-Hill Education books are available at special quantity discounts to use as premiums and
sales promotions, or for use in corporate training programs. To contact a representative, please visit
the Contact Us pages at www.mhprofessional.com.

CONTENTS

CHAPTER 1

Introduction to Geriatric Physical Therapy
William H. Staples

CHAPTER 2

Musculoskeletal Cases

CHAPTER 3

Neuromuscular Cases

CHAPTER 4

Cardiovascular and Pulmonary Cases

CHAPTER 5

Integumentary Cases

CHAPTER 6

Medically Complex Cases

CHAPTER 7

Other Geriatric Issues

x

CONTENTS

Steven B. Ambler, PT, DPT, MPH, CPH, OCS
Assistant Professor, Coordinating Faculty USF-UWF Partnership
School of Physical Therapy & Rehabilitation Sciences
USF Health Morsani College of Medicine
University of South Florida, Tampa, Florida

Bill Anderson, PT, DPT, GCS, CEEAA, COS-C
Director, Therapy Practice
VNA Home Health Hospice
Eastern Maine Health System
South Portland, Maine

Stacey Brickson, PT, PhD, ATC
Assistant Professor, Physical Therapy Program
Department of Orthopedics and Rehabilitation
University of Wisconsin–Madison, Madison, Wisconsin

James S. Carlson, MPT, CCS
Cardiopulmonary Residency Specialist, William S Middleton VA Hospital
Honorary Associate/Fellow, Department of Orthopedics and Rehabilitation
Doctor of Physical Therapy Program
University of Wisconsin–Madison
Madison, Wisconsin

Cathy H. Ciolek, PT, DPT, GCS, CEEAA
Assistant Professor, Department of Physical Therapy
University of Delaware, Newark, Delaware

Mitchell L. Cordova, ATC, PhD, FNATA, FACSM
Professor and Dean, College of Health Professions and Social Work
Florida Gulf Coast University
Fort Myers, Florida

James R. Creps, PT, DScPT, OCS, CMPT
Associate Director, Post-Professional Education
Assistant Professor, Department of Physical Therapy
School of Health Professions and Studies
University of Michigan-Flint, Flint, Michigan

Linda M. deLaBruere, PT, GCS
Physical Therapist, Mercy Hospital Rehabilitation Department
Eastern Maine Health System
Portland, Maine

Sarah Dudley, MPT, GCS, CEEAA
Physical Therapy Lead, VNA Home Health Hospice
Eastern Maine Health System
South Portland, Maine

Ahmed Elokda, PT, PhD, CLT, CEEAA, FAACVPR
Associate Professor, Department of Rehabilitation Sciences
Florida Gulf Coast University, Fort Myers, Florida

Christopher C. Felton, DO, ATC
Family Medicine
New Hanover Regional Medical Center
Wilmington, North Carolina

Meri Goehring, PT, PhD, GCS, CWS
Asssociate Professor, Physical Therapy
College of Health Professions
Grand Valley State University
Cook-DeVos Center
Grand Rapids, Michigan

Jana Grant, OT/L, MS
Occupational Therapist, VNA Home Health Hospice
Eastern Maine Health System
South Portland, Maine

Michael O. Harris-Love, PT, MPT, DSc
Deputy Director, Polytrauma/TBI Rehabilitation Research Fellowship
Director, The Muscle Morphology, Mechanics, and Performance Laboratory
Veterans Affairs Medical Center
Geriatrics and Extended Care Service
Washington, DC

Greg Hartley, PT, DPT, GCS, CEEAA
Assistant Professor, Clinical Physical Therapy
University of Miami, Miller School of Medicine
Coral Gables, Florida

Jill Heitzman, PT, DPT, GCS, NCS, CWS, CEEAA, FACCWS
Associate Professor, Physical Therapy Program
College of Health Sciences
Alabama State University
Montgomery, Alabama

Haniel J. Hernandez, PT, DPT
Research Fellow, Polytrauma/TBI Rehabilitation
Veterans Affairs Medical Center
Physical Medicine & Rehabilitation
Washington, DC

Katie Houghtaling, MSPT, GCS, CEEAA
Physical Therapist, VNA Home Health Hospice
Eastern Maine Health System
South Portland, Maine

Lucy H. Jones, PT, DPT, MHA, GCS, CEEAA
Owner, Rehabilitative Therapy Services
Adjunct Instructor, Geriatric Clinical Specialist
Drexel University, Philadelphia, Pennsylvania

Kyle Katz, PT, DPT
Alumnus, University of Indianapolis
HealthSouth Rehabilitation Hospital of the Woodlands
Conroe, Texas

CONTRIBUTORS

Timothy L. Kauffman, PT, PhD, FAPTA, FGSA

Kauffman Physical Therapy
Lancaster, Pennsylvania

Deborah A. Kegelmeyer, PT, DPT, MS, GCS

Associate Professor, Clinical Health and Rehabilitation Sciences
Physical Therapy Division
The Ohio State University
Columbus, Ohio

Julia Levesque LeRoy, PT, GCS

Physical Therapist, Community Health and Nursing Services, CHANS
Home Health Care, Mid Coast-Parkview Health
Brunswick, Maine

Amy M. Lilley, PT, GCS, CEEAA

Physical Therapist, VNA Home Health Hospice
Eastern Maine Health System
South Portland, Maine

Stacy Martin, PT, CEEAA

Physical Therapist, Cardiopulmonary and Telehealth Team
VNA Home Health Hospice
Eastern Maine Health System
South Portland, Maine

Lise McCarthy, PT, DPT, GCS

President, McCarthy's Interactive Physical Therapy
San Francisco, California
Assistant Clinical Professor, Department of Physical Therapy and Rehabilitation
University of California, San Francisco

Oseas Florencio de Moura Filho, PT (Brazil), MSc

Director, Physical Therapy Department
Physios - Clínica de Saúde Funcional Ltda.
Teresina, Piauí, Brazil

Erin N. Pauley, DPT, MS, ATC, CSCS

Texas Physical Therapy Specialists
San Antonio, Texas

Marangela Prysiazny Obispo, PT, DPT, GCS

Program Director, Physical Therapist Assistant Program
Keiser University Miami Campus
Miami, Florida

Rose M. Pignataro, PT, PhD, DPT, CWS

Assistant Professor, Department of Rehabilitation Sciences
Florida Gulf Coast University
Fort Myers, Florida

Ingrid Quartarol, PT, MS

Director, Pilates Contemporany (Brazil, Spain)
Professor, Unichristus University, Fortaleza, Ceara, Brazil

Elysa Roberts, OTR, PhD

Senior Lecturer, Department of Occupational Therapy
School of Health Sciences, Faculty of Health & Medicine
University of Newcastle, Callaghan
New South Wales, Australia

Eric Shamus, PT, DPT, PhD

Chair & Associate Professor, Department of Rehabilitation Sciences
Florida Gulf Coast University
Fort Myers, Florida

Jennifer Shamus, PT, DPT, PhD

Market Manager, Select Physical Therapy
Pembroke Pines, Florida

Nikki Snyder, PT, DPT, OCS, CSCS

Staff Physical Therapist, Orthopedic Clinical Specialist
Certified Strength and Conditioning Specialist
North Florida South Georgia Veteran's Administration
The Villages, Florida

Wendy Song, DO

Family Medicine Resident
Beth Israel Medical Center
New York, New York

Linda R. Staples, RN, BS, MA

Clinical Nurse Specialist, Retired

William H. Staples, PT, DHSc, DPT, GCS, CEEAA

President, Academy of Geriatric Physical Therapy
Associate Professor, Physical Therapy
Krannert School of Physical Therapy
University of Indianapolis
Indianapolis, Indiana

Arie J. van Duijn, PT, EdD, OCS

Associate Professor and Director, Doctor of Physical Therapy Program
Department of Rehabilitation Sciences
Florida Gulf Coast University
Fort Myers, Florida

Natalie V. Wessel, DO, MPH

Resident Physician, Department of Obstetrics and Gynecology
UC Davis Medical Center
Sacramento, California

PREFACE

I began teaching at the University of Indianapolis in 2003. With an expertise in geriatrics, I was anxious to teach in the lifespan sequence (two semesters) to our entry-level Doctor of Physical Therapy students. One area I found lacking was how to relate general knowledge to the aspect of direct care. I found case studies a great way to have the students see that aging changes accompany the older adult and are not separate issues. While this text took only a year to compile and edit, a lifetime of learning and planning went into this endeavor.

This text is meant to serve several purposes. This text is designed to be utilized as an adjunct throughout the Doctor of Physical Therapy curriculum. This text can be used with a general pathology course, an aging, lifespan, or gerontology (geriatric physical therapy) course. This text can also be a helpful study guide for the licensing exam, or even the geriatric specialty exam. The cases run the gamut from simple to challenging to complex that require advanced learning and study. The case studies or vignettes here are designed to have students investigate several aspects of a specific primary diagnosis. Students and even experienced clinicians moving into the field of geriatric physical therapy need to know and understand how to assess the functional ability of the older adult and why a focus on function is important. They will need to know how to perform a comprehensive geriatric assessment including strategies to enhance communication with their older patients in order to develop an overall plan for treatment and long-term follow-up.

I look forward to hearing from users of the text for updates, additional information, and even new cases for any future editions. I hope that my love and passion for this specialty area of practice can be appreciated and followed.

ACKNOWLEDGMENTS

I want to acknowledge all of my former patients who have taught me more about the practice of physical therapy and what it means to age than I would have discovered on my own. I am grateful to all of you. Most of the cases I have written are based on actual patients who have become part of this text. My desire is to impart that knowledge acquired from those patients to the next generation of geriatric physical therapists.

I want to thank all the authors of the cases presented in this text; without their assistance and dedication this book would not have made it to a publisher. More specifically, I would like to thank Jill Heitzman, PT, DPT, GCS, NCS, CWS, CEEAA, FACCWS, Deborah A. Kegelmeyer, PT, DPT, MS, GCS, and Meri Goehring, PT, PhD, GCS, CWS as lead writers. A special thanks also to James R. Creps, PT, DScPT, OCS, CMPT, and Eric Shamus, PT, DPT, PhD, for their special additions to this text.

To all my former and current coworkers, thank you for your help along my professional journey. To my former and current students, I hope to generate a passion for working with the older adult. You have pushed me to become a better teacher, a better scholar, and a better therapist. I hope that some of my passion rubs off onto you and you take up a career with providing services to older adults.

Lastly, to my wife Linda, and my two daughters Catherine and Courtney, thank you for being part of my life to enable me to complete this project.

ABOUT THE EDITOR

William H. "Bill" Staples, PT, DHSc, DPT, GCS, CEEAA, has demonstrated service to the physical therapy profession at the component and national levels, with a focus on progressing clinical practice, ensuring quality in the physical therapy licensure process, and advancement of the Academy of Geriatric Physical Therapy (AGPT, formerly the Section on Geriatrics).

Currently, he is an Associate Professor in the entry-level Doctorate of Physical Therapy Program of the Krannert School of Physical Therapy, the Doctor of Health Sciences, and for the Center for Aging and Community at the University of Indianapolis. Dr Staples has previously served as the Program Director of the university's Physical Therapist Assistant Program. He has also held an academic role with Ivy Tech State College (PTA program) in Muncie, Indiana. Staples received his Doctor of Health Science (DHSc) and Doctor of Physical Therapy (DPT) from the University of Indianapolis, an MS and Certificate in Physical Therapy from Columbia University, and BA in Zoology from Ohio Wesleyan University.

Over the past 20 years, Staples' leadership and service has resulted in such honors as the Academy of Geriatric Physical Therapy's Distinguished Educator Award, the President's Award, and the Joan M Mills Award. In 2014, he received the Lucy Blair Service Award from the APTA for exceptional service to that organization. He also received the Outstanding Faculty (University of Indianapolis) Award for Exceptional Service to the University in 2014.

He was highly involved in the Geriatric Specialty Council and the Board of ABPTS, with work that included the development of the specialty certification process and a significant increase in the numbers of clinical specialists. In addition, Staples has served on the Specialization Academy of Content Experts and is currently a lead reviewer for APTA clinical residency and fellowship programs, including the evaluation of multiple new clinical residency programs over the past 4 years. He served on the Item Bank Review Committee of FSBPT for 6 years and chair for 3 of those years. He has demonstrated commitment to enhancing clinical practice through increasing clinical practice knowledge through presentations and contributions to research. Since 1984, he has given more than 50 presentations in a variety of settings, with written contributions in texts, peer-reviewed journals, and PTNow that have contributed to evidence-based practice.

An APTA member since 1979, Staples has served the Academy of Geriatric Physical Therapy since 1984, and is a member of the Neurology Section since 2004 and Home Health Section since 1989. He has been involved with the Indiana Chapter of the APTA since 1990, and in 2012 received the Chapter's Anthony D. Certo Award "for distinguished contribution of time, energy, and expertise toward furthering physical therapy as professional practice." He is currently President of the Academy of Geriatric Physical Therapy and has served on the Board of Directors for 9 years, 6 as Treasurer. In 2008, he was inducted into Sigma Phi Omega, a national professional society for gerontology.

Dr Staples has lectured nationally on a variety of geriatric physical therapy issues and is an instructor in the Certification for Exercise Experts for Aging Adults program offered by the AGPT. His research has investigated exercise and Parkinson disease, fear of falling, and attitudes toward working with patients with dementia. He maintains his clinical skills by working part-time in home health care.

1

Introduction to Geriatric Physical Therapy

WILLIAM H. STAPLES, PT, DHSC, DPT, GCS, CEEAA

Case studies are utilized as a way for students to learn the principles of geriatric assessment including physical, cognitive, social, psychological, and environmental assessments. Goals are to promote wellness, independence and successfully maintaining or improving the quality of life for the patients who we see. As physical therapists we focus on function and mobility performance (gait, balance, transfers). In today's payment situation, we must be efficient in our ability to perform rapid screens to identify target areas for examination and then intervention. But in the older population we must at the same time be vigilant so that complications from comorbidities, "yellow" or "red" flags, do not escape us.

EXAMINATION OF THE GERIATRIC PATIENT

The core to determining what interventions need to be performed is first performing a comprehensive evaluation and examination. This is necessary for all patients. This chapter is not a guideline about how to perform an evaluation but some special thoughts to consider with older individuals. As we age, the incidence of chronic diseases and wear-and-tear injuries add to the normal aging changes, requiring in-depth questioning and use of functional tests and measures. As people age, it becomes more difficult to adapt to stresses placed on the body, our organ system's capacity decreases, function decreases, and impairments and disabilities increase. The geriatric physical therapy examination must consider all biopsychosocial realms of the patient both internal and external that may not affect the outcomes in the same way as some younger individuals. The elderly individual who comes to physical therapy is usually dealing with many physical, social, and psychological changes. Environmental factors including housing, home safety, transportation will affect how the older clients' needs will be addressed. As an example think about the patient seen by a physical therapist who may be going under a great deal of stress and is justifiably concerned about the illness of a spouse or the potential of becoming institutionalized themselves. For treatment techniques taught in physical therapy school, students are often taught in silos, meaning that they learn range of motion (ROM), manual muscle testing (MMT), sensation, transfers, etc, without adequate synthesis of these procedures into older adults. For instance, measuring ROM and performing MMT on fellow students may translate into the students believing that all older adults are not "normal."

How does the evaluation of a geriatric client differ from a middle-aged adult? The middle-aged patient may be coming to physical therapy for a specific problem, perhaps carpal tunnel. The therapist would try to determine the mechanism of injury and then determine how to prevent further worsening of the condition and how to resolve that specific condition. The therapist would typically not need to worry about many other factors that affect the older adult. The geriatric physical therapist may need to consider that the patient also has osteoarthritis in the contralateral knee and is using a cane in the painful wrist (which may even be the cause). Without the use of the cane the patient would be unable to safely ambulate and increase the risk for a fall, but use of the cane would make the primary condition more severe. Add to this a metabolic or heart condition and one could see how a simple orthopedic problem becomes complex.

Some problems are more common or expressed more severely in older adults. Falls or the fear of them, syncope, urinary incontinence, spinal stenosis, osteoporosis, postural hypotension, accidental hypothermia, or hip fractures are frequently seen in older adults and rarely considered in younger patients. Chronic diseases also make their appearances as people age.

To engage in a comprehensive geriatric assessment the therapist should try to control the environment by being in a well-lit room (but no glare) and avoid backlighting, minimize extraneous noise such as background music, and minimize complex situations such as a crowded gym or interruptions. The older person generally has diminished senses and proper environmental conditions are important for the patient to remain focused. Always introduce yourself, address the patient by last name, face the patient directly, sit at or squat to eye level, speak slowly in a deep tone, and ask open-ended questions such as, "What would you like me to do for you?" or "Why are you here today?" The exception to this would be a patient with dementia, in which case yes/no questions would work the best. With older adults the therapist will need to determine if hearing deficits are present. The therapist may need to raise voice volume accordingly and speak with a lower tone and more distinctly. If necessary, write questions in large print and make sure to allow ample time for the patient to answer.

The complete physical assessment of an older client should include not only functional status, physical therapists are great about that, but also medications, nutrition, hydration, vision, and hearing. Asking about medications may lead you to find a diagnosis the patient forgot to tell you about. For instance a patient taking a diuretic, a β-blocker, and an ACE inhibitor might tell you "no" when asked if they had hypertension. The patient is not lying, the patient thought that control of the disease was the same as not having the condition, or perhaps worse, did not know or remember why they were taking the drugs. Older adults take many medications (polypharmacy) that can cause interactions between them, resulting in additional problems. Patients with advanced life-limiting illness commonly take a number of disease-specific medications as well as medications for symptoms and comorbidities.[1]

Polypharmacy is the excessive and/or unnecessary use of medications that can result in a geriatric patient receiving large numbers of drugs that are unnecessary or perhaps even harmful. Polypharmacy can be associated with increased risk of adverse events, decreased quality of life, and increased financial burden.[2] Discontinuing unnecessary medications may improve the patient's overall well-being, but determining which medications may be safely discontinued can be difficult.[3,4] A number of textbooks and Web sites contain vital information concerning medications and many of the cases within this text can be utilized to understand side effects and possible drug interactions. A variety of websites have been utilized in this text to familiarize students and therapists, but this author has a preference for Drugs.com which is used extensively, but the author encourages each individual to choose their preference.

Polypharmacy can be seen in the use of drugs to treat adverse reactions to primary medications, or concurrent use of synergistic medications or the use of duplicate medications to obtain a positive result, and sometimes the use of medications to counteract the side effects of another drug. Concurrent use of interacting medications or use of contraindicated medications can also occur.

Alterations in drug response can be attributed to differences in the way the body handles the drug (pharmacokinetic changes), and differences in the way the drug affects the body (pharmacodynamic changes). Pharmacokinetic changes with age alter how the drug is absorbed, distributed, metabolized, and excreted. Age-related changes play the largest role in pharmacokinetic changes with age due to decreased absorption through the gastrointestinal tract, decreased total body water, decreased total body mass, decreased plasma protein concentrations, and increased fat affects lipid and water soluble medications. As people age there is a reduced ability of the kidneys to excrete drugs. The total drug metabolizing capacity of the liver decreases as we age so drugs remain active longer. Reduced ability of the kidneys to excrete drugs due to declines in renal blood flow, renal mass, and function of the renal tubules also causes drugs to stay in the body longer. Lipid-soluble drugs may build up and be stored in the fat and cause problems when released. The cumulative effect of the pharmacokinetic changes of aging is that drugs are often allowed to remain active for longer periods of time or deliver more drugs to the receptor site, thus prolonging drug effects and increasing the risk for toxic side effects. An example of this would be the half-life of drugs like benzodiazepines (Valium, Xanax), which can be extended by as much as fourfold.[5] An example of more drugs being delivered is aspirin which normally binds to plasma proteins, making it less active. In older adults this will produce a greater response from the aspirin since more aspirin will actually reach the target tissue as there are less plasma proteins available to bind to the aspirin.[6] Drug distribution changes can be substantial with aging, and with more drugs the risk of adverse drug reactions do not just multiply, they increase exponentially.

Pharmacodynamics is how the drug affects the body. The aging process may induce more or less sensitivity to particular medications. This is especially noteworthy for medications that affect the cardiovascular and central nervous systems. Changes that may affect pharmacodynamics include deficits in homeostatic control of circulation (decreased baroreceptor sensitivity, decreased vascular compliance) which may, for example, change the response of older adults to cardiovascular medications. Pharmacodynamic processes are set in motion when the drug reaches the target tissue sites. Effects can be presynaptic or postsynaptic in the nervous system, or involve enzyme inhibition. Reuptake inhibitors, such as SSRI antidepressants, are examples of drugs that act at presynaptic sites. Acetylcholinesterase inhibitors used for people with Alzheimer disease (donepezil, galantamine, and rivastigmine) are examples of enzyme inhibitors.[6,7] "Although elderly patients experience greater drug effects than younger patients, the reason is not always clear. The differences in drug responses can be attributed either to different baselines or to different sensitivities."[7]

Pharmacology is a needed issue to discuss because as the aging population increases, so does the use of drugs for two main reasons. First, multiple medical problems lead to multiple prescriptions, and second multiple doctors can lead to multiple prescriptions. Another less common occurrence, seen by this author, is the use of multiple pharmacies due to lower prices of certain medications, which prevents computerized findings of possible drug interactions. Patients also contribute to polypharmacy by incorrectly and inappropriately using prescribed or over-the-counter medications. Older adults may be more inclined to share drugs with a spouse or other friends who complain of similar symptoms. Some prescriptions may be expired and dates need to be checked. Older adults may also be more likely to forget when or how to take their medications. Many medications look alike and with diminished eyesight patients may unintentionally take the wrong pill. Individuals or family members are more likely to assume side effects of drugs are normal because the patients are older and some side effects mimic aging problems (incontinence, confusion), or ignore them all together. Physicians contribute to polypharmacy when they use drug therapy where a nondrug therapy could have been used.[3,4]

This increased incidence of adverse drug effects in the elderly is caused by two factors. Older adults take more medications and there is an altered response to the drug therapy due to aging changes. In general, the elderly are two to three times more likely to experience an adverse drug reaction. Older adults compose just 13% of the population but consume up to 33% of all drugs, and also rely on over-the-counter drugs that may go unrecorded by physicians or other health care providers.[8]

What things can physical therapists do about medications? Therapists can schedule therapy sessions around drug dosage schedule so medications that decrease performance in gait or balance activities such as sedatives or medications that cause dizziness can be minimized. If the performance will be enhanced or promote a synergistic effect, then physical therapy should be coordinated with peak drug effects such as with Parkinson medications or pain medications if the treatment would be painful such as following a total knee replacement. Therapists can also improve education and compliance with drug therapy by reinforcing the need for adhering to prescribed regimen and help monitor whether or not drugs have been taken as directed. In addition, educating patients, families, and caregivers as to why drugs are indicated and about their side effects can be very helpful.

Therapists must be aware of the drug regimen used by each patient and have a basic understanding of the beneficial and adverse effects of each medication. Therapists must also be cognizant of how specific drugs can interact with various rehabilitation procedures, which is especially true for geriatric patients receiving physical therapy. Older adults are generally more sensitive to the effects of drugs and the adverse effects may impede progress in therapy. An adequate understanding of the patient's drug regimen can help the physical therapist recognize and deal with these adverse effects as well as capitalize on the beneficial effects of drug therapy. Therapists need to avoid potentially harmful interactions between therapy and medications. Some therapy interventions used in the elderly could potentially have a negative interaction with some medications. An example of this would be the use of heat that causes peripheral vasodilation, which may produce severe hypotension in patients receiving certain antihypertensive medications.

We have an obesity epidemic in this country.[9,10] Americans are more obese than ever with more than 50% of adults being overweight or obese. People have become heavier around their waists, which is the least healthy place to keep weight. Obesity is linked to many chronic illnesses, although we are unsure if it is weight alone, or other factors related to weight.[9] People who are obese may actually be malnourished, especially older adults who need additional nutrients such as during wound healing. Being able to advise our patients on proper nutrition is just not vital to overall health; it is a significant factor in the rehabilitation process because of higher nutrition requirements. Malnourished people use body tissues for energy, have slower metabolic rates and reduced function of immune system. Older adults are often malnourished because of difficulty eating, shopping, and preparing food, they are isolated, or they lack appetite. Poor nutrition leads to much higher medical costs for chronic diseases (sarcopenia, DM, osteoporosis, cachexia, heart disease), longer hospital stays with complications, DVTs, weakening of immune system (wounds, infections, pneumonia), fatigue, frailty and confusion, low RBC count, weakness, falls, depression, dependence, and increased mortality.[9,10]

Proper nutrition is a component that is vital but often overlooked in the rehabilitation process. Therapists are generally not educated in this arena. Therapists should screen for malnutrition with a visual inspection along with measuring height, weight, body mass index, or if there has been any unintentional weight loss greater than 10 pounds in the last month. Poor nutrition may reflect a medical illness, depression, functional losses, or a financial hardship. Be aware of these factors so that you can respond appropriately if your clients bring up issues related to nutrition. They often do, especially in the home health arena. Remember just because the packaging states that the food or supplement is "natural" and/or "herbal" does not mean it is either safe or good for the patient. You should know how to read the nutritional information on the packaging.[11-13]

People get plenty of calories, but are often deficient in nutrients like calcium, which is especially true in the elder population. An example of the need for understanding nutrition would be for the therapist who has a patient who has recently increased their calcium intake per physician advice due to new diagnosis of osteoporosis or have had a recent fracture to know what might positively or negatively affect calcium absorption. The patient stays indoors all day, and may benefit from some outdoor activity in sunlight (not midday) to allow the body to produce vitamin D to help absorption. Conversely, a therapist may observe your patient drink three cups of coffee in an hour while you are in their home. The patient also has a box of salted fiber-added crackers on the kitchen counter. The therapist would want to educate the patient that some foods negatively impact calcium absorption such as caffeine, sodium, and fiber. While this patient may benefit from a dietician consult, it may not be reimbursable, so it usually falls to the nurse or therapist for education.

According to the State of Hunger in America report, almost one in six seniors faced the threat of hunger.[13] Food insecurity is associated with a host of poor nutrition and health outcomes among seniors, and that these high rates of food insecurity will likely lead to additional public health challenges for our country. This study suggests that a key potential avenue to stem the growth of health care expenditures on older Americans is to ameliorate the problem of food insecurity.[14] Causes of malnutrition can be poor dentition (tooth loss), decreased sense of smell, gum tissue atrophy, poor fitting dentures, decreased saliva, less efficient absorption, earlier satiety, restricted diet (salt, fat, sugar, protein which can cause food to lose taste), or from medication side effects (dry mouth, loss of taste, appetite suppression, nausea). Risk factors include low income, poor education, poor oral health and dentition, polypharmacy, mobility impairments, chronic health problems, and changed mental status (depression, confusion, or dementia). How can a therapist look for signs of malnutrition? Ask about eating habits or about alcohol intake. Do you observe poor wound healing, or are they easily bruised? Do they have dental difficulties (poor fitting dentures, loose when they speak or chew, not wearing them)? Do clothes fit too loose indicating weight loss? Are bowel movements infrequent?[11-13]

Another problem that older adults may face is dehydration. Loss of just 1% to 3% of body weight can cause symptoms. Risk factors in older adults include diminished thirst, loss of mentation, water metabolism changes, loss of physical function, visual problems, medications (diuretics, laxatives, sedatives), dysphagia, vomiting

and diarrhea (especially if acutely ill with the flu), decreased food intake, fear of incontinence, and/or lack of attention/knowledge from caregivers. The effects of dehydration may manifest itself as hypotension, elevated body temp, constipation, decreased urine output, tachycardia, headaches, dry tongue, loss of skin turgor, and/or changes in concentration or mentation, lack of skin rebound with skin pinch test, dark colored urine, dry, sticky mouth, fatigue or weakness, and/or chills.[15]

Cataracts, glaucoma, macular degeneration, and abnormalities of accommodation worsen with age. A therapist can assess vision difficulties by asking about everyday tasks such as driving, watching television, or reading. More practically, can they read their medication bottle? Asking about the last time they got a new prescription for classes may clue the therapist as to whether the glasses are adequate or not. More formally, a Snellen chart or Jaeger card can be used to assess eyesight. Hearing loss is also common among older adults. Impaired hearing can lead to depression and social withdrawal. A therapist can screen for hearing loss with tuning-fork test, finger-rub test, or whisper test. If hearing loss is suspected, then a referral to an ENT physician, speech therapist, or audiologist may be appropriate to formally test for hearing with an audioscope, assess for cerumen impaction, and determine the need for an ear cleaning. Hearing aids should be regularly checked and cleaned as well.

Functional outcome testing is vital to achieving successful rehabilitation of our patients. In addition to the psychometric properties of the test or measure, physical therapists must consider the clinical utility of each tool and its particular purpose. For instance, physical therapists consider the precision of the data yielded by a test or measure and whether it will meet the needs of the situation. Some measurements are only gross measurements which may be useful for a population screen but may not be useful for identifying a small change in status after intervention. The measurements used by the physical therapist should be sensitive enough to detect the degree of change expected as a result of intervention. Sensitivity and specificity are important components in choosing the "best" test available. Ideally, the metrics of any test or measure should have been studied within the population in which the therapist is using it to measure the function of the patient. Many measures are validated and have psychometric properties investigated for use in different populations or environments. For instance, a test utilized in community-dwelling older adults may not be an effective or validated tool for people living in a long-term care facility.

Some tests may be better used to screen for functional loss or to cast a wide net to determine if skilled intervention is required. This may determine whether the therapist provides the patient or caregiver education, or that direct hands-on intervention is required. Therapists cast this wide net to identify who might have the problem/pathology, so that they can then go back for more detailed testing to confirm that diagnosis/problem. This is especially true if the consequence of missing someone on a screen is high, such as missing someone at high risk of falling, not intervening, and then the person falls and breaks a hip.

Cognitive health needs to be considered with our patients. Therapists need to screen for cognitive loss because of the prevalence of Alzheimer disease as this should affect how the therapist will instruct and interact with the patient. Mentation may not just affect if the patient can follow directions or remember to perform a home exercise program. Cognition can also affect nutrition and hydration and therefore affect the entire rehabilitation process as mentioned earlier. Many people with dementia do not complain of memory loss, and cognitively impaired older persons are at risk for accidents, delirium, medical nonadherence, and increased disability. There are several cognitive screens that can be readily utilized including the Mini Mental Status Exam (MMSE), Mini-Cog,

Montreal Cognitive Assessment (MoCA), or St Louis University Mental Status (SLUMS) examination. Undiagnosed depression is quite common in older adults. The therapist can screen for depression with the two-question depression test or PHQ-2.[16,17] Or simply ask, "Do you often feel sad or depressed?" If the patient responds, "Yes," then the Geriatric Depression Scale might be appropriate. Also, the therapist should watch for signs of anxiety or bereavement. If the therapist believes that a screen yields a possible case of depression, the therapist should ask the patient if they want help with this problem and refer to the appropriate mental health practitioner. This author would also strongly suggest asking the patient if they are thinking about hurting themselves. From personal experience this author has yielded two positive answers to this question, necessitating a 911 call for emergency hospital admission.

No assessment of an older adult would be complete without investigating whether they have incontinence. This is not a part of normal aging but is a very common problem and major health issue. Incontinence can be assessed and treated successfully with physical therapy. There are two broad categories of incontinence: acute and chronic. Acute or transient is usually caused by a medical condition such as a urinary tract infection (UTI), kidney stones, cerebral vascular accident, or constipation. Acute incontinence can also be caused by consumption of foods and/or beverages that irritate the urinary system such as caffeinated beverages, alcohol, spicy, or acidic foods. An acronym to remember these causes is DIAPERS. This consists of delirium, infection, atrophy, pharmaceuticals, excessive urine output, restricted mobility, and stool impaction.[18]

Chronic or persistent incontinence is frequently seen due to changes or damage to the genitourinary system including the pelvic floor. Changes from pregnancy, childbirth, and menopause can affect the ligamentous and muscular structures that support the bladder.[18] There are four primary types of chronic incontinence. Stress incontinence is the most common type of incontinence due to loss of pelvic floor control. Mild to severe urine leakage can occur with activity, lifting, exercising, laughing, or sneezing.[18] Urge incontinence is caused by excessive activity of the detrusor muscle. This is also called an "overactive" bladder. Small amounts of urine in the bladder, cold exposure, change in position, or hearing running water may trigger the bladder to empty and the "urge" to empty the bladder occurs very quickly. Overflow incontinence is a result of underactive detrusor muscle activity. The inability to effectively and completely empty the bladder can lead to "dribbling" of urine. Overflow, or outlet obstruction, is more common in older men due to prostrate hyperplasia. Functional incontinence is the inability to get to the bathroom in time to void appropriately. This can be due to a loss of functional mobility or due to side effects of medications. Lastly, there is mixed incontinence which is a combination of two or more of the types of incontinence.[18]

Social assessment should include availability of the patient's personal support system including family, relatives, friends, and social system (church, cards, book club, golf, etc). Caregiver burden should be assessed for anyone caring for a patient with a chronic disease, especially Alzheimer disease. Economic well-being may not be an easy question to ask, but is important to assess ability to get physical assistance, make environmental changes, or purchase medical equipment not covered under Medicare or private insurance. Social workers and areas on aging systems can be great assets to physical therapy intervention. Driving ability may need to be assessed because of reduced vision, limitations in movement of neck or trunk rotation, shoulders, hips, and ankles, foot abnormalities including loss of sensation, confusion, poor coordination, reaction time, or alertness due to medication. Lastly, if suspected, elder abuse may need to be investigated.

According to the World Health Organization (WHO), an aging adult is someone 60 and older. WHO defines aging as: "The ageing process is of course a biological reality which has its own dynamic; largely beyond human control. However, it is also subject to the constructions by which each society makes sense of old age."[19] This varies among countries and includes loss of roles, or no longer an active contributor, and loss of physical function. This may be linked to established retirement age, or based on economic and political factors.[20]

In summary, the focus of geriatric assessment is on function. A successful assessment promotes wellness and independence. Strategies that enhance communication with older patients should be used. The comprehensive assessment includes physical, cognitive, psychological, and social aspects of health. The demographics or proportion of the population that is older is increasing compared to absolute numbers. Getting older affects all aspects of life and therapists need to understand and reflect on the education, culture, economics, entertainment, and medical care at a variety of facilities, government and payment policies, and how these interact with treatment plans.

GENERALIZED CHANGES DUE TO AGING

There are basic assumptions of the aging process. Aging takes place over time and does not suddenly occur magically once one turns 65. However, old age is actually a new concept. At the turn of the 20th century, the average person's life expectancy was in the 40s. An important differentiation to make is that aging is different from disease. Research has not yielded any absolute answers as to why we age and eventually die, but there are some key points to consider when working with older adults. Changes associated with aging are gradual, but the more complex the function, the more decline is seen. Individuals age at different rates which may be due to changes in the adaptability of the system to the stressors encountered. Other factors to consider are homeostasis and resilience. Two people with the same medical diagnosis may function much differently and have different outcomes. Aging is changes in adaptability of the system or individual to apoptosis, disease, stressors, and/or toxins.

The distinction between aging and disease (pathology) may be difficult and somewhat arbitrary and is a matter of degree. When changes impact a person's ability to function, these changes are described as a disease. Prior to loss of function, losses are considered "normal" changes of aging. There is not a clear line distinguishing these changes and much research is aimed at defining what is normal or expected versus an abnormal process.

In general all tissues tend to lose water, and increase the percent of insoluble collagen. Increases in the number of cross-linkages lead to decreased flexibility and increased resistance to movement. Tissues become more susceptible to shear forces, repetitive cyclic loading (overuse injuries), and microtraumas, which increases the vulnerability to injury and decreases recovery time. There is also a decrease in mitochondria with aging, which results in decreased energy production. Approximately 50% of decreased function can be attributed to pathology rather than the normal aging process. As a general rule, organ systems decline at 0.75% to 1.0% per year after age 30.[21,22]

The total number of cells decreases with age, as does their rate of replication. Cellular changes occur within the cells, making them less able to perform their programmed functions of producing necessary enzymes or proteins. Cells become less alike in structure and less organized in functions. An increased deposition of lipofuscin (a brownish pigment waste product from the breakdown and absorption of damaged blood cells) occurs and is found particularly in the heart, smooth muscle, and brain tissue. Lean muscle tissue decreases and there is an increase in fat concentration. Almost all organs decrease in size and mass except the prostate.[21,22]

Connective tissues have increased crisscrossing or cross-linking of collagen and elastin fibers. The collagen gets denser and stiffer; this impairs movement of nutrients and waste. Elastin becomes more rigid and may be replaced by collagen. This reduction of the amount of elastin in tissues results in wrinkles (integumentary fragility), loss of joint flexibility, and stiffening in arteries and bronchioles, making them all more susceptible to injury.[21]

The musculoskeletal system has a decrease in range of motion, speed of reaction time, and strength, which is similar to what is seen in disuse atrophy. A decrease in glycoproteins leads to a decrease in fluid retention, which then leads to dehydration. When cartilage dehydrates it becomes stiff and thin. Additionally, there is a loss of lubrication within the joints including a decrease in hyaluronic acid, which leads to decline in ease of movement of connective tissues and tissue degradation. Thankfully, exercise can increase hyaluronic acid production, whereas inactivity leads to increases in fibrinogen, which can cause joint adhesions.[21,22]

Muscle performance is affected as strength peaks around age 30 and noticeable declines begin at age of 50, although some elderly have strength values equal to those of young individuals at their peak. A change in force production occurs due to the reduction in size and number of fibers (especially type II fibers). In both aged and denervated muscle we see a decrease in the number and size of muscle fibers and fiber grouping. As we age, an increased recruitment of motor units for the given task is required. In other words, it takes more to do less.[22]

Strength training can increase muscle performance in older adults. The aspect of muscle performance most greatly affected in older adults is power. This is due to a decrease in the number of neurons per fiber and alterations in neurotransmission. Power decreases more because of the difficulty in developing torque at faster speeds.[21,22]

Skeletal changes include loss of bone density greater in women than men (due to loss of estrogen) and can cause osteopenia or osteoporosis. Skeletal changes can influence changes in posture which then affects mobility and function. Posture changes, along with changes in strength and flexibility, will also affect gait and mobility. Pathologic causes of strength declines include arthritis, cardiovascular disease, stroke, etc.[21,22]

Changes in energy availability that limit endurance are due to a decrease in myosin ATP activity, and a decreased number of mitochondria. The maximum VO_2 is decreased so endurance decreases at higher levels of activity. Endurance is unchanged in absence of a pathological condition with slower, lighter levels of activity. There is a decrease in ability of the cardiac system to deliver O_2 and nutrients and this is outlined in more detail in the cardiopulmonary chapter.[21,22]

Neurological changes are found in both the central and peripheral neurologic systems. Brain mass decreases in the cerebral cortex and cerebellum. Nerve impulse transmission is delayed due to a decline in neurotransmitters (dopamine, serotonin, GABA). Conduction velocity decreases especially in the posterior spinal column tracts that provide for reflex positive righting response, which put people at higher risk for falls. Older adults are more dependent on vision for balance. Older adults often cannot maintain balance when vision and somatosensory are removed due to normal degeneration of the vestibular system. Declines in balance and coordination decrease the ability to react to changes and can lead to injury. Pathological conditions include several types of dementia (Alzheimer, vascular, frontotemporal, and Lewy body dementias) and Parkinson disease.[21,22]

The acuity of all the sensory systems including hearing (presbycusis), vision (presbyopia), smell, taste, and touch diminishes with age. Each of the senses contributes a specific type of information necessary for the person to adapt, function, and adjust to the environment. Sensory declines may thereby compromise an individual's ability to maintain independence in their environment.[21,22]

Presbycusis is a sensorineural hearing loss. Changes in the inner ear or auditory nerve prevent transmission to the brain and cause loss of the higher and lower frequency levels. Speaking slowly and distinctly and allow the patient to visualize your face, not necessarily speaking louder will assist you to communicate with your patients. Conductive (peripheral) hearing loss occurs when sound transmission to inner ear is lost because signal intensity is insufficient. The sound received by inner ear can still be analyzed because inner ear itself is not affected. Causes of conductive dysfunction can be due to impacted cerumen, perforation of tympanic membrane, serum or pus in middle ear, or otosclerosis. Hearing aids may be effective for this condition.[21,22]

Changes in vision are due to losses in acuity, visual field, dark adaptation, accommodation (presbyopia), and color/depth perception. Vision is also limited by illumination and glare. Pathologies in vision may include glaucoma (caused by an increase in intraocular pressure), cataracts (due to increased density of the lens), macular degeneration (which is a pigmentary change of the macular area of the retina, caused by small hemorrhages), lens yellowing (cannot tell blue and green apart), and floaters (which are a benign clustering of collagen material in vitreous body of the eye).[1,2]

Sweat production declines, which can lead to overheating, but there is concomitant loss of the subdermal fat layer that leads to inability to contain body heat. Tactile sensation, touch, kinesthesia, and pain receptors all decrease.[21,22]

Senses of taste and smell become less acute with age with as much as 80% of the taste buds atrophying. There is a reduction in saliva flow. Olfactory bulb demonstrates cell loss associated with decreased perceptions of various smells. These may all combine to lead to the decline in appetite often seen in the elderly.[21,22]

Gastrointestinal changes also occur including a decline in motility of the esophagus and people may experience a substernal sensation of fullness that delays food entry into the stomach. Hiatal hernias are common due to relaxation of the lower esophagus (pathology). There is also reduction in motility of the stomach, colon, and small intestine. Nutrient absorption is hindered. Older adults tend to be constipated and may become impacted if immobile or dehydrated, which can lead to a medical emergency. Ulcerative disease is common pathology in the elderly and can be caused by certain medications.[21,22]

Liver mass and blood perfusion decline, which means that the metabolism of many drugs is decreased. Protein binding of medications may also be decreased. Changes in pancreatic function can lead to a decreased ability of the peripheral tissues to use the available insulin. The decreased ability of the pancreas to increase insulin production in response to increased blood glucose may lead to diabetes mellitus. The kidney declines in size, resulting in a 30% to 40% decline in functioning nephrons by age 85. An increase in residual urine in the bladder may lead to increased risk of infection.[21,22]

Overall, our bodies age in many ways, producing challenges for the people themselves and the health care providers who care for them. Some things we can change, and others not too much. It is the hope that this text will explain what happens as we age and how physical therapists can have a positive effect on the aging process.

REFERENCES

1. Currow DC, Stevenson JP, Abernethy AP, et al. Prescribing in palliative care as death approaches. *J Am Geriatr Soc.* April 2007;55(4):590-595.
2. Holmes HM, Hayley DC, Alexander GC, Sachs GA. Reconsidering medication appropriateness for patients late in life. *Arch Intern Med.* March 27, 2006;166(6):605-609.
3. Bain KT, Holmes HM, Beers MH, et al. Discontinuing medications: a novel approach for revising the prescribing stage of the medication-use process. *J Am Geriatr Soc.* October 2008;56(10):1946-1952.

4. Holmes HM, Min LC, Yee M, et al. Rationalizing prescribing for older patients with multimorbidity: considering time to benefit. *Drugs Aging*. September 2013;30(9):655-666.

5. Benzodiazepines. Drugs.com. http://www.drugs.com/drug-class/benzodiazepines.html. Accessed April 25, 2015.

6. Jacobsen S. Effects of pharmacokinetic and pharmacodynamic changes in the elderly. *Psychiatric Times*. http://www.psychiatrictimes.com/geriatric-psychiatry/effects-pharmacokinetic-and-pharmacodynamic-changes-elderly. Accessed April 13, 2015.

7. Bowie MW, Slattum PW. Pharmacodynamics in older adults: a review. *Am J Geriatr Pharmacother*. 2007;5:263-303.

8. Older adults. National Institute on Drug Abuse. http://www.drugabuse.gov/publications/research-reports/prescription-drugs/trends-in-prescription-drug-abuse/older-adults. Accessed June 21, 2015.

9. The obesity epidemic. Centers for Disease Control and Prevention. Obesity Epidemic. http://www.cdc.gov/cdctv/ObesityEpidemic/. Accessed April 24, 2015.

10. Obesity. Centers for Disease Control and Prevention. http://www.cdc.gov/obesity/adult/causes/index.html. Accessed April 24, 2015.

11. Furman EF. Undernutrition in older adults across the continuum of care. *J Gerontol Nursing*. 2006;32(1):22-27.

12. Visvanathan R, Chapman IM. Undernutrition and anorexia in the older person. *Gastroenterol Clinics North Am*. 2009;38:393-409.

13. DiMaria-Ghalili RA, Amella E. Nutrition in older adults: intervention and assessment can help curb the growing threat of malnutrition. *Am J Nursing*. March 2005;105(3):40-50.

14. Ziliak J, Gundersen C. The State of Senior Hunger in America 2012: an annual report. Report submitted to National Foundation to End Senior Hunger. 2014. http://www.feedingamerica.org/hunger-in-america/impact-of-hunger/senior-hunger/senior-hunger-fact-sheet.html. Accessed April 25, 2015.

15. Faes MC, Spigt MG, Rikkert O. Dehydration in geriatrics. *Geriatr Aging*. 2007;10(9):590-596.

16. Sheeran T, Reilly CF, Raue PJ, et al. The PHQ-2 on OASIS-C: a new resource for identifying geriatric depression among home health patients. *Home Healthc Nurse*. February 2010;28(2):92-104.

17. Li C, Friedman B, Conwell Y, Fiscella K. Validity of the Patient Health Questionnaire 2 (PHQ-2) in identifying major depression in older people. *J Am Geriatr Soc*. 2007;55(4):596-602.

18. Urinary incontinence. MayoClinic.org. http://www.mayoclinic.org/diseases-conditions/urinary-incontinence/basics/definition/con-20037883. Accessed June 21, 2015.

19. Ageing. World Health Organization. http://www.who.int/ageing/about/facts/en/. Accessed April 11, 2015.

20. Definition of an older or elderly person. World Health Organization. http://www.who.int/healthinfo/survey/ageingdefnolder/en/. Accessed April 11, 2015.

21. Guccione A, Wong R, Avers D. *Geriatric Physical Therapy*. 3rd ed. St Louis, MO: Elsevier; 2012.

22. Kauffman T, Scott R, Barr JO, Moran ML. *A Comprehensive Guide to Geriatric Rehabilitation*. 3rd ed. China: Churchill Livingstone; 2014.

CHAPTER 2

Musculoskeletal Cases

INTRODUCTION

AGE-RELATED CHANGES IN THE MUSCULOSKELETAL SYSTEM

James R. Creps, PT, DScPT, OCS, CMPT

Aging presents the human body with many challenges as it relates to the musculoskeletal system. There is a progressive loss of skeletal tissue muscle mass and strength with aging. This process is referred to as sarcopenia and invariably leads to decreased functional ability in the aged.[1] The reduction in muscle mass is most prominent in the lower extremities and is characterized by a preferential atrophy of type 2 muscle fibers.[2,3] The loss of muscle mass can be significant and has been reported to be approximately 30% in several studies.[2] In addition, over the course of an individual's lifespan, the muscle fiber loss noted as a consequence of aging results in a decline of between 25% and 40% of the cross-sectional area of the muscles of the thigh.[4] Multiple mechanisms have been hypothesized as potentially leading to the age-related loss in muscle mass and strength that is characteristically seen.

Increased apoptosis, or the process of programmed cellular death, may be a contributing factor.[5] In apoptosis, biochemical events lead to characteristic changes in cellular morphology. Specifically, in relation to muscle tissue, it appears nuclear fragmentation may lead to cellular death and subsequent tissue atrophy.[6] Apoptosis is different from necrosis, which involves some form of cellular trauma, and the resulting apoptotic bodies are engulfed and removed by phagocytic cells before they can cause damage to surrounding tissue.

Oxidative stress and inflammation in muscle tissue has also been implicated in the loss of muscle power and mass that is characteristically seen with aging.[7] Oxidation is the precursor to inflammation and is simply the interaction between oxygen molecules and human tissue. When oxygen is metabolized, it creates "free radicals" which steal electrons from other molecules, causing cellular damage. Oxidative processes stimulate inflammation and the cascade of biochemical reactions associated with it. The cytological changes seen in muscle tissue represent some of the adverse effects of the body's inflammatory reaction to oxidation.

Sarcopenia is a syndrome characterized by progressive and generalized loss of skeletal muscle mass and strength. This loss of muscle mass causes risks of poor outcomes including poor quality of life, disability, and early death.[8]

Finally, neuromuscular changes in the elderly also contribute to muscle wasting and weakness.[9] Muscle fiber denervation occurs, although it is not clear whether denervation precedes muscle wasting or is a result of it. In addition, reduced numbers of motor units,

as well as a decrease in the conduction velocity of the motor axon, are also partly responsible for the decrease in muscle function seen with aging.[10,11] Finally, the excitability of both spinal and cortical tissues decreases with age, and this is complicit in the age-related decline seen in skeletal muscle function.[12] All of the neuromuscular changes listed above are complicit in the movement dysfunctions seen in the elderly population. These dysfunctions, accompanied by changes in reaction time and perceptual deprivation, make this population at great risk for falls.

Similarly, tendons undergo changes with the aging process and demonstrate an increased incidence of injury with senescence.[13-15] Tendon repair and recovery requires lengthy periods of recuperation and rehabilitation in the elderly. The exact mechanisms that result in this increased propensity to injury and degeneration in this population are poorly understood; however, there appears to be a connection to an altered turnover rate and response in the cellular matrix.[16] Clearly, something associated with aging is affecting the ability of this tissue to maintain homeostasis, resulting in a diminished regenerative response.[17]

Recent research appears to indicate that tendon stem progenitor cells exhibit a profound deficit at self-renewal and decelerated motion with aging. This in turn results in a slower turnover of actin filaments. Essentially, the supply of tendon stem progenitor cells becomes exhausted in terms of both size and functional fitness with aging.[18] This concept of tissue-specific, age-associated shortages in number, stress resistance, and repair capacity of adult stem cells is not new.[19] In fact, multiple studies on human aging and age-associated conditions indicate that reduced regenerative potential is linked to a functional decline in the pool of available stem cells.[20,21]

In addition, it has been demonstrated that aging induces structural degenerative changes to capsular, fascial, and ligamentous structures. These changes occur mainly as a result of the decrease in elastic fibers responsible for resistance.[22]

Finally, there are also significant age-related changes that occur in osseous structures. Some of these occur as a result of chronic conditions, such as osteoporosis, although this condition can be accelerated due to reduced calcium intake over time secondary to dietary choices, or even as a result of medication interactions that decrease calcium absorption.[23-25] Osteoporosis is a significant metabolic disorder that causes pain in the elderly.[26] Deficiencies in vitamin D will also impair normal differentiation and proliferation of bone cells, setting the stage for this chronic disease. The elderly, faced with the challenges of maintaining a well-balanced balance diet in conjunction with adequate activity levels out of doors, are especially susceptible to long-term demineralization of bone and fracture as a result of this.[27-30]

Bone density decreases significantly after age 50, so maintaining mineral bone density through adequate nutrition and activity decreases the risk of fracture and should be a primary health objective in the elderly population.[31-32] Changes in bone health, in conjunction with old injuries and overuse, also cause osteoarthritis. Clearly, osteoarthritis is a major contributor to pain and dysfunction in the elderly.[26]

These changes in muscle and bone architecture, and changes in the mechanical properties of the tendons and ligaments can lead to an increase in injury and decreased function for the older adult. With pain and dysfunction come poor health outcomes as a result of sedentary behavior.[33] As a result of all of these physical changes in the geriatric population, exercise and adequate activity remain critically important in maintaining proper musculoskeletal health. With a proactive response to exercise and nutrition, many of the adverse changes seen in the musculoskeletal system can be managed. This is critically important in maintaining the functional independence of the elderly population and in reducing fall risk. Physical therapists are uniquely positioned to provide a wellness approach to overall health in the geriatric population so that the need for acute intervention in the face of illness and injury is mitigated.

REFERENCES

1. Sayer AA, Robinson SM, Patel HP, Shavlakadze T, Cooper C, Grounds MD. New horizons in the pathogenesis, diagnosis, and management of sarcopenia. *Age Ageing*. 2013;42(2):145-150.

2. Janssen I, Heymsfield SB, Wang ZM, Ross R. Skeletal muscle mass and distribution in 468 men and women aged 18-88 yr. *J Appl Physiol*. 2000;89:81-88.

3. Nilwik R, Snijders T, Leenders M, et al. The decline in skeletal muscle mass with aging is mainly attributed to a reduction in type 2 muscle fiber size. *Exp Gerontol*. 2013;48:492-498.

4. Klitgaard H, Mantoni M, Schiaffino S, et al. Function, morphology and protein expression of ageing skeletal muscle: a cross-sectional study of elderly men with different training backgrounds. *Acta Physiol Scand*. 1990;140:41-54.

5. Buford TW, Anton SD, Judge AR, et al. Models of accelerated sarcopenia: critical pieces for solving the puzzle of age-related muscle atrophy. *Ageing Res Rev*. 2010;9:369-383.

6. Marzetti E, Calvani R, Bernabei R, Leeuwenburgh C. Apoptosis in skeletal myocytes: a potential target for interventions against sarcopenia and physical frailty-a mini-review. *Gerontology*. 2012;58:99-106.

7. Thompson LV. Age-related muscle dysfunction. *Exp Gerontol*. 2009;44(1-2):106-111.

8. Cruz-Jentoft AJ, Baeyens JP, Bauer JM, et al. Sarcopenia: European consensus on definition and diagnosis: report of the European working group on sarcopenia in older people. *Age Ageing*. 2010;39(4):412-423.

9. Jang YC, Van Remmen H. Age-associated alterations of the neuromuscular junction. *Exp Gerontol*. 2011;46(2-3):193-198.

10. Campbell MJ, McComas AJ, Petito F. Physiological changes in ageing muscles. *J Neurol Neurosurg Psychiatry*. 1973;36(2):174-182.

11. Dalpozzo F, Gerard P, De Pasqua V, Wang F, Maertens de Noordhout A. Single motor axon conduction velocities of human upper and lower limb motor units. A study with transcranial electrical stimulation. *Clin Neurophysiol*. 2002;113(2):284-291.

12. Oliviero A, Profice P, Tonali PA, et al. Effects of aging on motor cortex excitability. *Neurosci Res*. 2006;55(1):74-77.

13. Tuite DJ, Renstrom PA, O'Brien M. The aging tendon. *Scand J Med Sci Sports*. 1997;7:72-77.

14. Smith RK, Birch HL, Goodman S, Heinegard D, Goodship AE. The influence of ageing and exercise on tendon growth and regeneration-hypotheses for the initiation and prevention of strain-induced tendinopathies. *Comp Biochem Physiol A Mol Integr Physiol*. 2002;133:1039-1050.

15. Rees JD, Wilson AM, Wolman RL. Current concepts in the management of tendon disorders. *Rheumatology (Oxford)*. 2006;45:508-521.

16. Peffers MJ, Thorpe CT, Collins JA, et al. Proteomic analysis reveals age-related changes in tendon matrix composition, with age and injury-specific matrix fragmentation. *J Biol Chem*. September 12, 2014;289(37):25867-25878.

17. Liu L, Rando TA. Manifestations and mechanisms of stem cell aging. *J Cell Biol*. 2011;193:257-266.

18. Kohler J, Popov C, Klotz B, et al. Uncovering the cellular and molecular changes in tendon stem/progenitor cells attributed to tendon aging and degeneration. *Aging Cell*. 2013;12:988-999.

19. Sharpless NE, DePinho RA. How stem cells age and why this makes us grow old. *Nat Rev Mol Cell Biol*. 2007;8:703-713.

20. Rando TA. Stem cells, ageing and the quest for immortality. *Nature*. 2006;441:1080-1086.

21. Sahin E, DePinho RA. Linking functional decline of telomeres, mitochondria and stem cells during ageing. *Nature*. 2010;464:520-528.

22. Barros EM, Rodriques CJ, Rodriques NR, Oliveira RP, Barros TE, Rodriques AJ. Aging of the elastic and collagen fibers in the human cervical interspinous ligaments. *Spine J*. January-February 2002;2(1):57-62.

23. Dietary supplement fact sheet: calcium. National Institutes of Health (US)Web site. http://ods.od.nih.gov/factsheets/Calcium-Health Professional. Accessed June 26, 2015.

24. Institute of Medicine Standing Committee on the Scientific Evaluation of Dietary Reference Intakes (US). *Dietary Reference Intakes for Calcium, Phosphorus, Magnesium, Vitamin D, and Fluoride*. Washington, DC: National Academies Press; 1997.

25. Choi YS, Joung H, Kim J. Evidence for revising calcium dietary reference intakes (DRIs) for Korean elderly. *FASEB J*. 2013;27:1065.28.

26. Mediati RD, Vellucci R, Dodaro L. Pathogenesis and clinical aspects of pain in patients with osteoporosis. *Clin Cases Miner Bone Metab*. 2014;11(3):169-172.

27. Maier GS, Seeger JB, Horas K, Roth KE, Kurth AA, Maus U. The prevalence of vitamin D deficiency in patients with vertebral fragility fractures. *Bone Joint J*. January 2015;97-B(1):89-93.

28. Yang YJ, Kim J. Factors in relation to bone mineral density in Korean middle-aged and older men: 2008-2010 Korea National Health and Nutrition Examination Survey. *Ann Nutr Metab*. 2014;64:50-59.

29. Hong H, Kim EK, Lee JS. Effects of calcium intake, milk and dairy product intake, and blood vitamin D level on osteoporosis risk in Korean adults: analysis of the 2008 and 2009 Korea National Health and Nutrition Examination Survey. *Nutr Res Pract*. 2013;7:409-417.

30. Peterlik M, Boonen S, Cross HS, Lamberg-Allardt C. Vitamin D and calcium insufficiency-related chronic diseases: an emerging world-wide public health problem. *Int J Environ Res Public Health*. 2009;6:2585-607.

31. Rice BH, Quann EE, Miller GD. Meeting and exceeding dairy recommendations: effects of dairy consumption on nutrient intakes and risk of chronic disease. *Nutr Rev*. 2013;71:209-223.

32. Crandall CJ, Newberry SJ, Diamant A, et al. Treatment to prevent fractures in men and women with low bone density or osteoporosis: update of a 2007 report. *Comparative Effectiveness Reviews*, No. 53. Rockville, MD: Agency for Healthcare Research and Quality; 2012.

33. Thyfault JP, Mengmeng Du, Kraus WE, Levine JA, Booth FW. Physiology of sedentary behavior and its relationship to health outcomes. *Med Sci Sports Exerc*. 2015;47(6):1301-1305.

1

HIP OSTEOARTHRITIS—CONSERVATIVE TREATMENT STRATEGIES

Meri Goehring, PT, PhD, GCS, CWS

William H. Staples, PT, DHSc, DPT, GCS, CEEAA

Lewis, a 62-year-old male, presents to your outpatient clinic with a diagnosis of right hip osteoarthritis. He lives with his wife at their single-story ranch-style home with their two dogs. Lewis is an accountant and spends 8 to 10 hours each work day sitting at his desk working on his computer or talking with clients. Despite his sedentary role at work, he maintains an active lifestyle outside of the workplace. Lewis and his wife share many hobbies including hiking, mountain biking, downhill skiing, golfing, running, and walking their dogs. Lewis was a multisport athlete throughout high school and ran track and cross country for 2 years in college. He reports that pain in his knee has been gradually worsening over the past 6 months and in the last month it has been limiting his ability to participate in his usual recreational activities. He also states that in addition to his knee pain worsening, he has been experiencing anterior hip pain on his right side when he is sitting as well as when he is "up and on his feet for long periods of time." His primary goals are to be able to return to his normal lifestyle including recreational activities.

This patient's previous medical history includes that he was hit by a truck 15 years ago while out running and he sustained a dislocated right hip, fractured ribs 6 and 7 on the right side as well as a concussion. His hip was reduced upon arrival to the emergency room. Lewis did not receive physical therapy for his injuries which healed on their own over time. No other significant injuries or illness.

PHYSICAL THERAPY EXAMINATION

Height: 5 ft 11 in; weight: 175 lb; HR: 62 beats per minute; BP: 126/78; SpO$_2$: 99%

Lumbar spine: no reproduction of symptoms with lumbar spine testing

Hip: positive right hip scouring, Faber, Ober, and Thomas tests

Knee: unable to reproduce knee pain with any special tests or knee movements.

Lower extremity muscle testing:

Gluteus medius: R = 3+/5, L = 4−/5; hip IR: 4/5 bilaterally; knee extensors: R = 4/5, L = 5/5

Gluteus maximus: R = 3+/5, L = 4/5; hip ER: R = 4−/5, L = 4/5; knee flexors: R = 4/5, L = 5/5

ROM testing: decreased ROM right hip all planes of movement

No impairments in knee or ankle range of motion bilaterally

Balance: single leg stance (average of three trials): R = 22 seconds, L = 1 min+

Functional outcome measurements:

Lower Extremity Functional Scale: 46/80

■ CASE STUDY QUESTIONS

1. What is the incidence of osteoarthritis?
2. What risk factors present (if any) are indicative of osteoarthritis?
3. Is running a risk factor for osteoarthritis?
4. Could the muscle weakness in the gluteus medius be related to his osteoarthritis?
5. Does arthritis cause an increased risk for falls?
6. What tests could you use to determine that this individual is not at risk for falls?
7. Is the Lower Extremity Functional Scale an appropriate outcome measure in this case?
8. Why is Lewis a good candidate for conservative treatment rather than more invasive treatments such as a total hip arthroplasty? (Consider factors such as recreational activities, age, and post-surgical precautions.)
9. Develop an initial plan of care consisting of four to six interventions (ie, manual therapy, therapeutic exercise, etc).
10. Would you consider a weight reduction plan for this patient?
11. Describe the pain in the stages of osteoarthritis.

2

TOTAL HIP ARTHROPLASTY: CASE 1

Meri Goehring, PT, PhD, GCS, CWS

William H. Staples, PT, DHSc, DPT, GCS, CEEAA

George is a 74-year-old male retired mechanic who volunteers at the front desk of the local YMCA. He currently lives with his wife in a two-story home with five steps to enter with one hand rail on the right-hand side. His bedroom and bathroom with a shower are located on the second floor with 12 steps. The bathroom has no grab bars for toilet but has one grab bar for the walk-in shower. George has poor vision (20/60) but otherwise was independent in his activities of daily living but required assistance with grocery shopping requiring a motorized cart to propel him as he was limited in walking long distances due to pain prior to his surgery. Prior to his hip replacement, George was experiencing hip pain intermittently for 5 years until 6 months ago when the pain became constant and unbearable 8/10 when standing or ambulating.

George is being seen in the acute care setting post-op day 1 from a cemented total hip arthroplasty performed with a lateral approach (also known as a Hardinge approach). He complains of 4/10 pain in his right hip and around his surgical incision. George appears to be in good health with a lean, well-nourished physique and a BMI of 25. He was able to get up to the bedside commode yesterday with moderate assistance ×2 with nursing. He has not attempted to walk except for the sit-to-stand transfer and take two steps to the bedside commode. Upon a systems review, you find in supine his resting heart rate was 67 beats per minute, blood pressure of 127/67 mm Hg, and respiratory rate of 15 breaths per minute. Upon sitting, the systems review reveals a heart rate of 72 beats per minute and blood pressure of 122/70 mm Hg. The patient was able to come to sitting with moderate assistance, and sit with no loss of balance and no dizziness.

Strength testing in sitting revealed normal strength in bilateral upper extremities and left lower extremity (5/5 grossly). The right lower extremity was limited by pain with 3+/5 strength for knee flexion and extension, and 4/5 strength for plantar flexion and dorsiflexion. The hip was not tested. Upon standing, George appeared pale in the face and states that he is feeling a bit dizzy. Heart rate and blood pressure were taken and found to have a heart rate of 84 beats per minute and a blood pressure of 109/65. Upon standing for a few minutes and having a drink of water, George reports feeling much better and willing to walk to the bathroom. A recheck of blood pressure revealed his blood pressure was 123/74 mm Hg. Upon arrival to the bathroom, George was a moderate assistance ×2 for safety for toilet transfers. He was only able to ambulate 20 ft in total with two standing rest breaks of 30 seconds with moderate assistance ×1. George was educated on his hip precautions and placed back to bed with leg exercises to perform.

Day 2 postoperation: George was able to come to sitting from supine position with minimal assistance and perform elevated toilet transfer with moderate assistance ×1, recite all of his hip precautions, and ambulate 80 ft with minimal assistance with one standing rest break of 30 seconds.

■ CASE STUDY QUESTIONS

1. Why is surgery indicated for George?
2. Describe the surgical approach used for this patient.

3. Why would the therapist need to know post-surgical approaches are used and how do they differ?

4. What are the possible complications of this surgery?

5. What are the "standard hip precautions?"

6. If George has been given standard hip precautions, what education would provide to the patient to prevent hip dislocation?

7. Does it make a difference that this patient has had a cemented total hip?

8. What are some of the standardized tests that can be utilized with this patient?

9. What type of interventions will be used during the hospitalization?

10. When can George return to his volunteer work?

3

TOTAL HIP ARTHROPLASTY: CASE 2

Meri Goehring, PT, PhD, GCS, CWS

Margaret is an 83-year-old female retired homemaker. She lives at home with her 89-year-old hard of hearing husband in a handicap accessible first floor apartment. They have a walk-in shower with a shower bench for her husband that she is currently using for her grooming/showering. There is one grab bar next to the toilet along with a countertop if needed for assistance. Margaret currently reports that she is using an elevated toilet seat for assistance to avoid violating her hip precautions.

Prior to her surgery, Margaret was independent in all her activities of daily living and her instrumental activities of daily living. She also assisted with the care of her husband, Ronald, such as making his meals, performing housekeeping and laundry, and assisting him with getting him to his doctor's appointments. Her husband, Ronald, accompanies her on her appointment with you today, and appears to be in fair health, but much larger of a man than Margaret, estimating his height to be approximately 5 ft 10 in, and weighing approximately 275 lb. Prior to her hip replacement, Margaret was experiencing left hip pain for approximately 10 years intermittently, but in the last 2 years has been constant (7/10) whenever she was walking or active throughout the day.

Margaret had an anterolateral (Watson-Jones) approach surgery that was cemented. Margaret appears to be in fair health with a well-nourished physique, and a BMI of 29.5.

Margaret is being seen in the subacute setting at a local skilled nursing facility. She is post-op day 4 and complains of 5/10 left hip pain when she is sitting and 8/10 pain when she performs a sit-to-stand transfer to the bedside commode. She complains of pain in her left hip and along her surgical incision site, located in the posterior aspect of her leg, along the gluteus maximus. The wound appears red and inflamed, but no apparent excess seepage is present at this time. She requires a moderate assistance ×1 with a standard walker for sit-to-stand transfers (to and from the bedside commode). She was able to ambulate 30 ft with a standard walker and moderate to maximal assistance ×1 with a wheelchair follow, requiring only one standing rest break for 20 seconds.

With lower extremity manual muscle testing for strength, Margaret scores a 2/5 left abductor strength, 3+/5 with left hip flexors and extensors with increased pain; right hip is 4/5; bilateral 3+/5 knee extensors and knee flexors, and 4/5 ankle plantar flexion and dorsiflexion. With upper extremity, Margaret scored a 3+ to 4−/5 grossly bilaterally. Margaret was educated on her hip precautions multiple times throughout the evaluation. Lastly, she was able to perform the TUG test in 27.64 seconds.

Day 4 postoperation (day 2 in subacute facility): Margaret is concerned that she is not at home to assist her husband at this time. He has never had to spend more than a day by himself; this is day 4 for him. She was unable to remember her hip precautions. She ambulated 45 ft with decreased pain but increased reliance on standard walker with one standing rest break. She continues to require moderate assistance ×1 for sit-to-stand transfers. When she was placed in a chair, she would frequently attempt to cross her legs, stating that if she would be able to do that, she would be able to get comfortable as this was a position she repeatedly sat in at home. Additionally, she repeatedly tells you (the therapist) that she is concerned that her hip is painful and that she is afraid it is going to give out on her, stating it feels very weak.

■ CASE STUDY QUESTIONS

1. Why is surgery indicated for Margaret?

2. Describe the surgical approach used for this patient.

3. Why would the therapist need to know post-surgical approaches are used and how do they differ?

4. What are the possible complications of this surgery?

5. What is the survivability rate of a person following surgery at 25 years?

6. What are the "standard hip precautions?"

7. If Margaret has been given standard hip precautions what education would provide to the patient to prevent hip dislocation?

8. Why are these precautions in place, and how long do they remain in place?

9. Does it make a difference that this patient has had a cemented total hip?

10. What are some of the standardized tests that can be utilized with this patient?

11. What type of interventions will be used during the subacute (nursing home) rehabilitation?

12. When can Margaret return home and resume her caregiver role?

13. Is there anything that can be done now to help Ronald?

14. How long will the hip replacement remain functional?

4

HIP FRACTURE: CASE 1

Meri Goehring, PT, PhD, GCS, CWS

Marsha is a 91-year-old widowed African American woman who is a retired librarian. Marsha has osteoporosis with a DEXA score of −2.6. Marsha also is hard of hearing and has poor vision. Marsha enjoys reading large print books and is active in her church. Marsha lives in a retirement community with family in the area. Marsha was independent in her activities of daily living and used a cane for community ambulation. Marsha reports that she fell 10 days ago on her way to the bathroom. Marsha was unable to get up from the floor due to severe pain in her groin. She was wearing her life alert button and was able to get help quickly. She reports that her hip broke, which caused her fall. Marsha is now being seen by physical therapy in a skilled nursing facility 5 days post-open reduction internal fixation (ORIF) of her left hip to address an intertochanteric hip fracture. Marsha's hospital stay was uncomplicated and unremarkable.

The examination begins with a systems review. Marsha is oriented to person, place, and time. Marsha's vital signs are a blood pressure of 124/84, heart rate is 80 beats per minute and regular, respiratory rate is 17 breaths per minute, and oxygen saturation is 96%. Marsha is taking tramadol (Ultram) 100 mg every 6 hours and paracetamol (acetaminophen) 500 mg every 6 hours. Strength and range of motion of the right lower and both upper extremities are within functional limits. The left hip is 2+/5 for hip flexion, abduction, and adduction, hamstrings and quads are 4/5, and ankle is 5/5. Light touch sensation is intact throughout; the surgical incision shows no sign of infection. Marsha's left hip pain is 3/10 with rest and 7/10 at worst. Marsha is 50% weight bearing on her left lower extremity. Marsha is able to ambulate with a standard walker for 35 ft. Her 10 m fastest gait speed is 0.35 m/s using the walker nonweight-bearing (NWB) left lower extremity.

CASE STUDY QUESTIONS

1. Where on the femur do these type of fractures typically occur?
2. How common are hip fractures?
3. What factors make hip fractures more likely?
4. What is the mortality rate for people having a fractured hip?
5. What types of morbidity can be expected?
6. Why were the medications prescribed?
7. Other than oral medications, what is another common method of pain relief?
8. Will a delay in surgery cause any potential complications?
9. How would a fear of falling after fracture influence this patient?
10. Does this patient have osteoporosis?
11. What types of hip fixation failures might occur?
12. What are the rehabilitation options for this patient?
13. What would a typical post-hospital discharge therapy program entail?
14. Are there any hip precautions for this patient?
15. What are some standardized tests/functional outcome measures that can be utilized for patients following hip fracture?

5

HIP FRACTURE: CASE 2

Meri Goehring, PT, PhD, GCS, CWS

Ron is an 89-year-old retired automotive factory worker. He has severe osteoarthritis in both of his hips, knees, and hands. He lives alone in his two-bedroom, one-bath, single-story ranch-style home. His wife passed away 5 years ago following a heart attack. He has lived in this home for the last 56 years and has no intentions of leaving as he feels this is only place he is comfortable. Ron was independent in all of his activities of daily living and instrumental activities of daily living and had no previous falls prior to his fall 3 days ago that left him with a fractured left hip. Ron was walking the trail near his house, the same trail that he has walked nearly every day for the last 23 years since he retired from the factory. He tripped on a tree root that left him falling on his left hip and in extreme, agonizing pain. Fortunately, another pedestrian was walking on the trail and found him within 10 minutes of his fall and called for the ambulance. Prior to his fall, Ron walked with only a walking stick on the trail and a straight cane in the community when needed. He reports he did not use any assistive devices at home prior to his fall. Ron is being seen by physical therapy in an acute hospital setting 1 day after his open reduction internal fixation with three long screws of his left hip due to a subcapital hip fracture. He was disappointed not to get a total hip arthroplasty but the orthopedic surgeon was concerned about his age and his overall health.

The examination begins with a systematic review and shows a resting heart rate of 93 beats per minute, a sitting blood pressure of 136/87 mm Hg, and respiratory rate of 21. Upon standing, Ron's blood pressure was 109/68 mm Hg. Ron is oriented to person, place, and time and appears to have intact light touch sensation to the surgical incision site on his left hip. He verbalizes that he is at 2/10 at rest for pain and 5/10 in standing for pain. Strength is 2−/5 for hip flexion, 3/5 for hip adduction, 2/5 for hip abduction, hip extensors are 3/5. Per physician orders Ron is allowed up to 25% weight bearing on his left leg and requires cueing not to increase his weight bearing more than 25%. He was able to ambulate 27 ft with a standard 4-point walker with increased reliance and weight bearing through UEs, and on his right LE, assistance was needed for walker management notably during turns. A TUG test was performed; he was able to complete the test with the walker in 29 seconds.

After 3 days in the hospital Ron is able to ambulate up to 80 ft with a standard walker 25% weight bearing and no longer requires cueing. Transfers are independent from bed, chair, and toilet. Ron is adamant about not being sent to a nursing home for further rehabilitation, which is what the social worker has recommended.

CASE STUDY QUESTIONS

1. What is a subcapital hip fracture?
2. What would the visual and radiographic changes appear like following a subcapital hip fracture?
3. What is the major complication of an intracapsular hip fracture?
4. What are some of the gender differences regarding hip fractures?
5. What are some of the major comorbidities that can cause death after hip fracture?
6. What percentage of community dwelling adults who have a hip fracture end up dwelling in a long-term care facility due to the fracture?
7. What are some of the rehabilitation options after hip fracture?
8. What types of information can help you determine a good outcome/prognosis?
9. What types of information can help you determine a poor outcome/prognosis?
10. Should Ron go to the skilled nursing home or home to receive further rehabilitation?
11. What types of standardized tests might you incorporate?
12. What are the most commonly used interventions in home health services for a hip fracture?

13. What is the mean number of home care visits following a hip fracture?

14. Are there any hip precautions for this type of fixation?

MINIMALLY INVASIVE ANTEROLATERAL TOTAL HIP ARTHROPLASTY

Julia Levesque LeRoy, PT, GCS

Linda M. deLaBruere, PT, GCS

The patient is a 66-year-old female who has undergone a minimally invasive surgery (MIS) anterolateral approach right total hip arthroplasty (THA) today. She has an order for a physical therapy consult the day of surgery, for gait training weight bearing as tolerated (WBAT) right lower extremity (RLE), with no exercises except ankle pumps, gluteal and quadriceps sets. Physical therapy was also requested to make recommendations regarding discharge disposition since she does live alone.

The patient is 5 ft 5 in tall, weighs 168 lb. She has had right hip pain for about 3 years. Pre-surgical radiographs of her right hip showed moderate to severe degenerative joint disease with osteophytes in inferior margin of acetabulum. She has failed conservative therapy of steroid injections times four, which temporarily reduced pain for 3 months per injection, and outpatient physical therapy for pain modalities, exercise, and activity modification. She was unable to ambulate more than 50 ft without significant pain (8/10 on numeric scale) in her hip and she has opted to undergo a total hip replacement. Preoperative examination states her blood pressure is 140/95, RR 18 to 20, HR 92 beats per minute. Her right hip range of motion (ROM) was 90° flexion, hip abduction was 0° to 30°. She climbed stairs step to step and was unable to climb step over step. She underwent a right minimally invasive (MIS) anterolateral approach total hip arthroplasty (THA) this morning.

Comorbidities include a left "frozen shoulder," depression, anxiety, hypertension, and osteoarthritis in her hips. Her medications include lisinopril 20 mg; Lexapro 10 mg; lorazepam 0.5 mg; glucosamine 2000 mg; fish oil 1200 mg (she was asked to discontinue the glucosamine and the fish oil 1 week prior to surgery).

Current living situation: The patient is divorced and lives alone in a two-story house with bed room and bathroom upstairs (the stair case has a railing on the right side); she does have a half bath downstairs as well as a spare room. There are three steps with bilateral rails to enter into the home. She works at an office job and usually ambulated without an assistive device but over the past 3 months required the use of a straight cane due to increased pain. She drove and was independent with all ADLs and household chores. She was having increased difficulty with donning and doffing shoes and socks so has been wearing slip-ons. She has hired help to do yard work. Her daughter lives nearby with a new grandson and she has lots of friends and support from her church. Her best friend is taking a week off of work to assist the patient at home postoperatively. She did attend a Joint Camp at the hospital, which is a preoperative education class to learn about what to expect following surgery. She has had premade meals in her freezer, cleaned and shopped before surgery. She has already purchased a front-wheeled walker and a raised toilet seat.

EXAMINATION

The patient is seen post-op day #0 following right MIS THA. The ROM of the right hip functionally is 90°, and 10° of hip abduction. No passive ROM was tested due to surgery. Manual muscle testing (MMT) was not done due to recent surgery; however, she did require minimum assistance to maneuver the RLE in and out of bed. Vital signs are: BP in supine 110/70 HR 85; sitting BP 98/65 HR 90; standing BP 95/60 HR 96; O$_2$ saturation 98% pre- and postmobility. The patient has no complaints of light-headedness or dizziness. Her supine to/from sit bed mobility requires minimum assist of one to move the right leg with the head of bed slightly elevated. Transfers require verbal cues for hand placements and contact guard assistance (CGA) of two for sit to/from stand with the front-wheeled walker. Her gait required CGA of 2 with the wheeled walker with a step-to gait pattern for 10 m (32.8 ft), and verbal cueing on walker management and weight-bearing status. Further mobility training is to be deferred until post-op day 1. She feels she is well prepared for going home and is highly motivated for returning home by tomorrow afternoon. She is willing to be discharged post-op day 2 if needed. Her long-term goal is to keep up with the grand kids and help take care of them.

The patient was educated regarding the lack of specific hip precautions. She had heard about posterior precautions and was not aware that they did not apply to her. Therapeutic exercise of ankle pumps, gluteal and quadriceps sets were also done 10 repetitions each and patient instructed on doing them every waking hour.

ASSESSMENT

The patient presents with decreased functional ROM and strength of the right hip, impaired functional mobility, and abnormal gait postoperatively. Pain is not a limiting factor at this point and despite the blood pressure being low for this patient she was asymptomatic. She has made arrangements prior to surgery for assistance and is very motivated to return home postoperatively. She would benefit from skilled physical therapy for 1 to 2 days in acute care to address above impairments as well as perform stairs and car transfer to determine needs for a safe discharge home. Recommend home physical therapy safety assessment especially with stairs and gait with appropriate assistive device.

■ CASE STUDY QUESTIONS

1. How common are total hip arthroplasties?

2. What are the differences between anterior and posterior hip replacements: for instance, precautions, therapeutic exercises, preparations required prior to surgery?

3. How can a patient prepare for surgery?

4. Are there any benefits to getting up post-op day 0 versus post-op day 1?

5. What is the average length of stay for an MIS anterior/lateral total hip replacement?

6. What type of exercises are beneficial post-THA?

7. In regard to discharge recommendations, what are the benefits of home versus inpatient rehab?

8. What are the benefits of home PT/OT/RN for this type of surgery?

9. Are there any post-op complications the patient should be aware of?

10. Are there any benefits to a walker to cane versus use of crutches for an assistive device?

11. When can this client expect to return to normal activity (drive, go back to work, etc)?

HIP PAIN

William H. Staples, PT, DHSc, DPT, GCS, CEEAA

A 62-year-old male presents to physical therapy with a complaint of right hip pain that started 6 weeks ago. He was seen by his primary care physician 5 weeks ago and underwent radiographic imaging that was negative for fracture and degenerative changes. The physician suggested Advil for reducing pain and inflammation and told the patient to remember to stretch before exercising. In addition, he suggested to the patient that he take up a less demanding exercise regime. The patient is also taking irbesartan (30 mg daily) for mild hypertension and Flovent (110 μg, 2 puffs bid) for asthma.

The patient scheduled this physical therapy appointment due to his inability to run. The patient is an avid runner and had been completing 30+ miles per week prior to the onset of his hip pain. Over the past several years, he has averaged four to five sub-2-hour half-marathons a year. In addition, he has been playing competitive soccer since college. He had seen another therapist at the hospital clinic 3 weeks ago who told him he had a tight piriformis muscle and gave him a stretching program. The patient reports that the stretching feels good, but that it has not enabled him to run.

The patient reports that his hip pain began when he was playing soccer and stretched out into full hip flexion with knee extension trying to reach a ball. He reports that he felt and heard a distinct pop in the back of his hip. He states there was immediate 6/10 pain, and that he thought he had torn a hamstring. Initially, the patient had trouble walking without pain (antalgic gait pattern) for the first week, but now states the pain has subsided unless he tries to run. The patient complains of groin pain (4/10), and pain "in the hip joint" (6/10), when running or weight bearing. He is only able to jog a mile before having to stop due to pain or the hip "giving way." He is frustrated that the stretching exercises did not help, and has come to consult with another therapist for further assessment.

Range of motion tests within normal limits, with slight limitation in internal rotation. Passive hamstring range is limited to 75°, but equal bilaterally, and did not elicit any pain. Strength is 5/5 for all hip, knee, and trunk movements. There is no clicking of the hip during movement. A pedal pulse is intact, and a neurological screening is negative. The patient denies any history of cancer, night sweats, or recent loss in weight. Hip pathology is suspected, and the therapist begins specialized tests.

■ CASE STUDY QUESTIONS

1. What would degenerative hip changes appear as in a radiograph?

2. Would a loss of hip internal rotation be an important finding?

3. What is the first test you would utilize?

4. Describe the test position for this first test.

5. Would you measure for a leg-length discrepancy? How?

6. Is the piriformis muscle of concern? If so how would you test it to see if it is the source of the pain?

7. What is the Stinchfield Resisted Hip Flexion Test?

8. Could the iliotibial band be causing this problem? How would you test for that?

9. What other tests might you consider to make a differential diagnosis?

10. How would you test for an anterior hip labral tear?

11. How would you test for a posterior hip labral tear?

12. After a positive response to the last test you suspect a posterior labral tear. How can a definitive diagnosis be made?

13. What would be the treatment of choice for this patient if a posterior labral tear diagnosis is made?

14. Are labral tears common in older adults?

OSTEOARTHRITIS OF THE KNEE: PART 1

William H. Staples, PT, DHSc, DPT, GCS, CEEAA

A 60-year-old man comes to your clinic with a diagnosis of left knee pain. He is the head chef at a local restaurant and spends 8 to 10 hours a day on his feet. He complains of medial knee pain of mild 2/10 in the morning that worsens to 5/10 by the evening meal service. The pain is more intense when standing and he reports that he has been taking more breaks during the day to sit due to fatigue and to take weight off the leg. He is taking ibuprofen (Motrin) 400 mg four times a day by mouth. His physician told him he had osteoarthritis (OA) and gave him a corticosteroid injection in his knee yesterday and his primary care physician has recommended that he seek physical therapy to help his condition.

Examination reveals no other significant medical history or other medication use. He is 6 ft, 1 in tall and weighs 195 lb. His vital signs are heart rate 74 beats per minute, blood pressure 138/86 mm Hg, and a respiratory rate of 18 beats per minute. He states that he does not have time for exercise and that "my work is my exercise." Active range of motion (ROM) is limited in the left knee to 117° of flexion, passive ROM of the left knee is limited to 125°. Crepitus is noted in the mid-range through the end range. Radiographic films show diminished joint space in the medial compartment of the left knee. He states that he first hurt his knee playing basketball in college and has had two subsequent surgeries including a meniscectomy 30 years ago. Neurological, cardiopulmonary, and integumentary systems were screened and found no deficits. There is no family history of OA. He states he drinks two glasses of wine with dinner every night.

■ CASE STUDY QUESTIONS

1. How common is OA?

2. What is the most common joint occurrence for OA?

3. What are the most common factors contributing to OA?

4. What type of medication is this patient taking?

5. Are there any side effects to the medicine he is taking?

6. What would you expect the patient to experience after the corticosteroid injection?

7. Are there any precautions due to the recent corticosteroid injection?

8. What recommendations would you make for this patient?

   a. Footwear

   b. Bracing

   c. Modalities

   d. Exercises

   e. Weight loss

   f. Education

9. What specific exercise or activity programs would benefit this patient?

10. Are there any precautions that you would take?

9

OSTEOARTHRITIS OF THE KNEE: PART 2

William H. Staples, PT, DHSc, DPT, GCS, CEEAA

Three years have passed since you first saw this patient as an outpatient in your hospital. You have recently transferred to the hospital's home health agency and received a referral to see this patient at home. He is now a 63-year-old man who is status post left total knee replacement (TKR) 2 days ago. He is still the head chef at a local restaurant and must spend 8 to 10 hours a day on his feet. The pain was getting so bad that by the end of his shift (8/10) that he made the decision to have surgery. Prior to surgery he was taking ibuprofen (Motrin) 600 mg four times a day by mouth and had been receiving corticosteroid injections in his knee three to four times per year with good but short-lived (2 months) pain relief. He states that he wore the brace every day but only followed the home exercise program only for about three to four months after seeing you last time.

Examination now reveals a medical history of hypertension for which he is taking Avapro (irbesartan) 300 mg by mouth, daily. New medications following surgery include Norco (hydrocodone bitartrate and acetaminophen) 10 mg every 4 hours and Xarelto (rivaroxaban) 10 mg daily for 8 days. Orders include physical therapy three times per week and he is weight bearing as tolerated (WBAT) on the left lower extremity. He was given a rolling walker in the hospital. Nursing is to remove the staples in 10 days.

He is 6 ft, 1 in tall and weighs 215 lb. His vital signs are heart rate 74 beats per minute, blood pressure 134/82 mm Hg, and a respiratory rate of 18 beats per minute. The incision has staples in place with no drainage covered with a sterile gauze pad. He is wearing bilateral TED hose. Left knee pain at rest is 3/10, with passive range of motion (ROM) 7/10. Active ROM is limited in the left knee to 3° to 67° of flexion; passive ROM of the left knee is limited to 1° to 75°. He is able to perform a straight leg raise but has a 12° extensor lag. Neurological, cardiopulmonary, and integumentary systems were screened and no red flags were found. Family history is negative OA but positive for cardiovascular disease as his father passed away from a stroke suffered 2 years ago. He states he drinks two glasses of wine with dinner every night.

The restaurant owner has given the patient 3 weeks off to recover before he needs to return to work.

■ CASE STUDY QUESTIONS

1. Why was he only receiving three to four corticosteroid injections per year?

2. Why is he taking Xarelto (rivaroxaban)? Are there any side effects to this medication?

3. Are there any side effects to the other medicines he is currently taking?

4. What postoperative recommendations would you make for this patient?

   a. Footwear

   b. Bracing

   c. Modalities

   d. General exercises

   e. Weight loss

   f. Education

5. What specific exercises would benefit this patient?

   a. Passive ROM techniques

   b. Active exercise

   c. Resistive exercises (open and closed chain exercises) (eccentric and/or concentric)

6. How would you progress his gait pattern?

7. Are there any additional treatments or precautions that you would take now?

8. Is there any evidence that a continuous passive motion (CPM) would help this patient improve?

9. What would the long-term plan be for this patient?

10. What outcome measures would be best to utilize long-term success?

10

KNEE OSTEOARTHRITIS

Nikki Snyder, PT, DPT, OCS, CSCS

Joe is a 75-year-old male who was referred to physical therapy (PT) for right knee osteoarthritis (OA). Joe joined the army at 18 years old and served for 5 years. While in the army, Joe had a right knee injury with a subsequent medial meniscectomy surgery. He reports a full recovery after the surgery with return to active army duty tasks. After discharge from the army, he obtained a print and dye position with the local newspaper. Joe's work involved walking in the print room, operating heavy equipment, monitoring the printing machines, and climbing ladders. Joe retired as the supervisor of the print room 3 years ago. Joe gained 20 lb since retiring and his current body mass index (BMI) is 38. During the physical therapy (PT) screening, Joe's vital findings were blood pressure 158/85, heart rate 75, respiratory rate 18, and oxygen saturation 99%. Joe takes medication for hypertension and high cholesterol, but is otherwise healthy. Joe does not exercise regularly, but enjoys golfing two times per week with his friends. Joe is divorced, lives alone, and has two grown-up children who live 800 miles away. His home is 1000 sq ft on one level. Joe's home does not have steps or stairs into or out of the house. He is currently taking Tylenol extra strength four times per day.

Physical therapy evaluation reveals right knee range of motion measured 0° extension and 119° of flexion otherwise within normal limits all four limbs. The right lower extremity knee manual muscle test was 4/5 extension and 5/5 flexion; hip strength was 4/5 with flexion, extension, and abduction; and ankle strength was 5/5 with plantar flexion and dorsiflexion. His left-leg strength was 5/5 throughout. Joe demonstrated a normal gait pattern without significant deviation, but could not control going up or down a step with the right leg and reports right knee pain with sit-to-stand transitions. He has generalized right knee pain of 2/10 during most of the day that increases with activity. Further PT testing revealed the following: pain (4/10) in the medial right knee with McMurray testing, right single leg stance eyes open for 3 seconds, 30 seconds on the left, and point tenderness on the medial joint line of the right knee.

■ CASE STUDY QUESTIONS

1. What comorbidities are contributing to Joe's osteoarthritis?

2. How does the Centers for Disease Control and Prevention define obesity?

3. What is the best diagnostic test to determine the bone structure present in Joe's right knee?

4. What clinical testing is recommended to further screen for the presence of an internal derangement?

5. What is the potential that Joe had a meniscal tear in the right knee?

6. Is further diagnostic testing recommended to rule out the presence of an internal derangement?

7. What functional tests are indicated to demonstrate improvement in Joe's knee with physical therapy treatment?

8. What physical therapy treatments are recommended for Joe's knee OA pain?

9. What is the prognosis with PT treatment for knee osteoarthritis in an older adult?

10. What is the current pharmacological recommendation for the arthritis pain for this patient?

11. Would you recommend that this patient take chondroitin sulfate and glucosamine?

11

UNICOMPARTMENTAL KNEE REPLACEMENT

William H. Staples, PT, DHSc, DPT, GCS, CEEAA

You are seeing a 66-year-old male patient in the hospital this afternoon following a minimally invasive partial (unicompartmental) knee replacement surgery performed this morning. He has a history of right medial knee compartment osteoarthritis (2 years) and was supplied with a deloading brace at that time. The pain continued to worsen that led him to be more sedentary over the last year. Prior to the pain increase he was quite active. Prior to surgery he was taking Celebrex 200 mg twice a day, and Tylenol (acetaminophen) 325 mg every

4 hours. On evaluation the right knee is bandaged with a post-op splint (immobilizer). The immobilizer is removed and range of motion measures of knee flexion/extension are active 5° to 75° and passive 3° to 92°. The patient is able to straight leg raise but has a 5° extensor lag. Left lower and bilateral upper extremities are within normal limits for strength and ROM. Current medications include Percocet 10/325 (oxycodone-APAP 10-500 mg) and he has a morphine sulfate pump (patient-controlled analgesia). Intravenous fluids were discontinued in the last hour. Vital signs are heart rate 66, blood pressure 126/84, respiratory rate 14, and oxygen saturation (SpO$_2$) 99%. You make the clinical decision to get the patient up and begin gait training.

■ CASE STUDY QUESTIONS

1. What is different in this surgery compared to the "traditional" total knee replacement?

2. What are the advantages of the minimally invasive partial (unicompartmental) knee replacement surgery?

3. What are the disadvantages of a partial knee replacement?

4. Which patients are appropriate for this surgery?

5. Is this too early to start physical therapy?

6. What precautions would you take today?

7. What are some typical exercises that could be given to this patient as a home exercise program?

8. How would you progress the exercises after three to four weeks?

9. What could the final stages of a rehabilitation program encompass?

10. Are patients allowed to kneel following unicompartmental knee arthroscopies?

11. Is the ability to kneel following knee replacement improved or worsened following surgery?

12. What is Percocet (oxycodone-APAP)?

13. What is patient-controlled anesthesia?

12

MENISCAL TEAR

William H. Staples, PT, DHSc, DPT, GCS, CEEAA

An active 64-year-old comes to your clinic on a Wednesday complaining of right knee pain following a soccer game on Sunday. He believes he was hurt performing a sliding tackle but did not notice any pain immediately. After the game he was enjoying a few beers with his teammates and noticed a "twinge" in his knee when he got up to leave. The pain has been gradually worsening over the past 3 days. The right knee is slightly swollen (about 1 cm larger in circumference than the left) and slightly warm to the touch. There is tenderness along the medial joint line. He usually runs 20 miles per week, but yesterday could only walk for about 30 minutes until he stopped due to increasing pain. He can walk with only minimal pain now, although the pain increases with squatting, lifting, or rising from a seated position. His vital signs are heart rate 60, blood pressure 114/78, respiratory rate 12, and pulse oximetry 99%. He is taking Aleve (naproxen) two 220 mg pills three times per day. You decide to perform some tests to determine the integrity of the knee joint.

■ CASE STUDY QUESTIONS

1. What are some signs and symptoms of a small meniscal tear?
2. What tests would you perform to determine if this patient has a meniscal tear?
3. How would you perform an Apley test?
4. How would you perform a McMurray test?
5. If the Apley and the McMurray tests were both negative for a meniscal tear, what other diagnoses would need to be ruled out, or to determine if other structures were also injured?
6. If both the Apley and McMurray tests are positive for a meniscal tear would you recommend that the patient see an orthopedic surgeon?
7. Would you recommend arthroscopic surgery if both the Apley and McMurray tests are positive for a meniscal tear for this patient?
8. Are older adults more susceptible to meniscal tears?
9. What exercise recommendations would you provide for this patient?
10. Are there any other recommendations you would make?

13

TOTAL KNEE ARTHROPLASTY: CASE 1

Meri Goehring, PT, PhD, GCS, CWS

William H. Staples, PT, DHSc, DPT, GCS, CEEAA

Jim is a 70-year-old male who is a retired fisherman. He lives in a two-story home with his wife who is in fair health but unable to physically assist her husband. His bedroom is on the second floor and there are 25 steps to the second floor. He was independent in all activities of daily living prior to his knee arthroplasty. Jim had delayed the right knee arthroplasty for 3 years but the pain was 7/10 with golfing and sailing on his 30 ft sailboat. Jim was a high jumper and long jumper in college and is now slightly overweight with a BMI of 26 and has been having right knee pain for the past 35 years. He had undergone a conservative course of medications and exercise but his condition continued to deteriorate.

Jim is now being seen in the acute care hospital day 0 postoperation. The patient is very groggy, had an indwelling catheter, and his wife is present during the initial evaluation. The systems review included a medical history, blood pressure of 110/55, heart rate of 55 beats per minute, numbness around the incision site and right lower extremity. Jim has a past medical history of osteoarthritis and a left torn rotator cuff 20 years ago. The patient was given a spinal nerve block for the surgery. Jim is able to sit on the edge of bed independently without nausea and slight decrease in blood pressure of 100/50. Jim has good strength in his upper extremities and left lower extremity. Upon a standing trial his blood pressure dropped to 95/47 and Jim felt light-headed and dizzy. Blood pressure increased when Jim returned to bed. There is a 7-cm difference in anthropometric measure at the mid-joint line with right greater than left. Jim's passive knee flexion is 74° and extension is 7° away from neutral into flexion. Jim was helped back into bed laying supine with his right leg in a continuous passive motion machine set from 0° to 120°.

Day 2 postoperation: Jim is up and out of bed ambulating 150 ft with a two-wheeled walker. The catheter has been removed and a standard knee arthroplasty range of motion protocol has been implemented with Jim. Jim receives physical therapy twice per day while he is in the hospital.

■ CASE STUDY QUESTIONS

1. Why was surgery recommended for Jim?
2. How common are total knee replacements?
3. Why has there been such a dramatic increase in total knee procedures in the last 20 years?
4. What are the odds of someone age 25 developing osteoarthritis?
5. What is the average age for someone undergoing a total knee replacement?
6. What are the potential complications after surgery for Jim?
7. Who is at the highest risk of developing complications?
8. What type of ADL outcomes might be expected after surgery?
9. What type of activities outcomes might be expected after surgery?
10. What type of employment outcomes might be expected after surgery?
11. What type of physical therapy interventions would be used to treat this patient?
12. What standardized tests/functional outcome measures would be utilized to document progress with this patient?
13. When will most improvements be made and end?

14

TOTAL KNEE ARTHROPLASTY: CASE 2

Meri Goehring, PT, PhD, GCS, CWS

William H. Staples, PT, DHSc, DPT, GCS, CEEAA

Betty is a 68-year-old female seamstress who owns her own alterations shop and specializes in wedding dresses. She lives alone in an apartment on the first floor with only two steps to enter her building. She has no rails in her apartment complex and has no adaptive equipment at this time. Her two daughters live nearby in a town approximately 20 minutes from where she lives but otherwise has no assistance when she is at home as her husband of 45 years recently died due to lung cancer. Prior to her surgery, which lasted under 2 hours, she was independent in all activities of daily living and instrumental activities of daily living. She walked on a treadmill three mornings a week before work at the local senior center and played cards there the other two afternoons a week in the same building. Prior to surgery her anesthesiologist rated her as an ASA physical status 2 level. She states that she has had mild left knee pain for the last 20 years or so, with a WOMAC score of 36. Upon observation she is a moderate overweight individual with a BMI of 30 but no other chronic diseases. Today her daughter was able to bring her to therapy but the remaining visits it will be her grandson who will be taking her to therapy until she is cleared to drive from the orthopedic surgeon. Betty ambulated into the clinic with her standard walker with an antalgic gait and only toe touch weight bearing on the left leg due to increased pain. She states that she tries to perform her home exercises from the hospital but due to the pain she is inconsistent with them.

Betty is 7 days post-op cemented left total knee arthroplasty and is being seen for the first time in the outpatient orthopedic clinic since being discharged from the hospital 3 days ago. She is very upbeat about getting to work with therapy, as she feels very stiff and limited at this point in her recovery. She complains of excessive drainage from her bandage and increased tenderness along the surgical incision site. You note that she has redness along the knee joint with swelling and a combination of clear and light bloody drainage. She states that she woke up last night "freezing" and since then has not been able to warm up. Betty reports that she has been able to walk in her home two or three times a day with a standard walker or uses her furniture when need be or for more assistance, most notably when she stands up from a sitting position. She has not slept in her bed since the surgery and has only had sponge baths, as she is afraid of getting in and out of the tub shower without assistance or a grab rail at this time. Betty has a past medical history of skin cancer on her forehead, broken right femur 8 years ago from a motor vehicle accident that has healed fully per patient report, and osteoarthritis.

Betty has 4/5 gross strength in her right lower extremity, 4+/5 strength in her bilateral upper extremities overall. On her left leg, she presents with 3+/5 hip flexor strength, 3/5 quadriceps strength with pain in left knee joint, 3−/5 hamstring strength with pain in left knee joint, and 4/5 plantar flexor and dorsiflexion strength overall. Upon circumferential measurement, you find that the patient has a 9 cm difference between the surgical left leg and the right at the joint line. Betty's passive knee flexion is 83°, passive extension is 6° away from neutral into flexion, and both motions were limited to pain. Betty's active knee flexion was 78° limited by pain and active knee extension was 9° from full extension, again limited by pain. The patient was able to complete the TUG test using the walker in 22.6 seconds. Her vital signs are heart rate 78, respiratory rate 18, blood pressure 148/86, oxygen (SpO$_2$) 96, and temperature 100.9°F.

■ CASE STUDY QUESTIONS

1. What is the WOMAC?
2. Is it possible that Betty did not need a knee replacement?
3. Are there alternatives to surgery?
4. What are more common knee or hip replacement surgeries? Why?
5. What are the potential complications after surgery for Betty?
6. What is the American Society of Anesthesiologists' (ASA) scale?
7. Is Betty at high risk of developing complications?
8. Does Betty have any possible signs of complications?
9. What type of ADL outcomes might be expected after surgery?
10. What type of activities outcomes might be expected after surgery?
11. Will Betty be able to return to work following her therapy?
12. What typical physical therapy interventions would be used to treat this patient in the first 4 weeks?
13. What typical physical therapy interventions would be used to treat this patient in the next 4 weeks?
14. What typical physical therapy interventions would be used to treat this patient after 8 weeks?
15. What standardized tests/functional outcome measures would be utilized to document progress with this patient?

15

TOTAL KNEE ARTHROPLASTY: CASE 3

William H. Staples, PT, DHSc, DPT, GCS, CEEAA

The patient is a 65-year-old Caucasian female who underwent cemented left total knee replacement (TKR) surgery due to progressively worsening osteoarthritis with subjective reports of pain varying from 5 to 7/10 on a verbal analog scale. The pain had limited her mobility and the ability to complete functional activities such as housework. The patient's past medical history is significant for hypothyroidism, gastroesophageal reflux disease (GERD), osteoarthritis in both knees, vitamin D deficiency, and obesity (BMI 30). The patient lives with her retired husband, who has taken over much of the household duties, in a one-story home that has two steps to enter (no handrail) and has a basement which requires her to navigate 12 steps where the laundry is done. This patient has adopted a sedentary lifestyle during the previous years, secondary to increased pain and decreased range of motion in both knees. Prior to surgery, the patient was independent with all ADLs including cooking, cleaning, driving, navigating stairs, and all transfers. The patient's primary goal for physical therapy is to reduce pain and be able to return to prior levels of activity such as standing for prolonged periods of time to cook, ambulating stairs to be able to do the laundry and the occasional babysitting of her grandchildren.

The patient is seen 1 day postsurgery with the knee bandaged, drain in place, and knee in an immobilizer. The surgical dressing is removed to inspect the incision on anterior left knee that is approximately 10 in (25 cm) long with surgical staples intact. The incision line is reddened with a small amount of blood. The joint is swollen and measures 8 mm larger than the right. The patient reports pain in the left knee of 8/10, and presents with increased left knee edema, gross left lower extremity strength of 4/5 except for quadriceps which is 2/5 with a 25° extensor lag. Knee range of motion (immobilizer removed) is 7° to 52° active extension and 4° to 63° passive extension, which is very painful. She has decreased bed mobility, requiring moderate assist, and difficulty with standing bedside (moderate assistance) or transfers, which require max assist from the bed to a chair. The immobilizer is to be used when not receiving physical therapy to maintain knee extension or ambulating with a walker at the beginning of the rehabilitation process to protect the incision and due to preoperative weakness. She has an IV line, is receiving antibiotics and a morphine on-demand pain pump. Her vital signs are: heart rate 82, respiratory rate 18, blood pressure 132/84, and an oxygen saturation (SpO$_2$) of 96%. Other medications include Xarelto (rivaroxaban), Vicodin (hydrocodone and acetaminophen), Nexium (esomeprazole), and Synthroid (levothyroxine).

On day 2 gait training is commenced with weight bearing as tolerated (WBAT) orders from the physician. The therapist chooses to leave the immobilizer on during gait training. She transfers sit to stand with moderate assistance. She ambulates about 20 ft, four times with moderate assistance in the parallel bars. The immobilizer was removed for active, active assistive, and passive range of motion exercises, which are painful (8/10) and isometric exercises of the hamstrings, quadriceps, and hip extensors and ankle pumps. Her vital signs were consistent as day 1.

On day 3 the patient is in better spirits, the morphine pain has been discontinued and the patient is anxious to return home. She transfers with minimal assistance. During gait training with a rolling walker and no immobilizer the following gait deviations are noted. During stance phase on the left she lacks full knee extension at heel strike and is apprehensive with approximately 50% weight bearing with a flat foot. During the swing phase of the left leg she exhibits decreased knee flexion during swing and shortened stride length. Today the patient only requires minimal assist to ambulate with a rolling walker 50 ft times 4 with a 3- to 4-minute rest period to recover. Her knee range remains quite limited and she continues to have significant pain (7/10) with range of motion exercises and physically resists knee flexion.

On day 4 the patient is much improved and able to ambulate up to 125 ft with only stand-by assistance (SBA) with the rolling walker with approximately 75% weight bearing on the left. The patient is able to ambulate 0.6 m/s as measured using the 10-Meter Walk Test using a rolling walker. She is unable to safely negotiate stairs without moderate assistance. A care plan meeting is called for that afternoon with the social worker leading the meeting. A discussion about whether to use a continuous passive motion machine (CPM) occurred during the meeting. A decision is made with your professional judgment that the patient should be able to go home tomorrow following therapy with a referral for home health care and a couple of environmental changes.

■ CASE STUDY QUESTIONS

1. What is the difference between a cemented and noncemented total knee replacement?

2. Why would the surgeon choose cemented over noncemented prosthesis?

3. What is rivaroxaban (Xarelto) and what is the typical dose?

4. Which knee ligaments are typically preserved or sacrificed during a total knee arthroplasty?

5. Would you recommend a continuous passive motion machine (CPM) to assist with gaining range of motion in the knee?

6. Is there any evidence that support using a continuous passive motion machine to lower the risk of a deep vein thrombosis?

7. What is an extensor lag?

8. On day 2, was the therapist's decision to leave the immobilizer on during gait the correct one? Why or why not?

9. On day 3, was the therapist's decision to remove the immobilizer on during gait the correct one? Why or why not?

10. What is one of the most important clinical outcome measures?

11. Why was the 10-Meter Walk Test performed?

12. Why did the therapist believe that this patient could go home versus going into a skilled nursing facility?

13. What environmental changes might have to be made at the patient's home?

14. What equipment might also benefit this patient?

15. Is there any other intervention that would assist this patient's recovery?

16

CHONDROMALACIA PATELLA

Eric Shamus, PT, DPT, PhD

Erin N. Pauley, DPT, MS, ATC, CSCS

A 68-year-old female presents with a recent onset of anterior right knee pain. The pain is described as dull and aching, and is present with climbing stairs and sitting for prolonged periods.

The patient states she is unable to pick up objects off the ground due to knee pain. The patient denies any recent trauma or history of injury to the knee, but states she has been kneeling on the floor when cleaning. Her past medical history was unremarkable and neurological screening including dermatomes, myotomes, and deep tendon reflexes were all within normal limits. Quadriceps flexibility was moderately limited on the right leg, and manual muscle tests revealed limitations in knee extension (4−/5) and hip extension (4/5). The patient had general crepitus throughout the range of motion. The McMurray test and ligamentous stress tests were negative. The patient had a positive Clarke sign and discomfort with general compression onto the patella.

After your evaluation you determine that you need to do more research for this disorder to determine your treatment approach. Please answer the following questions based on your research.

■ CASE STUDY QUESTIONS

1. What is chondromalacia patella?

2. What populations are at the greatest risk of experiencing chondromalacia patella?

3. What are common symptoms of chondromalacia patella?

4. What are possible causes of chondromalacia patella?

5. What special tests are appropriate to make a differential diagnosis of chondromalacia patella?

6. How is the patellar apprehension or Fairbank test performed?

7. How is the patellar grind test (Clarke sign) performed?

8. What exercises might be included in this patient's plan of care?

9. What are appropriate stretches for patients with chondromalacia patella?

10. What are appropriate treatment options for patients with chondromalacia patella?

11. What other conditions might present with anterior knee pain?

17

TIBIAL PLATEAU FRACTURE

Meri Goehring, PT, PhD, GCS, CWS

Mary is a 65-year-old female who teaches mathematics on a part-time basis at the local community college. She is retired from full-time teaching, but continues to teach one class a semester to supplement her retirement income. She has been married for 40 years and her husband owns and manages a liquor store. They have traveled extensively over the years and enjoy food and wine. They live in a small community with excellent public transportation. Ten days ago, Mary was running to catch the bus when she stepped off a curb and twisted her left knee. She had immediate, severe pain. She went to see an orthopedic surgeon who did radiologic imaging (x-ray). The x-ray imaging did not show any fractures and the physician felt the knee may have a torn meniscus or strained ligament and injected the knee with cortisone. The physician recommended physical therapy and you are seeing her in an outpatient clinic.

You examine Mary and perform several tests. First, your screening examination indicates Mary has high blood pressure 175/90. Her BMI is 32, so Mary is classified as obese. She is 6 ft tall and says she has always been heavy. She admits that she and her husband enjoy wine and that she drinks three to four glasses of wine a day, sometimes more on weekends. She tells you she does not exercise regularly but that she walks to the bus 5 days a week, which is about a 10-minute walk twice daily. She has no problems with her skin, and her neurologic screen is negative. However, she tells you she has had several falls last winter on the ice when walking to the bus. You decide to do a balance test and find that her Berg balance score is 38/56.

She tells you that the cortisone shot did not help much and that the knee is still very painful, sometimes waking her up at night. She says she has still been going to work, but walks very slowly. You note as she walks into the clinic that she has an antalgic gait with a very short stance time on the left leg and a quick right step.

Your musculoskeletal evaluation reveals the following:

Strength and ROM right LE are within normal limits all joints.

Strength and ROM left LE at hip and ankle are within normal limits. The left knee has normal ROM but painful at end range of flexion. Strength of left knee is 4/5 in extension, 5/5 in flexion.

You administer the WOMAC to determine the patient's baseline.

The results of special orthopedic tests of the left knee are as follows: varus-valgus stress test negative; anterior-posterior drawer tests negative; posterior sag test for posterior collateral ligament negative; rotary instability tests negative; pivot shift test painful; patellar stability tests normal; McMurray test painful; and Apley test painful. A tuning fork applied to the proximal anterior tibia elicits a positive pain reaction, and use of a stethoscope yields little sound distally.

Mary refuses to try climbing stairs saying that her knee is just too painful for stairs at this time.

You suspect that Mary may have a torn meniscus, but suspect that it could be something else due to her level of pain and night pain, which is unusual. The cortisone injection did not reduce her pain and this is also a concern. So, you provide Mary with crutches and instruct her in a weight bearing as tolerated, 3-point gait on level and stairs. She is very appreciative that you gave her crutches as she feels she is too young for a walker, but is able to walk much further with the crutches without as much pain.

You call the orthopedist, inform him of your findings in regard to blood pressure and knee pain and tests performed. The orthopedist then orders magnetic imaging and finds that Mary has a nondisplaced tibial plateau fracture and recommends nonweight-bearing gait for 6 weeks.

■ CASE STUDY QUESTIONS

1. What causes a tibial plateau fracture?
2. Would her obesity be a problem?
3. Might her history of alcohol consumption have any relationship to the fracture?
4. Why is it important to report Mary's high blood pressure to the physician?
5. What is the WOMAC?
6. What does the WOMAC measure?
7. Is the WOMAC considered valid and reliable in this case?
8. What other kinds of tests could be used?
9. What key symptoms indicated that this may not be a meniscus tear, but may be caused by some other musculoskeletal issue?
10. Why was this not diagnosed via radiograph?
11. Why was a tuning fork utilized to detect a fracture?

18

ACHILLES TENDONITIS
William H. Staples, PT, DHSc, DPT, GCS, CEEAA

You are seeing a new 63-year-old male patient in your outpatient clinic who decided to take up jogging 1 month ago as a way to decrease weight and increase his cardiovascular fitness at the urging of his physician. He is 5 ft 8 in tall and weighs 190 lb but reports that he has lost almost 5 lb since he began his new exercise regime. His vital signs are heart rate 74, respiratory rate 18, blood pressure 142/90, and oxygen saturation 97%. He reports that he is having pain behind his left ankle and distal calf muscle. Pain at present is 3/10 on a verbal analog scale, but increases to 5/10 after about 1 mile of jogging. The calf musculotendon junction and the Achilles tendon are tender to palpation. The patient states that he had just increased his distance from 2 to 3 miles this past week and is discouraged that he will have to give up running.

Strength and range of motion are within normal limits in both lower extremities. The patient is wearing his "street shoes" but has his running shoes in his car, which you ask him to retrieve for you to inspect. You observe his gait both in his running shoes and barefoot. You observe bilateral overpronation in both feet in weight bearing, greater in the left. You determine that this patient has Achilles tendonitis.

His medications consist of Avapro (irbesartan) 300 mg once daily in the morning, and a "baby" aspirin (81 mg) with dinner. No other significant medical history is present.

■ CASE STUDY QUESTIONS

1. What is the medical term for "flat feet?"
2. What examination test might you use to determine the amount of pronation that is present?
3. What interventions would decrease the pain at this time?
4. What advice would you give the patient about his current running program?
5. What interventions would be of long-term assistance in preventing the continued Achilles tendonitis for this patient?
6. What is this patient's body mass index (BMI)?
7. Why is it important to inspect the patient's shoes?
8. Why would you want to observe the patient's barefoot gait?
9. What is Avapro?
10. Are you concerned about his vital signs at rest?
11. Is there any other information that could be provided about decreasing his blood pressure?

19

PLANTAR FASCIITIS: CASE 1
Meri Goehring, PT, PhD, GCS, CWS

George is a 62-year-old man who just recently retired as a high school history teacher, and now lives with his wife in their ranch-style home. George is an upbeat positive guy, but gets tired taking care of his wife, who is rather ill and needs help with most daily activities. As a result, George does not partake in much physical activity and is on the low end of being obese (BMI = 30). He has noted a gradual pain in his right foot over the last couple of months, and is now coming to see you in your outpatient clinic for management of the pain. He tells you that the pain in his foot is much worse with the first few steps in the morning, and is worse during the day after standing or walking for a prolonged time. The pain is described as a sharp pain, and he points to his medial tubercle of the calcaneus to show where the pain is. He has been taking ibuprofen for the pain, but he has found that it only dulls the pain a bit. He wants a more permanent form of treatment.

Performing a systems review on George reveals a resting HR = 88, BP = 132/80, and RR = 26. George is cognizant and oriented ×3. He has a well-healed scar on his right knee from a total knee arthroplasty he had 5 years ago, and he is able to squat to 90° of knee flexion before his right heel lifts off the ground. George's right ankle PROM dorsiflexion is 5° shy of neutral and has limited inversion/eversion, compared to his left ankle, which is able to just go past neutral into dorsiflexion (by about 5°). He has pes cavus in standing and during gait. Additionally, both forefeet overpronate, right more than left when ambulating. He is unable to walk on his heels, and can hardly maintain balance enough to walk on his toes beyond three steps. When you have him stand for 3 minutes, the pain gets sharper and he requests to sit down. A slump test was negative.

■ CASE STUDY QUESTIONS

1. How might plantar fasciitis change George's functional mobility?
2. Will plantar fasciitis have any effect on George's balance?
3. Why is this condition potentially more dangerous in older adults than in younger individuals?
4. What other diagnoses should you rule out?
5. Is there a specific gold standard for diagnosing plantar fasciitis?
6. What are the most common symptoms?
7. Is there a known etiology for this condition?
8. What kind of nonsurgical treatment is available?
9. Has physical therapy been found to be an effective treatment?
10. What standardized scale might you use when examining this patient?
11. Is surgical intervention a possibility?

much of the time, but also walks some to rearrange and stock the used clothing. Over the last 2 months, she has worked an average of 5 days per week, sometimes 6 days per week, 8 hours per day. Within the last two weeks she has developed pain on the bottoms of both of her feet that is much worse in the morning and gets better as she walks. She says if she sits down at all, it is very painful to begin walking again. She says the pain is in the heel area but that the entire soles of both feet are painful. She needs to continue working as she is trying to help her adult children with some of their expenses. The pain is described as a sharp pain, and she points to the medial area of the heels to show where the pain begins. She is taking ibuprofen for the pain, which helps, and tells you she also has osteopenia and is taking over-the-counter calcium, but no other medications.

Performing a systems review on Mary reveals a resting HR = 88, BP = 140/80, and RR = 26. Mary is cognizant and oriented ×3. She is able to squat to 80° of knee flexion before her heels lift off the ground. Mary's ankle PROM dorsiflexion is 5° shy of neutral on both feet. She has pes cavus in standing and during gait, and both forefeet overpronate during stance. She is unable to walk on her heels or her toes beyond three steps. When you ask her to stand in place for 3 minutes, she reports pain is present. She says if she stays busy and walks some, the pain is not as bad.

■ CASE STUDY QUESTIONS

1. Are Mary's symptoms typical of plantar fasciitis?
2. What might you do if Mary does not make any improvement in a reasonable time frame?
3. Mary asks why this occurs. Is there a specific etiology?
4. What types of treatments have undergone randomized clinical trials?
5. Has manual therapy and exercise been shown to be effective?
6. Would you recommend orthotic devices?
7. What are some of the intrinsic and extrinsic factors that can contribute to the development of this condition?
8. What is the function of the plantar fascia?
9. Is there any emerging information regarding physical therapy treatment for this condition?
10. Are there any other suggestions you make to Mary?
11. What types of standardized measures might you use to determine outcomes?

20

PLANTAR FASCIITIS: CASE 2

Meri Goehring, PT, PhD, GCS, CWS

Mary is a 73-year-old female who works for her church thrift store 3 days a week. She lives alone in a small, ground floor apartment. Mary is active and participates in an exercise group at the local YMCA at least 5 days per week. She is at a normal weight for her height with her BMI at 28. She comes to you after a referral from a physician who feels she may have plantar fasciitis.

She states she has been working a lot more over the last 2 months because the thrift store manager has been recovering very slowly from a motor vehicle accident. She says she stands at a cash register

21

GOUT: CASE 1

Meri Goehring, PT, PhD, GCS, CWS

George is a 72-year-old male (retired truck driver) who is experiencing an attack of gout of the left first metatarsal-phalangeal joint. He states that wearing shoes and weight bearing (especially walking) is painful, and he also experiences pain during the night. George is obese, has diagnosed hypertension, diabetes mellitus, and hypercholesterolemia. George also has a history of alcoholism, describes occasional dark spots and blurry vision, obstructive sleep apnea, polyuria, bilateral knee pain, low back pain, and altered sensation in his feet/lower legs. His physician prescribed nonsteroidal anti-inflammatory drugs (NSAIDs) and a corticosteroid injection for the gout.

Upon physical therapy examination at an outpatient clinic, George's left foot displayed a red, hot, swollen first MTP joint. George described pain with pressure and mobilization of the joint. Other than lack of movement in the MTP range of motion is within normal limits throughout. He is unable to bear weight on the left foot for greater than 2 minutes due to pain, and is limited in walking distance, also due to pain. George shows apparent cardiovascular deconditioning due to a sedentary lifestyle, and displays many lower extremity strength deficits due to said lifestyle. Vital signs are: HR 80; RR 20; BP 144/90; SpO$_2$ 95%; Temp 98.7°F. Strength is grossly 4/5 throughout.

■ CASE STUDY QUESTIONS

1. What is gout?
2. What is the incidence of gout?
3. Why is gout painful?
4. With proper medical treatment, how long does this take to resolve?
5. In this case, why are medications so important?
6. What are the risk factors for gout?
7. What other specific conditions might you have suspected in this case?
8. What are some signs that George may have uncontrolled diabetes?
9. While the patient is experiencing acute pain, what type of physical therapy treatment is indicated?
10. What are some appropriate goals for George?
11. What kind of modalities might you provide?
12. What kind of exercise might you recommend?

22

GOUT: CASE 2

Meri Goehring, PT, PhD, GCS, CWS

Tracy is a 58-year-old male factory worker who complains of left-sided posterior ankle pain. He was referred to your outpatient clinic from an orthopedic surgeon with a diagnosis of Achilles tendonitis and/or bursitis. He states that weight bearing (especially walking) is extremely painful and any movement causes pain. He rates his pain as 4/10 at rest, 8/10 with weight bearing of any kind. Tracy is overweight, but not obese, with a BMI of 30. There is no history of alcoholism, but Tracy admits to drinking a few beers most evenings. Tracy has a history of bilateral knee pain due to osteoarthritis, but he states this pain is different than his previous pain, which he describes as a dull ache that would get worse during the day and would reduce when he would rest. The orthopedic surgeon prescribed nonsteroidal anti-inflammatory drugs (NSAIDs) for pain that have not been working well.

Tracy reported no history of trauma. Upon physical therapy examination, you find strength and range of motion of the ankle and foot to be within normal limits and painful only upon resisted plantarflexion of the foot. You find some swelling over the calcaneal tuberosity and there is a hard nodule that has a bony feel and is tender on palpation. There is no pain with palpation of the Achilles tendon.

There is no improvement after three treatments of ice, massage, and exercise. In fact, after massage the patient reported an increase in pain. You continue to ask the patient questions regarding his pain and about family history as you suspect there may be some other issue. The patient informs you that there is a family history of gout. You decide to contact the patient's family physician to inform the physician of your findings and discuss the possibility as gout as a contributing factor. Further physical therapy was stopped and the patient was advised to limit weight bearing on the foot until the patient could be returned to his family physician. The physician finds that the blood urate levels were high and the patient was started on medications. Symptoms were reduced within 48 hours.

■ CASE STUDY QUESTIONS

1. Is gout a form of arthritis?
2. What other specific conditions might you have suspected in this case?
3. Why was careful observation and palpation important in this case?
4. Is there a specific name for the nodule that you found?
5. How are these nodules best visualized with diagnostic imaging?
6. Why was continued subjective questioning important in this case?
7. What risk factors does Tracy have for gout?
8. Does gout only affect one joint?
9. Is Tracy's osteoarthritis of the knees a factor in his gout?
10. What goals might you develop for Tracy?

23

SHOULDER IMPINGEMENT

Meri Goehring, PT, PhD, GCS, CWS

Hank is a 64-year-old man who is retired from working as head of maintenance in the local school system. He lives with his wife, and they enjoy playing in couples' golf and tennis leagues year round. Hank also still does some handyman work for neighbors in the area to keep busy. Two weeks ago he was working on some plumbing under a neighbor's sink when he felt a sharp pain on the superior portion of his right shoulder. He tried golfing a few days later, and his shoulder did not bother him, so Hank thought it was fine. But when he went to his tennis league the next day, he had quite a bit of pain while playing, most notably with serving. Since then, he has been avoiding overhead reaching and handyman jobs in odd positions so that he does not get the sharp pain in his shoulder.

Hank has a history of hypertension, atrial fibrillation, and low back pain. He is currently taking Microzide (hydrochlorothiazide), imipramine (Tofranil) also known as melipramine, Rythmol (propafenone hydrochloride), Coumadin (warfarin sodium), and ibuprofen as needed for the pain.

When you see Hank in your outpatient orthopedic clinic, he rates his pain as 2/10 at rest, and a 5/10 with any glenohumeral movements. The pain is worst at a 7/10 with overhead movements. His systems review is recorded with HR = 72, BP = 124/70, RR = 14. He is oriented and appropriate. When you ask Hank to take off his shirt so that you may examine his shoulder, you notice a large, asymmetrical mole at the base of his neck that has some minimal bleeding around the edges and make a note of it in the chart. His posture shows forward head, he has moderately rounded shoulders with internal rotation at the right glenohumeral joint and both scapulae are abducted from the spine at rest. He is grossly a 4/5 on the right, compared to 5/5 on the left for upper extremity movements at the glenohumeral and elbow joints. Hank tests positive with painful arc, the Hawkins-Kennedy Test, Neer test, and Feagan test for instability. He is tender to palpation on the superior and anterior aspects of his humeral head.

■ CASE STUDY QUESTIONS

1. How common is shoulder pain?
2. What is the most frequent cause of shoulder pain?
3. What are the symptoms of subacromial impingement syndrome?
4. What is causing the pain?
5. What are some of the intrinsic factors that can cause this problem?
6. What are some of the extrinsic factors that can cause this problem?
7. Can physical therapy benefit someone with subacromial impingement syndrome?
8. What other conservative treatments are available for shoulder impingement syndrome?
9. Is there information regarding which is best, either injection with corticosteroids or physical therapy?
10. What are some common tests to rule in or out an impingement syndrome?
11. What other problems would be involved to rule out in a differential diagnosis?
12. Is surgery an option for this problem?
13. Does the mole concern you?

24

SHOULDER PAIN

Meri Goehring, PT, PhD, GCS, CWS

Mary is a 50-year-old female who works as a secretary at a local university. She lives alone and has never been married. Mary has been in good health, but reports that she knows she is overweight. She has a BMI of 32. Mary reports that she does not get much exercise and prefers to read or watch movies for entertainment. She also likes to cook. Mary states she had some sharp pains in the front of her left shoulder about 6 weeks ago that she thought were associated with some overhead lifting she did while rearranging her kitchen cabinets. She now tells you that she has pain reaching behind her back, over her head, and across her body. She reports increased pain at night, increased pain while lying on her left arm, and pain that is easily made worse with movement. She reports pain with any movement of the shoulder.

Mary was given the Shoulder Pain and Disability Index (SPADI) and scored a 70. The examination begins with a systems review. Her blood pressure is 155/85, heart rate is 90 beats per minute, respiratory rate was 28. Light touch sensation was intact in all extremities and cervical; thoracic and contralateral shoulder ranges of motion are within functional limits. DTRs are 2+ in the upper extremities. Strength in her right upper extremity was 5/5 throughout and range of motion is without limitation. Upon examination of her left shoulder, there is a range of motion loss in external rotation, abduction, and internal

rotation and is limited by a springy end feel and pain. External rotation was measured at 5°, abduction was 20°, and internal rotation was 13°. Her strength in external rotation, abduction, and internal rotation are 2+/5 within her available range of motion. Joint play assessment reveals a restriction in all directions. She has pain 8/10 with a cross arm test, is able to touch the pocket on the back of her pants, and is unable to touch the back of her neck with the affected arm.

■ CASE STUDY QUESTIONS

1. What diagnosis do you suspect in this case?
2. What are the common signs and symptoms of this diagnosis?
3. Is there single, agreed upon diagnostic reference standard for this diagnosis?
4. What motions are often restricted?
5. What is a capsular pattern?
6. What is the mechanism of injury for this disorder?
7. What is the epidemiology of this disorder?
8. Is the SPADI developed for an inpatient- or outpatient-type setting?
9. Is there one agreed upon diagnostic reference for this condition?
10. What is the medical term for a frozen shoulder?
11. Are there conditions that can appear similar but are actually different?
12. What standardized tests have been shown to be specifically reliable and valid in their determination of a diagnosis?
13. What types of rehabilitation interventions can be utilized?
14. Are there medical interventions for this disorder?

25

ROTATOR CUFF TEAR: CASE 1

Meri Goehring, PT, PhD, GCS, CWS

Leon is a 72-year-old man who enjoys playing golf and chess with his grandchildren. He is retired from managing a local business, and still follows the details of the economy avidly. He is still very independent, and lives alone. When out in the community, Leon ambulates with a single-point cane in his left hand. About a month ago, Leon was golfing with his son and granddaughter when he felt a brief pain in his left shoulder. In the week following, he had a moderate pain in the shoulder, and he felt weaker with any shoulder movements and walking with his cane. Leon normally sleeps on his left side, but the pain grew sharper and more severe after laying on it, and it would even wake him up at night.

After seeing his physician, imaging showed a full thickness rotator cuff tear. Leon wanted to try conservative treatment prior to exploring surgical means, and his physician referred him to your outpatient clinic. He also injected two shots of triamcinolone acetonide into his left shoulder. Leon has a history of high cholesterol, hypertension, and atrial fibrillation. He is currently taking Lipitor, HCTZ daily, and nitroglycerine as needed.

When you go through Leon's systems review, he is oriented ×3 and very chatty, has no noticeable integument issues, and his radial pulse is weak but regular with HR = 72, BP = 126/70, SpO_2 = 96%, and RR = 14.

His strength records are as follows: shoulder flexion R 4+/5 L 3+/5, abduction R 5/5, L 4/5; external rotation R 5/5, L 3+/; internal rotation R 4+/5, L 3+/5; elbow flexion R 5/5, L 4/5; elbow extension R 5/5, L 5/5.

His left shoulder AROM is moderately limited in shoulder IR/ER and abduction. Leon's goals for PT are to get back to golfing and playing with his grandchildren, and to be able to carry his groceries without pain.

CASE STUDY QUESTIONS

1. Name the four muscle tendons that support/stabilize the gleno-humeral joint.
2. What are the main functions of these tendons?
3. How common is tendinopathy present with complaints of shoulder pain?
4. What are considered some of the main reasons for rotator cuff tears to occur?
5. At what age are these most likely to occur?
6. What are the most common clinical manifestations of a rotator cuff tear?
7. What functional skills are difficult?
8. What type of diagnostic imaging will confirm a rotator cuff tear is present?
9. When is surgery indicated?
10. When is conservative treatment best?
11. What is HCTZ?
12. What is triamcinolone acetonide?

26

ROTATOR CUFF TEAR/REPAIR: CASE 2

Meri Goehring, PT, PhD, GCS, CWS

Lorenzo is a 69-year-old recently retired automobile factory worker who lives with his wife in a two-story home. He has five steps to enter his home with a rail on the right-hand side (when ascending the stairs) and a rail on his left-hand side when ascending to his second floor in his home. He has a half bathroom downstairs with his full bathroom upstairs with a walk-in shower but no grab bars. His wife recently retired as well and they enjoy going out to the movies, seeing their grandchildren, and volunteering at the local homeless shelter once a month.

Lorenzo recently underwent a rotator cuff repair for his left supraspinatus muscle he tore while picking up a box above his head to prepare for the upcoming holiday. He felt sudden pain after he got the box down and decided to go to the doctor as he felt intense pain that persisted for several days. The MRI showed a full-thickness tear of his supraspinatus tendon. Lorenzo decided to opt for surgery due to the immense pain he was experiencing, as he did not think physical therapy would work.

You are seeing Lorenzo 3 days after his operation. The orthopedic surgeon's precautions for Lorenzo are no passive range of motion. The surgeon has prescribed Codman/pendulum exercises only for the first 3 weeks after surgery. Following his 3-week consult, Lorenzo can begin active assisted range of motion for 1 week (fourth week postoperatively) and then begin active range of motion the following week (fifth week postoperatively). Lorenzo walks in to the outpatient clinic wearing an arm abduction sling. Active external rotation is not allowed until the seventh week postoperatively.

You begin the initial evaluation with a systems review and this is what you find: Vital signs are BP: 126/94 mm Hg, HR: 73 beats per minute, RR: 16 breaths per minute, and SpO_2 of 92%. Light touch sensation appears intact throughout the upper and lower extremities. Right upper extremity strength and range of motion appear WNL. Left shoulder passive range of motion is severely limited with flexion is limited to 75°, abduction is limited to 72°, and internal rotation is limited to 25°. There are no limitations in the left elbow, wrist, or hand. He demonstrates decreased handgrip strength on his left 28 lb when compared to his right, 52 lb, using a dynamometer. Lorenzo scored an 87 on his DASH score.

CASE STUDY QUESTIONS

1. What is the goal of rotator cuff surgery?
2. Should this patient wear a sling? Why or why not?
3. Should rehabilitation start immediately? Why or why not?
4. Is use of joint mobilization appropriate? When and what type?
5. When should a sling be removed and when should some type of exercise begin?
6. What are the goals for physical therapy treatment when surgery has not been performed?
7. If surgery is indicated, what are the options?
8. Why are there different types of immobilization positions?
9. What are the differences in outcomes between surgical and non-surgical interventions?
10. What is the typical rehabilitation protocol postsurgery?
11. What are the common factors that influence outcomes?
12. What standardized outcome measures may be indicated and what is the criteria for return to normal activity?
13. What is the Constant Shoulder Score?
14. What are the criteria for return to normal activity?

27

HUMERAL HEAD FRACTURE

Meri Goehring, PT, PhD, GCS, CWS

Mary is a 65-year-old substitute teacher who served as an international missionary for 15 years but has been stateside for the past 7 years taking care of her elderly mother. She has osteopenia (DEXA score of 1.75), slight thoracic kyphosis, and some fungus on her fingernails and toe nails. Mary stays active doing yoga two times a week and jogs 2 to 3 miles 5 to 6 days a week. On Mary's last run, Mary slipped on the ice falling onto her left shoulder and sustained a left humeral head fracture that was 50% displaced. Mary is left-hand dominant. The doctors suggested Mary have surgery but Mary did not have medical insurance and wanted to try conservative treatment without surgery.

Mary is being seen in an outpatient orthopedic setting on a pro bono basis through a local hospital. Mary is 9 weeks postinjury and radiographs show a bone callous formation over the break. Her physician has given her permission to start physical therapy.

The physical therapy examination began with a systems review. Her blood pressure was 110/65, heart rate was 67 beats per minute, respiratory rate 14, oxygen saturation 98%. Sensation to light touch was intact throughout, and deep tendon reflexes were normal (left upper extremity not tested). Mary has been immobilized in a sling for 9 weeks and has moderate swelling in her hand, wrist, forearm, and upper arm. Mary's pain at rest in her shoulder is 0/10 and 4/10 with active movement at the end of range. Mary's finger and wrist pain ranges from 2 to 6/10 at rest and the pain usually decreases with activity. Mary appears anxious with shoulder range of motion and is limited in all directions. Mary's active shoulder flexion is 30° and active shoulder abduction is 25° using shoulder elevation to compensate. Forearm supination is moderately limited to 45°, finger extension to neutral is moderately limited, and elbow extension is mildly limited by 7°. She was able to provide some resistance during manual muscle testing within her available range of motion. Mary's hand and wrist are stiff and painful. Mary scored a 48 on the QuickDASH. Mary just started antibiotics to reduce the inflammation and takes a wide variety of supplements to promote bone healing.

Mary was given a home stretching and range of motion program for her shoulder, elbow, wrist, and fingers.

■ CASE STUDY QUESTIONS

1. What type of fracture is likely?
2. Will this require surgery?
3. What are the common risk factors for this type of fracture?
4. What has a protective effect against this type of fracture?
5. What are the common clinical problems reported by patients with this type of fracture?
6. What are the stages of bone healing?
7. Approximately how long does each healing stage last?
8. If surgery is needed, what types of surgical repair might be used?
9. If surgery is not needed, what treatment may be indicated?
10. What functional limitations may be present?
11. Why might this patient be fearful?
12. When can the patient expect to return to normal function?
13. What are the possible complications that could occur?
14. What would a typical rehabilitation protocol entail?
15. What shoulder motions required for various feeding tasks?
16. What are standardized measures/functional outcomes for this condition?
17. When can the patient return to work?

28

HUMERAL NECK FRACTURE

Meri Goehring, PT, PhD, GCS, CWS

Ethel is a 77-year-old retired secretary of 42 years. She lives alone in a two-bedroom ranch-style home with two steps to enter and a flight of stairs that goes to her basement where her laundry room is located. She has osteopenia, arthritis in her knees, shoulders, and wrists, moderate thoracic kyphosis, and diabetes mellitus type 2.

Ethel stays active by going to a senior citizens Zumba class called Zumba Gold where she is able to perform chair aerobics for 1 hour once a week. During the last snowstorm, Ethel was shoveling the sidewalk by her front door when she slipped on some ice and fall onto her outstretched right arm. Luckily her neighbor was outside and saw this happen. The neighbor quickly came to the rescue and found that she was in a great deal of pain after landing on her right shoulder. Ethel was taken to the emergency department by the neighbor to find out that she had a minimally (1.5 cm) displaced fracture of her right humeral neck. For now, the orthopedic surgeon elected not to proceed with surgery stating that he feels that she can recover from this utilizing a more conservative approach. Ethel is being seen in outpatient physical therapy 1 week postfracture.

The examination began with a systems review and Ethel's blood pressure was 146/85, heart rate was 86 beats per minute, respiration 16 breaths per minute, pulse oximetry 94%. Neurologically sensation to light touch was intact and reflexes were 2+ bilaterally on both the upper extremity reflex testing sites and lower extremity reflex testing sites. Ethel has been immobilized for 1 week thus far with noticeable moderate swelling in the left elbow and mild swelling in left wrist and hand. Elbow range of motion appears to be moderately limited noticeable in elbow extension, and wrist range of motion appears mildly limited most notably in extension and radial deviation. She was unable to provide any resistance during the manual muscle testing of the elbow due to pain. Ethel states that she was given wrist exercises to maintain mobility in her wrist as well as to keep the swelling down in her left arm. She states that she has not done these exercises the last 2 days due to pain. Ethel states that at rest her shoulder is a 3/10 pain, at best her shoulder is a 1/10, and this typically occurs when she sits in her chair with her arm supported and a hot pack on her shoulder. At worst, Ethel states that her shoulder is an 8/10 pain. "The only thing worse is child birth!" Ethel filled out a QuickDash and scored a 74.

■ CASE STUDY QUESTIONS

1. How common is this type of fracture?
2. Which is more common: surgical intervention or conservative treatment?
3. What is the most common cause of this kind of fracture?
4. What are the risk factors for proximal humeral fractures?
5. What specific disease processes can predispose individuals to this type of injury?
6. What can decrease the risk for a fracture?
7. Does hand dominance make a difference?
8. What are the general clinical manifestations of acute fractures?
9. What are some of the possible surgical interventions for a severely displaced proximal humerus fracture?
10. What are the most common functional limitations noted with proximal humeral fracture?
11. When might this patient expect to return to normal function?
12. What are the possible complications?
13. What is the typical rehabilitation protocol?
14. When can the patient expect to regain shoulder function?
15. How much shoulder motion is necessary in order for this patient to eat normally?
16. What types of standardized measures might be included in your examination?
17. When will the patient be able to return to work?
18. What is the Neer four-part classification system for proximal humeral fractures?

29

SHOULDER DISLOCATION

Eric Shamus, PT, DPT, PhD

Steven B. Ambler, PT, DPT, MPH, CPH, OCS

A 69-year-old patient is being seen in the clinic with a chief complaint of right anterior shoulder pain that began after a shoulder dislocation 1 week ago. He states that he injured the shoulder when he fell to the ground and dislocated his right shoulder. He was taken by the ambulance to the hospital emergency room where it was relocated.

The patient has been wearing a sling since the injury. The patient is taking naproxen 500 mg two times a day and has no pain at rest at this time. He does have 4 to 5/10 pain when he wakes in the morning and when he has to reach overhead. He denies numbness and tingling and has no other complaints at this time. The patient is currently retired and is keeping the arm in the sling. He is left handed and would like to be able to get back to yard work and other activities around his house.

Vital signs: HR 72, RR 15, BP 154/89, SpO_2 97%, temp 98.6°F.

ROS (review of systems): Unremarkable for integumental or neurological problems.

PMH: diabetes mellitus type 2, diagnosed 9 years ago, and has an elevated A1C (7.5).

After your evaluation you determine that you need to do more research for this disorder to determine your treatment approach. Please answer the following questions based on your research.

■ CASE STUDY QUESTIONS

1. What direction of shoulder dislocation is most common and why?

2. What direction of humerus movement will cause an anterior dislocation?

3. What are associate pathologies?

4. What are some potential activity and participation limitations for this patient after a shoulder dislocation?

5. What is the difference between a subluxation and a dislocation, and what are the common signs of a subluxation?

6. What are the contributing factors for a subluxation or dislocation of the shoulder?

7. What type of imaging is first used for a dislocation and why?

8. What are differential medical diagnoses?

9. What are the issues with relocating a dislocation?

10. The patient returns to your facility in 1 week. What structure specific tests and movement test(s) would be beneficial to conduct on this patient?

11. What is appropriate treatment when the patient returns in 1 week?

12. What is the prognosis following a dislocation?

13. What factors for this patient would moderate the prognosis positively or negatively?

30

TOTAL SHOULDER ARTHROPLASTY: CASE 1

Meri Goehring, PT, PhD, GCS, CWS

William H. Staples, PT, DHSc, DPT, GCS, CEEAA

Carolyn is a 72-year-old Caucasian woman who underwent a right total shoulder arthroplasty (TSA) 2 weeks ago. Carolyn underwent the TSA secondary to pain and stiffness and her orthopedic surgeon chose to perform a TSA instead of a hemiarthroplasty. Prior to surgery she noted extreme difficulty when participating in recreational activities like bowling on the Wii, as well as daily activities such as sweeping the floor and getting dressed. Following the TSA, Carolyn started physical therapy in the hospital, but since being admitted to a skilled nursing facility, refused therapy for at least 2 weeks. Carolyn has signs of cognitive impairment with an "abnormal" score on the Mini-Cog test. Previously, Carolyn was ambulating, driving, and performing daily activities without any assistance as she was living alone in a small ranch home. Carolyn does not have any children and enjoys her independence. She was admitted to the local skilled nursing facility because she is now unable to drive, lives alone in an apartment, and has little social support.

Upon examination, Carolyn presents with increased swelling and redness at the right shoulder. Her incisions are healing well with no signs of infection. Currently her pain is a 5/10 on a verbal analog scale, but is receiving Lortab (10 mg/325 mg) for pain every 6 hours, which ease her pain level. She is unable to actively move her right shoulder as her right arm has been immobilized within the sling since her last therapy session 2 weeks ago. Active range of motion and strength testing is not performed at this time. Passive motion is restricted, especially external rotation.

■ CASE STUDY QUESTIONS

1. What is the most common pathological condition leading to a total shoulder arthroplasty (TSA)?

2. Why did the surgeon most likely choose a TSA over hemiarthroplasty?

3. What are the common radiographic findings for a patient undergoing a TSA?

4. What is the Mini-Cog test?

5. What possible biopsychosocial concerns do you have working with Carolyn?

6. Do you expect any delays in her rehabilitation?

7. What physical therapy interventions are appropriate for Carolyn at this time?

8. What types of exercise are appropriate for Carolyn? How about in the first 4, 6, 12 weeks?

9. What are the main goals for Carolyn?

10. What will Carolyn need to be educated about?

11. Would you make any other referrals?

12. Will she be able to go home independently?

31

TOTAL SHOULDER ARTHROPLASTY: CASE 2

Meri Goehring, PT, PhD, GCS, CWS

William H. Staples, PT, DHSc, DPT, GCS, CEEAA

Colleen is a 72-year-old female (retired postal worker) who is 2 weeks status post unconstrained right total shoulder arthroplasty due to severe osteoarthritis of the right shoulder. Her rotator cuff is intact. She also has mild osteoarthritis in her left shoulder, and is a smoker (1 pack per day for 52 years). She had stopped smoking 3 days prior to surgery per her physician request, but started again last week. She reports no constitutional symptoms, wears glasses, and reports occasional sinus pain/stuffiness with seasonal allergies. She often produces a dry cough, experiences occasional heartburn, and has a history of hypothyroidism which is managed by the drug Synthroid (levothyroxine) 100 μg/day.

Currently, Colleen wears a sling during most of the day, but is weaning out of the sling while at home. She continues to take 5 mg Norco as needed three to four times per day, often at nighttime or before/after therapy. Her incisions display some peeling and dried blood, but not abnormally, and mild redness and swelling of the right shoulder are noted. Upon outpatient physical therapy examination, passive right shoulder range of motion showed limitations in all directions, most markedly in flexion, abduction, and external rotation. All directions displayed an empty end feel, limited by pain. Elbow, wrist, and hand range of motion was full and painless. She has been performing pendulum and assisted range of motion exercises at home, is not lifting anything heavier than a coffee mug, and is icing the shoulder two to three times per day as she was instructed in the hospital. She is able to perform shoulder isometrics into abduction, adduction, flexion, extension, internal and external rotation with no increase in pain. She could also sustain scapular isometrics into elevation, depression, upward and downward rotation. Colleen is experiencing difficulties in upper body dressing (especially bra fastening), bathing (ie, washing hair), and with her grooming. Her husband has been able to perform cleaning and cooking around the house, and has been driving her as well.

■ CASE STUDY QUESTIONS

1. What is Norco?
2. What are the possible side effects of Norco?
3. Do you expect any problems/delays in her rehabilitation?
4. What is an unconstrained total shoulder arthroplasty?
5. What therapeutic short-term goals (2-4 weeks) would you establish for Colleen during this phase 1 of therapy?
6. What interventions would you perform at this time?
7. What are the most common postoperative complications of a total shoulder replacement?
8. What motions or exercises should be avoided at this time?
9. Colleen is doing well and it is now 5 weeks postsurgery (phase 2, weeks 4-12). What interventions will you now perform?
10. The therapy is now entering the 13th week. What exercises do you teach the patient now?

11. Are there any precautions to monitor with a person taking Synthroid?
12. What would some signs and symptoms of someone with untreated hypothyroidism?

32

REVERSE TOTAL SHOULDER ARTHROPLASTY

William H. Staples, PT, DHSc, DPT, GCS, CEEAA

Eunice is a 75-year-old female (retired nurse) who is 2 weeks status post reverse right total shoulder arthroplasty due to severe osteoarthritis of the right shoulder. Her rotator cuff was not intact. She also has type 2 diabetes mellitus for which she takes metformin (Glucophage) 500 mg orally twice a day.

Currently, Eunice wears an abduction splint during most of the day, but is weaning out of the splint while at home. She has been taking 5/325 mg Norco as needed for pain four times per day. Her incisions display some peeling and dried blood, and mild redness and swelling of the right shoulder are also noted. Upon outpatient physical therapy examination, passive right shoulder range of motion showed limitations in all directions, most markedly in flexion, abduction, and external rotation. All directions displayed an empty end feel, limited by pain. Elbow, wrist, and hand range of motion was full and painless. She has been performing pendulum and assisted range of motion exercises at home when the splint is removed, is not lifting anything heavier than a coffee mug, and is icing the shoulder two to three times per day as she was instructed in the hospital. She is able to perform shoulder isometrics into abduction, adduction, flexion, extension, internal and external rotation with only minimal increase in pain. She could also sustain scapular isometrics into elevation, depression, upward and downward rotation. Eunice is experiencing difficulties in upper body dressing (especially bra fastening), bathing (ie, washing hair), and with her grooming. Her husband has been able to perform cleaning and cooking around the house, and has been driving her as well.

■ CASE STUDY QUESTIONS

1. What is the best time to take Norco?
2. What are the possible side effects of Norco?
3. Do you foresee any problems/delays in her rehabilitation?
4. What is a reverse total shoulder arthroplasty?
5. What muscle is the primary mover following a reverse total shoulder?
6. What therapeutic short-term goals (2-4 weeks) would you establish for Eunice during this phase 1 of therapy?
7. What interventions would you perform at this time?
8. What are the most common postoperative complications of a total shoulder replacement?
9. What motions or exercises should be avoided at this time?
10. Eunice is doing well and it is now 5 weeks postsurgery (phase 2, weeks 4-12). What interventions will you now perform?
11. The therapy is now entering the 13th week. What exercises do you teach the patient now?

12. Are there any precautions or side effects to monitor with a person taking Glucophage?

13. What are the guidelines for blood sugar for safe exercise?

33

ROTATOR CUFF INJURY WITH REVERSE TOTAL SHOULDER ARTHROPLASTY

James R. Creps, PT, DScPT, OCS, CMPT

Joe is a 77-year-old, right-handed male who remains very active. He is in a senior golf league and has been golfing as a hobby for over 50 years. Over the course of golf season, he noticed that he was having some soreness in his right shoulder and that it seemed to become weak. In addition, he felt pain in the joint if he attempted to sleep on his right side. Joe attempted to treat his symptoms with over-the-counter pain relievers and anti-inflammatory agents, but he noticed little improvement in his condition. Because of this, he called his primary care physician and was set up for an appointment.

MRI studies ordered by his physician revealed severe arthritis of the glenohumeral joint and a large tear of the medial rotator cuff. Muscle atrophy, lamellar dissection, and fatty infiltration could be seen in the area of the tear. His primary care physician decided to inject the joint to reduce inflammation and referred him to physical therapy for conservative care.

Upon evaluation, the physical therapist did a thorough examination of his shoulder, which revealed moderate tenderness to palpation of the distal supraspinatus tendon. All neurological tests were normal; however, Joe demonstrated severe right shoulder weakness into abduction and external rotation and a positive Drop Arm Test. Vital signs were HR: 68; RR: 16; BP: 132/74; SpO2: 98%; Temp: 98.7°F.

Joe's physical therapist attempted to treat his condition with manual therapy and therapeutic exercise, but his condition did not significantly improve. After 8 weeks of care, Joe was referred to an orthopedic surgeon. The surgeon felt that Joe was a good candidate for a reverse total shoulder joint arthroplasty. Joe underwent the procedure, although significant complications resulted in an extended hospital stay following surgery. Joe was eventually released from the hospital and attended 12 weeks of outpatient rehabilitation. He was reassessed after 6 months and demonstrated only mild shoulder pain. Joe returned to playing golf, but he never achieved the level of function he had preoperatively.

■ CASE STUDY QUESTIONS

1. Are rotator cuff tears a common cause of shoulder pain and dysfunction in the elderly?

2. Do rotator cuff tears in the elderly tend to be more severe?

3. Is fatty infiltration and muscle atrophy a common finding in chronic rotator cuff tears?

4. Is it unusual that Joe did not experience more pain given the severity of his rotator cuff tear?

5. Does an MRI substantially increase the cost of diagnosis of rotator cuff tear and is it possible to use other clinical indicators to determine who might be a surgical candidate for rotator cuff repair?

6. Are medial rotator cuff tears in the elderly usually associated with inferior long-term outcomes when managed conservatively as compared to lateral tears of the rotator cuff?

7. Has it been determined that the use of corticosteroid injections is effective in the management of rotator cuff disease?

8. Is there consensus among health care providers on whether conservative care or surgery is best for elderly patients with rotator cuff tears?

9. Does reverse total shoulder arthroplasty represent a possible treatment option for the patient's suffering from arthropathy deficient rotator cuff who failed conservative care?

10. Is there an increased rate of perioperative complications with reverse total shoulder arthroplasty when compared to total shoulder arthroplasty?

11. Is reverse total shoulder arthroplasty common for the treatment of rotator cuff tear arthropathy?

34

BICEP TENDON RUPTURE

Meri Goehring, PT, PhD, GCS, CWS

William H. Staples, PT, DHSc, DPT, GCS, CEEAA

George is a 77-year-old man who is a retired Marine sergeant having served in Korea. George lives alone in a bilevel home and enjoys fly-fishing and bike riding. Six weeks ago George had fallen from a ladder while cleaning his gutters and tore his right rotator cuff and sustained a superior labral tear from anterior to posterior (SLAP), which was confirmed by magnetic resonance imaging (MRI). George was able to immediately go in for surgery and they repaired his rotator cuff and the SLAP tear. George has a family history of heart attacks, high cholesterol, osteoarthritis, and hypertension. George had a lumbar fusion at L4/5 25 years ago, a right meniscectomy 35 years ago, a left rotator cuff repair 10 years ago and again 5 years ago, left knee arthroscopy 20 years ago, and left ankle fracture, 40 years ago. George does have arthritis and high cholesterol, which is controlled by Lipitor (atorvastatin calcium).

George is seen for initial evaluation 1 week following surgery in your outpatient clinic today. His blood pressure is steady around 120/70, his heart rate is 75 beats per minute, and respiratory rate is 16 breaths per minute. George complains of 6/10 pain with right should flexion and you can see a lump in the right upper arm that the patient reports developed over the last 3 days. He said that he felt a pop when he was carrying a gallon of milk and then there was a lump. He reports that his arm is not more painful than usual and actually is less painful with elbow flexion. A passive and active assist range of motion and isometric exercise program for the shoulder was initially implemented in the hospital.

Upon examination by you the physical therapist, you see an obvious "Popeye" deformity. Elbow and shoulder range of motion have not changed.

■ CASE STUDY QUESTIONS

1. What is the most common form of biceps tendon rupture?

2. What tendon is most commonly involved?

3. Is the biceps tendon considered superficial or deep?

4. Where specifically does the tendon rupture?

5. In what types of individuals is this injury most common?

6. Is significant history of shoulder problems associated with this injury?

7. What is the major impairment associated with this injury?

8. Does the previous rotator cuff injury have any significance?

9. What are the signs and symptoms of a ruptured biceps tendon?

10. How are biceps tendon ruptures best diagnosed?

11. What standardized functional examinations could be included?

12. Is surgery recommended to repair a biceps tendon?

13. What is the likely prognosis for recovery?

14. What type of education might this patient need?

35

WRIST FRACTURE: CASE 1

Meri Goehring, PT, PhD, GCS, CWS

Leonora is a 72-year-old female retired telemarketer. She is a heavier individual with a BMI of 32 kg/m². She lives with her daughter and three grandchildren in a four-bedroom, two-story house in the suburbs. Her bedroom is on the upstairs level with her daughter and two of her grandchildren. The house is "not even close to being handicapped accessible" according to Leonora. She is considered to have osteoporosis as she has a DEXA T-score of −2.9 standard deviations away from normal. She has recently consulted a dietician to manage her high cholesterol and diabetes by eating healthier through fruits and vegetables. She currently drinks four to five cups of coffee a day, five to six cans of soda a day, and typically one 8 oz glass of water before she goes to bed at night. Currently, Leonora is on Simvastatin, Metformin, Atenolol, Vicodin, a nicotine patch as she is trying to quit smoking, cyclobenzaprine, Naproxen, Zoloft, and Lunesta.

She recently fractured her left wrist when she was babysitting her grandchildren and she tripped over a toy that was on the floor. She states that she fell on an outstretch arm when she heard something pop. When she looked at her wrist upon the fall she noticed that her wrist was malaligned from her forearm, saying it looked "like a dinner fork!" You are currently seeing Leonora at an outpatient clinic 13 weeks after the injury. Leonora had an external fixation, because the fracture was displaced, on her left wrist for 7 weeks, then immobilization for 6 weeks. Imaging of the injury states that it is 85% fully healed.

You begin the examination process with a systems review and this is what you find: blood pressure 167/89, heart rate 84, respiratory rate of 21. Light touch sensation appears to be intact on the upper extremities, but has diminished light touch sensation in the lower extremities up to her knees bilaterally. Sharp/dull sensation is intact throughout her lower extremities. Her reflexes are 2+ bilaterally in the upper and lower extremities. Shoulder range of motion is WNL bilaterally. Elbow range of motion is 25% diminished on her injured left arm, wrist range of motion is limited to 5° of flexion, 3° of extension, 2° of radial deviation. She lacks 3 degrees of ulnar deviation actively. Passively, wrist range of motion was limited to 10° of wrist flexion with severe pain, 5° of wrist extension with severe pain, 3° of radial deviation with pain but not as severe as all other motions, and 2° of ulnar deviation with severe pain.

Leonora rates her pain at a 6/10 at rest and 10/10 with movement (at worst). Using a hand dynamometer, Leonora demonstrates 48 lb of pressure (strength) on her right hand and 8 lb of pressure on her left hand with severe pain. Upon palpation, severe swelling is noted in the fingers and hand, moderate swelling in the wrist, and

minimally swelling in the left elbow. An incision is located on radial border of her wrist that measures 3 in in length; it appears healthy and normal at this time. No manual muscle testing was performed at this time due to Leonora being in severe pain. Leonora scored a 92 on the QuickDASH assessing her left wrist, a 23.4 on the TUG test, and 21 seconds on the five times sit-to-stand test.

■ CASE STUDY QUESTIONS

1. What type of fracture is present?

2. What percent of fractures are wrist fractures?

3. What is the primary risk factor for wrist fracture?

4. What other factors are associated with risk for fracture?

5. What is the most common medical treatment for a wrist fracture?

6. Why are wrist fractures significant to older adults?

7. What is the most common mechanism of injury for wrist fractures?

8. Are wrist fractures related to hip fractures?

9. What are some intrinsic and extrinsic factors that can lead to low-trauma wrist fracture?

10. What are some of the long-term outcomes following distal radial fractures?

11. What are some of the complications that may occur?

12. What does the ongoing rehabilitation program entail?

13. Should therapy also exercise the nonfractured arm?

14. What types of standardized measures might you incorporate?

36

WRIST FRACTURE: CASE 2

Meri Goehring, PT, PhD, GCS, CWS

William H. Staples, PT, DHSc, DPT, GCS, CEEAA

Lonnie is a 79-year-old male retired insurance salesman. He lives with his wife, two dogs, and three cats in a two-story home. The master bedroom is located upstairs along with his study where he likes to read and play chess. The house has three steps to enter. Lonnie is a tall, slender man standing at 6 ft 5 in, demonstrates a moderate thoracic kyphosis, lean body mass with a BMI of 22. Lonnie was active going to the gym three times a week to lift weights and walking outside 3 days a week with Sundays being his rest days due to church activities. Lonnie was walking outside on the sidewalk when he tripped over a raised ledge on the sidewalk and fell on an outstretch arm. Due to this fall, Lonnie sustained a right wrist fracture with the fracture site approximately 3 cm proximal to the proximal carpal bones. Lonnie's right wrist was placed in a short arm cast and immobilized for 8 weeks. Lonnie is right handed. Lonnie's medications are Vicodin, acetaminophen, Lipitor, and Lopressor. He states he is a social drinker having a couple of beers at night.

Lonnie was referred to your clinic 2 days after casting to provide him a home program with the plan to return in 8 weeks for further rehabilitation.

Lonnie is now being seen in the outpatient orthopedic clinic 8 weeks postfracture and 1 week post-cast removal. Radiographs show that bone formation is occurring and a callous has formed over the fracture. Lonnie rates his pain 2/10 at best and 7/10 with movement. The examination begins with vital signs and a systems review. Lonnie's blood pressure is 127/86 mm Hg, heart rate is 75 beats per minute, and respiratory rate is 17 breaths per minute. Light touch sensation is intact throughout.

Lonnie demonstrates mild range of motion limitation in the elbow with extension limited by 8°. Wrist range of motion was limited to 5° of wrist flexion and 3° of wrist extension actively, 10° of wrist flexion and 7° of wrist extension passively. Ulnar deviation and radial deviation were both limited as well with 2° of ulnar deviation and −1° of radial deviation. Lonnie was unable to fully extend his fingers and hand, and unable to make a fist due to pain in his wrist, only able to make a first to hold a golf club. Hand dynamometer strength was tested and he measured with 67 lb on his left hand and 19 lb on his right hand. Moderate swelling is noted in his right hand, wrist, and fingers. Lonnie scored a 78 on the Disabilities of the Arm, Shoulder, and Hand (DASH). Lonnie was started with exercises and given home exercises, with a focus on wrist and hand range of motion.

■ CASE STUDY QUESTIONS

1. What kind of functional problems are most common with this type of injury?
2. What are some of the intrinsic and extrinsic factors that can contribute to this type of injury?
3. What are the treatment options for distal radial fractures?
4. What are some of the complications that may occur?
5. What would compromise the initial rehabilitation program following casting?
6. What precautions would you educate the patient about?
7. What does the ongoing rehabilitation program entail beginning at 8 weeks?
8. What does a score of 78 on the DASH tell you?
9. What is the Patient-Rated Wrist Evaluation (PRWE)?
10. Should this man be screened for osteoporosis, why or why not?
11. Do men commonly fracture bones due to osteoporosis?
12. How is osteoporosis diagnosed?
13. Are there medications that may help treat osteoporosis?

37

COLLES (WRIST) FRACTURE: CASE 3

James R. Creps, PT, DScPT, OCS, CMPT

Phyllis is an 85-year-old white female who fell in her home and was transferred to the hospital by ambulance. Upon evaluation in the emergency department, it was determined that she had injured her right wrist and suffered a Colles fracture of the distal radius. Orthopedics was called in for a consult, and Phyllis's wrist was manually reduced in a position of supination and a plaster cast was applied. The orthopedist determined that surgical fixation was unnecessary to ensure adequate stabilization of the fracture site despite poor alignment of the distal radius. Phyllis was released from the emergency department with discharge instructions and told to follow up with her orthopedist as directed.

Phyllis complied with the treatment plan as determined by the orthopedist, which included physical therapy following cast removal 8 weeks after the fracture for 3 days a week for 4 weeks. Upon discharge from physical therapy, she completed a self-assessment of her condition utilizing the Patient-Rated Wrist Evaluation (PRWE) tool. Three months following the initial wrist injury, she reported significant improvement in her ability to complete her activities of daily living, although she continued to have problems completing all of her homecare tasks. By 6 months, she reported that she felt she was essentially back to normal and was managing independent living without difficulty.

■ CASE STUDY QUESTIONS

1. Are falls resulting in this type of injury common in the elderly?
2. Are Colles fractures more common in men or women?
3. Does age increase the probability of fracture related to osteoporosis in patients with decreased bone mineral density (BMD)?
4. Can the incidence of these types of fractures be reduced in the elderly with the proper use of calcium, vitamin D, bone formation drugs, antiresorptive drugs, and dual-effect drugs?
5. Does external surgical fixation of distal radial fractures result in better outcomes than surgical fixation?
6. Does alignment of the distal radial fracture greatly influence clinical outcomes following Colles fracture?
7. Why is the forearm placed in supination during plaster fixation of this type of fracture?
8. Is Phyllis's return to her previous activity level consistent with the majority of patients who have suffered this type of injury?
9. Is the Patient-Rated Wrist Evaluation (PRWE) a reliable and valid instrument for measuring subjective outcome assessment in patients with this type of injury?
10. Describe a typical rehabilitation program for a Colles fracture.

38

DISTAL RADIUS FRACTURE

William H. Staples, PT, DHSc, DPT, GCS, CEEAA

An 84-year-old woman, who lives with her daughter, is seen 8 weeks after a fall that resulted in an open right distal radius type 4 intra-articular fracture. She fell with palm-down outstretched wrists. She underwent an open reduction with volar fixed-angle plating technique to reduce the fracture with a plaster cast. She had to spend 10 days in the hospital because she developed a bacterial infection in the wound site and had to undergo a course of intravenous gentamicin. She received a platform walker during physical therapy at the hospital and was given a home exercise program to "clench your fist as much as you can; straighten your fingers as much as you can and if complete active movement is not possible then the joints of the fingers should be passively moved through their full range of motion with the help of the uninjured hand and to move your shoulder through its full range of motion many times in a day, and the elbow joint should be moved through its full range of motion." Her cast was removed by the physician 2 weeks ago and a removable wrist splint is now being used. Her current medications include furosemide, acetaminophen 325 mg every 4 hours, Miacalcin nasal spray (calcitonin salmon), calcium, and a stool softener.

During your examination you determine that she is alert and oriented, normal eyesight corrected with glasses, but hard of hearing. When asked if she had hearing aids she states that her hearing has just recently gotten worse, which she attributed to the aging process. She also complains of tinnitus. She is wearing a wrist splint, which is removed for the examination. She states that she has been practicing her exercises. Except for her right wrist, her extremity strength is grossly 4/5 and her range of motion lacks 12°-15° of bilateral shoulder flexion and abduction. Her right wrist has 10° of active extension and 25° of active flexion. Pronation if full but lacks any supination past neutral. Passive range past any of the active ranges is quite painful. Fingers except the thumb have full active and passive range. Her thumb which was partially immobilized lacks approximately 50% of the normal range in all motions except extension. Grip strength using a dynamometer measures 2 kg of force on the right compared to the left, which measures 20 kg. She has a forward flexed posture with a forward head and a moderate thoracic kyphosis. During the last 4 weeks she has begun using a straight cane for gait in her home. A note from the orthopedic surgeon states that the patient's only restriction is "no weight bearing through the wrist joint until week 12 postsurgery."

■ CASE STUDY QUESTIONS

1. How common are distal radial fractures in the elderly?
2. What are some underlying causes of the fracture?
3. What is an open fracture?
4. What is a type 4 intra-articular fracture?
5. Describe the volar fixed-angle plating technique.
6. Is there a more common name for this type of fracture?
7. What is gentamicin?
8. What are some possible side effects of gentamicin?
9. What is tinnitus?
10. If the gentamicin caused the hearing loss, will it return?
11. What is Miacalcin and what is the usual dose?
12. How will the rehabilitation process proceed from here?
13. What is the proper technique for measuring grip strength?
14. Why is measuring grip strength important?

39

DEGENERATIVE JOINT DISEASE OF THE CMC JOINT

James R. Creps, PT, DScPT, OCS, CMPT

Nina is an 84-year-old, right-handed female who lives with her husband. She is very creative and has been quilting as a hobby for over 60 years. One week ago, she attended a weekend quilting bee with several of her close friends. When she got home, she felt an excruciating pain in the thumb of her dominant hand. She attempted to treat her symptoms with rest and ice; however, her pain continued to become more severe. Because of this, she called her primary care physician and was immediately scheduled for an appointment on the same day.

Upon evaluation, the physician did a thorough examination of her hand, which revealed significant tenderness to palpation at the base of her right thumb. All neurological tests were normal; however, Nina demonstrated difficulty with active abduction-adduction of the joint. MRI and radiological studies revealed severe arthritis of the CMC joint (Eaton and Littler Stage 4) with dorsal translation of the first metacarpal, as well as incompetency of the anterior oblique and intermetacarpal ligaments. Her primary care physician gave Nina a prescription for Naproxen, placed her thumb in a splint, and referred her to physical therapy for conservative care.

Nina's physical therapist attempted to treat her condition with manual therapy, therapeutic exercise, and taping, but her condition did not improve. After 6 weeks of care, and a return visit to her primary care doctor, Nina was referred to a surgeon. The surgeon felt that Nina was a good candidate for total joint arthroplasty with a noncemented prosthesis. Nina underwent the procedure without complication and was released by the surgeon after routine postoperative care. She was reassessed a year later and demonstrated improved hand function and pain based on the Patient-Rated Wrist Evaluation (PRWE) and Michigan Hand Questionnaire Score. She had returned to her prior level of function and was once again quilting.

■ CASE STUDY QUESTIONS

1. How common is degenerative joint disease of the CMC joint in the elderly?
2. Is this condition more common in men or women?
3. Is thumb range of motion universally affected or are certain movements more prone to restriction?
4. How common is the Eaton-Littler classification system used for radiographic staging of CMC joint arthritis?
5. Is dorsal translation of the first metacarpal common with this condition?
6. Does incompetency of the ligamentous stability of the joint frequently occur with this condition?
7. How effective is naproxen in reducing pain in this patient group?
8. Does bracing effectively stabilize the CMC joint in patients with severe arthritis?
9. Is manual therapy and exercise an efficacious choice for treating this condition?
10. If conservative physical therapy management of the condition fails, is surgery seen as an effective option?
11. Is Nina's return to her previous activity level consistent with the majority of patients who have had surgical treatment for CMC joint arthritis?
12. Is the Patient Rated Wrist Evaluation (PRWE) a reliable and valid instrument for measuring subjective outcome assessment in patients with this type of injury?

40

CERVICAL OSTEOARTHRITIS— CONSERVATIVE TREATMENT STRATEGIES

Meri Goehring, PT, PhD, GCS, CWS

Evelyn, a retired school teacher, is 98 years old and presents to your clinic with complaints of neck pain of unknown origin. She has had neck pain "off and on" her whole life but in the last few months it has been getting worse and more consistent, limiting her ability to participate in her usual daily and recreational activities. She complains of occasional mild to moderate posterior headaches, though they typically resolve with ibuprofen. She has a prescription for physical therapy that reads: "upper cervical osteoarthritis: evaluate and treat."

Her previous medical history is noncontributory to her current problem.

The patient lives in a small one bedroom condo in a retirement community. Prior to the increase in neck pain, she regularly participated in senior group fitness classes at least three times per week and she is also working part-time transporting mail from site to site within a large medical complex, requiring her to carry up to 20 lb.

A systems review finds that the patient is alert and oriented ×3, and has no neurological or cognitive impairments. The skin is dry but intact. There is gross bilateral upper extremity weakness, but myotomes and dermatomes are intact.

The patient has a height 4 ft 9 in and weight 106 lb.

Vital signs are HR: 50 beats per minute; BP: 102/68; RR: 18; SpO$_2$: 96%; temp: 98.5° F.

Cervical pain: 3-5/10 at rest and 6-8/10 with movement into extension.

Postural assessment (in standing) and movement quality screening: Moderate forward head and shoulders as well as thoracic kyphosis with decreased lumbar lordosis. Abnormal scapular rhythm and decreased movement quality.

ROM and muscle testing:

Motion Tested	MMT Score (R, L)	ROM (R, L)
Cervical flexion	4−/5	47°
Cervical extension	3+/5[a]	50°
Cervical lateral flexion	3/5[a], 3/5	35°[a], 40°
Cervical rotation	3−/5, 3/5	50°, 60°
Shoulder flexion	3/5, 3/5	100°, 101°
Shoulder abduction	3−/5, 3−/5	89°, 90°

[a] Painful with testing.

Balance: Single leg stance ≥20s bilaterally.

Functional outcome Measurements: Neck Disability Index: 25/50.

From the initial examination, you determine that the patient is not at a risk for falls and is a good candidate for physical therapy as a conservative treatment option.

■ CASE STUDY QUESTIONS

1. Is there another name for cervical spine arthritis?

2. What signs and/or symptoms from the patient history and examination support the diagnosis of cervical osteoarthritis?

3. Are there any findings that might lead you to believe the patient does have cervical osteoarthritis?

4. What is the etiology of cervical spine arthritis?

5. Are there any diagnoses you would want to rule out?

6. Is the Neck Disability Index an appropriate outcome measure in this case?

7. Is Evelyn a good candidate for physical therapy treatment?

8. Are this patient's headaches concerning to you as a physical therapist?

9. Are severe headaches typically associated with osteoarthritis?

10. Identify three to five impairments found in the physical therapy examination that can be treated with standard physical therapy interventions.

11. What types of physical therapy treatments are indicated?

12. Should a soft cervical collar be used for treatment?

41

OSTEOPOROSIS: CASE 1

Meri Goehring, PT, PhD, GCS, CWS

You are a home health physical therapist who is visiting a new patient for the first time at her home. Your patient, Nancy, is a 76-year-old African American woman who last month tripped over her cat while walking into her kitchen and fell to the floor with her right arm outstretched and sustained a fractured humerus (primary diagnosis). Her long-arm cast was recently removed, use of a sling was discontinued and physical therapy has been ordered. She has a secondary diagnosis of general deconditioning and impaired balance.

Her script reads: PT Evaluate and treat. Decreased right UE strength and ROM s/p immobilization.

SOCIAL HISTORY

Nancy's husband passed away 2 years ago and she has lived alone in their single-story home since. Nancy and her husband never had children, her neighbors and her two sisters who live several hours away check in on her from time to time but she says that it is not uncommon for her to go days without seeing or speaking with anyone. She admits that since her husband's passing she has been depressed and has lived a very sedentary lifestyle and has a difficult time leaving the house. Nancy is no longer able to drive herself around because of her failing eyesight, which she blames for her recent fall. She does not eat many fresh fruits or vegetables due to the difficulty to get to the store. She drinks five to six cups of coffee a day. She does not smoke or drink alcohol.

PAST MEDICAL HISTORY

Left wrist fracture as a child, HTN, and a history of migraines (~2/month). Left total hip arthroplasty 4 years ago. Diagnostic testing indicates the presence of osteoporotic changes. Her mother died after a fall and fractured her hip at age 82.

PRIOR LEVEL OF FUNCTION

Prior to her fall, Nancy was independent with all ADLs and ambulation around her home but required general household assistance 1 day each week for cleaning tasks and getting groceries. Community ambulation required a small based quad cane to assist with balance.

PHYSICAL THERAPY EXAMINATION

Height: 5ft 3in	Weight: 110 lb	BMI: 19.5

Vital signs: HR 70 beats per minute regular; RR 18 breaths per minute; BP: 134/82; temp 98.6°F; SpO$_2$ 96%.

Posture: moderate thoracic kyphosis, forward head and forward shoulder. Excessive forward trunk lean in standing.

Manual muscle testing: reveals gross weakness 3−/5 right UE, 3−/5, left UE 4−/5, right LE 3+/5, and left LE 3/5.

Range of motion: right UE—Shoulder is moderately reduced in all planes but able to perform ADLs; left UE has mild deficits in shoulder flexion, abduction, and external rotation.

Balance: Four Square Step Test (FSST): 18.5 seconds. Fall Efficacy Scale (FES-I): 80

Endurance: Two-Minute Step Test 38.

Mental status: The patient is alert and oriented ×4. Geriatric Depression Scale Score: 15

■ CASE STUDY QUESTIONS

1. What risk factors presented in this case may lead you to believe that Nancy may have osteoporosis?

2. Which of the risk factors from Question 1 are nonmodifiable?

3. Which of the risk factors from Question 1 are modifiable?

4. What diagnostic test is the gold standard for diagnosing osteoporosis? What does this test measure?

5. What intervention strategies can we offer as physical therapists to help treat patients with osteoporosis?

6. Is resistance training indicated in patients with osteoporosis? Why or why not?

7. Explain the principle of overload and how it relates to this case.

8. What is the FES-I, and what does it measure?

9. Why is improving balance and preventing falls a focus of concern for you with this patient?

10. What implications (if any) do her balance deficits have on your intervention plan?

11. What does the time of the Four Square Step Test indicate?

12. Write three functional goals for Nancy.

42

OSTEOPOROSIS: CASE 2

Meri Goehring, PT, PhD, GCS, CWS

As a physical therapist in an inpatient rehabilitation facility, you are scheduled to evaluate and treat Harold, a 70-year-old Caucasian male. Harold was admitted to the emergency room 5 days ago with severe back pain after he missed a step descending the stairs in his two-story home. Diagnostic imaging indicates the presence of spinal compression fractures in the L3 and L4 vertebrae. A DEXA scan confirmed suspicions of moderate osteoporotic changes of the patient's spinal column. Prior to hospitalization Harold lived at home independently. He was divorced from his wife 5 years ago. His home has three bedrooms and a bathroom upstairs and a bathroom downstairs but no bedrooms downstairs. There are three steps into the house with a railing on the right-hand side. He is a retired plumber and currently works part time at the local hardware store. Duties there include bending and stooping as well as reaching overhead when stocking shelves and retrieving items to help customers. Harold has a 10-year history of alcohol abuse and states that he has not eaten a proper meal since his divorce. Additional premorbid activities include walking, playing cards, and gambling on sporting events. The patient has not had any alcohol since his admittance to the emergency room. The patient also states that he is "motivated and ready to get his life back in order."

Medications: Flovent, prednisone during acute asthma episodes (3-4/year, 15-year use), lisinopril, Glucophage, acetaminophen

Past medical history: asthma, hypertension, hyperlipidemia, diabetes mellitus, osteoarthritis in both hips

PHYSICAL THERAPY EVALUATION

Height: 6ft 1 in, weight: 160 lb

Resting vital signs	Vital sign response to standing
– HR: 80	– HR: 96 *Pt states feeling of light-headedness
– BP: 130/90	– BP: 106/74
– RR: 24	– RR: 38

Postural assessment: The patient has decreased lumbar lordosis and increased thoracic kyphosis.

Range of motion: gross UE range of motion and strength are WNL but the patient complains of pain (3/10) in his low back at end-range shoulder flexion. Moderate back pain (6/10) is experienced with trunk flexion and mild back pain (2/10) with hip flexion but both are relieved with slight trunk extension and hip extension. Decreased bilateral hip range of motion was measured.

Strength: gross LE weakness (4/5) and marked core and hip abduction weakness were present (2/5).

Quality of life measure: QUALEFFO-41	54.4

Gait: The patient is able to walk 200 ft over level surfaces with a wheeled walker and stand by assist for balance.

Stairs: The patient is able to ascend and descend four stairs with hand rail and min assist of one.

■ CASE STUDY QUESTIONS

1. What diagnostic findings would lead to the diagnosis of osteoporosis?

2. Does Harold have primary or secondary osteoporosis?

3. What risk factors present with this patient are likely contributors to his osteoporosis?

4. Is this patient overweight?

5. Why should you take extra precaution with fall prevention with this patient? (Think about the effects of osteoporosis.)

6. Interpret this patient's vital sign response to standing. Is it normal or abnormal? Concerning?

7. Why is resistance training an encouraged intervention with this patient?

8. What is a QUALEFFO-41 and why was it used?

9. What psychosocial aspects of this patient may impact your ability to treat?

10. What are two key educational needs for Harold?

11. What criteria should be met before Harold can be discharged to home?

12. What other health care professionals will be working with this patient? Would you make any referrals?

43

OSTEOPOROSIS: CASE 3

Meri Goehring, PT, PhD, GCS, CWS

William H. Staples, PT, DHSc, DPT, GCS, CEEAA

Molly is a 76-year-old woman who worked for many years as a secretary to the president of a local insurance company prior to retiring about 10 years ago. She enjoys knitting, sewing, and reading in her retirement. She knows the importance of physical activity and tries to walk around the neighborhood regularly, but has noticed that she has been leaning over her rolling walker more than usual over the last few months. Last week while she was walking to a neighbor's house, she had a sharp stabbing pain in her back near the thoracolumbar junction. She also noted the pain radiating to her chest, and feared she was having a heart attack. When she went to see her physician, she tested negative for any cardiovascular events. She had radiographs taken of her thoracolumbar spine, and they discovered an anterior wedge compression fracture of her T12 vertebra. After having a dual-energy x-ray absorptiometry (DEXA), Molly was found to have osteoporosis with a T-score of −2.7. Molly was eager about approaching conservative treatment, and is now seeing you in your outpatient orthopedic clinic.

Upon clinical observation of Molly, you notice her very kyphotic posture in sitting and standing with moderate forward head and rounded shoulders. When she walks from the waiting room to the treatment room, you see that she increases her kyphosis by leaning forward extensively over her walker. She uses her accessory muscles noticeably for breathing. She mentions that her pain is worse when sitting or standing, at about a 6/10, but better in side-lying, that she rates 2/10.

In the systems review, you record that Molly's resting HR = 82, RR = 16, and BP = 130/75. Her bilateral shoulder flexion is 120° with 4−/5 strength when manually muscle tested. Her external and internal rotation at the glenohumeral joint is within normal limits. When you measure her spinal curves with the flexicurve, her index of kyphosis is 14.25 (using the formula thoracic width/length × 100). She has difficulty engaging her back extensors, and is unable to engage her transversus abdominis to brace her core.

No neurologic signs are present. The integument is intact.

■ CASE STUDY QUESTIONS

1. What diagnosis is commonly associated with vertebral fractures?
2. What percentage of fractures due to osteoporosis are vertebral fractures?
3. What methods are used to determine if someone has osteoporosis?
4. Do vertebral fractures occur in individuals without osteoporosis?
5. Where do these vertebral fractures most commonly occur?
6. What are the symptoms of a compression fracture?
7. If loss of height occurs, can this cause pain?
8. Can physical therapy benefit individuals with vertebral fractures?
9. What type of strengthening program should be incorporated into the treatment?
10. Will any type of orthotic device benefit an individual with a vertebral fracture?
11. When is the best time to treat osteoporosis?
12. Can surgery help?
13. What is a flexicurve?

44

OSTEOPOROSIS: CASE 4

Meri Goehring, PT, PhD, GCS, CWS

Jean is an 87-year-old woman who was a homemaker and is now a widow of 10 years. She has hypertension, osteoporosis, BMI of 17.5, "dowagers' hump," has a recent history of depression, and is highly anxious. Jean's daughter lives with her and was previously assisting Jean with meals, and supervision for ADLs. Jean is being seen in her home for physical therapy two to three times per week. Jean has a history of occasional falls (three times in last 6 months) and walks with a four-wheeled walker. Jean is on blood pressure medication and takes supplemental vitamins for her general health. Jean was having upper thoracic back pain (5/10) and radiographs showed a new vertebral compression fracture at T5, and an old fracture at T6 for which she had no previous complaint. She has a DEXA score of −2.8. Jean is fairly sedentary and does not participate in regular exercise.

The systems review showed that Jean's blood pressure was 140/73, heart rate was 70, she was intact to light touch, she denied numbness and tingling, reflexes were normal, breathing appeared to be normal, and some bruising was noted on the patient's arms and legs. Jean reports that she has very "thin skin," with several areas of senile purpura present. Jean's posture revealed moderate slumped posture with a forward head and shoulders, and increased kyphosis. Jean reported mid-thoracic pain today of 3/10 at rest and 5/10 with activity. Jean had a Barthel score of 65, Mini Mental Status Exam of 23, ABC score of 33%, and TUG time of 24 seconds. Jean's lower extremity strength was 4−/5 grossly. Jean's active range of motion in her lower extremities and upper extremities were within functional limits except shoulder flexion limited to 140°, and bilateral hamstring tightness.

■ CASE STUDY QUESTIONS

1. How common are vertebral compression fractures in the USA?
2. What is the difference between osteoporosis and osteopenia?
3. In what part of the spine do most vertebral compression fractures occur?
4. What associated problems might reduce quality of life?
5. What are the federally approved medications in the treatment of osteoporosis?
6. What type of physical therapy treatment should be initiated first?
7. Can back muscle strengthening exercises help?
8. What might be the benefits of a well-fit orthosis?
9. What type of orthotic device might you recommend?
10. Jean has very thin skin. What precautions might you take when recommending a brace?
11. What is senile purpura?

45

DORSAL KYPHOPLASTY: CASE 1

James R. Creps, PT, DScPT, OCS, CMPT

Martha is a slightly built 81-year-old white female who lives alone and is moderately active. She periodically takes steroid medication to control symptoms associated with rheumatoid arthritis. Two weeks ago, she was working in her garden and was attempting to pull the root of a large bush when she felt an excruciating pain in her lower thoracic spine. Any attempts at straightening up were met with increased symptoms, and Martha immediately got on her cell phone and contacted her son. He came to her home and transported her to the local emergency department when he realized how severe her symptoms were.

Upon admission to emergency services, the physician did a complete physical examination, which revealed significant tenderness to palpation at T10 and an inability to extend the spine to neutral.

All neurological tests were normal; however, Martha demonstrated difficulty with complete inspiration secondary to pain. Radiological studies revealed a compression fracture of T10, which was stable and did not involve the posterior margin of the vertebrae. The emergency room physician called for a consult with orthopedic surgery for consideration of appropriate management of the condition. Martha reported that her mother had suffered from a similar injury a few years before she had passed away.

The surgeon felt that Martha was a good candidate for balloon kyphoplasty to decrease her pain and stabilize her vertebral fracture, although he opted for conservative management initially. Martha was sent home with pain relieving medications, activity restrictions, and use of a thoracic brace. Upon follow-up 6 weeks later, Martha continued to have significant thoracic pain, difficult breathing, and a flexed thoracic posture. As a result, balloon kyphoplasty was scheduled for Martha with the intention of reducing her symptoms, improving her posture, and stabilizing her thoracic spinal segments.

■ CASE STUDY QUESTIONS

1. How common are thoracic fractures?
2. What was the most likely cause of Martha's vertebral compression fracture?
3. How common is this type of injury in the elderly?
4. What placed her at risk of compression fracture?
5. Is she at risk for additional vertebral fractures as a result of her care for this condition?
6. Was conservative management of this injury indicated?
7. If conservative management fails, has the effectiveness of balloon kyphoplasty been validated in the literature?
8. How common is balloon kyphoplasty used to treat thoracic compression fracture?
9. What are some of the risks associated with completion of balloon kyphoplasty?
10. What are some of the benefits associated with stabilizing a thoracic compression fracture using balloon kyphoplasty?
11. A return to what type of activity level can be expected following balloon kyphoplasty?

46

OSTEOPOROSIS: FRACTURED PUBIC RAMUS

Lucy H. Jones, PT, DPT, MHA, GCS, CEEAA

You have been asked to perform a home health evaluation for a new client. Delores is an 85-year-old woman with a primary diagnosis of osteoporosis. Her medical history includes hypertension and gastroesophageal reflux disease (GERD). She fell in the bathroom and fractured her right pubic ramus, was hospitalized for 3 days, and then spent 1 week in a rehabilitation unit. She has now returned home and lives alone in a split level ranch-style home, with 14 steps up to the second floor, and 3 steps with no railing out to the garage. She has a small dog. She is now able to ambulate up to 50 ft with a rolling walker, and sleeps on the sofa on the first floor. She transfers independently from the sofa to standing. Her muscle strength is grossly 4/5 all four extremities, except for the right hip, which is 3/5 for

all motions. She currently does her own wash on the first floor, and can reheat meals in a microwave

Her primary goal is to get up the steps to her bedroom. Her second goal is to be able to leave the house to visit her daughter who lives 30 minutes away. Her pain level is now 6/10 with the Visual Analog Scale (VAS) with pain in the right groin. Medications include aspirin, Dyazide (hydrochlorothiazide), Lopressor (metoprolol tartrate), MiraLAX (polyethylene glycol 3350—OTC), Prilosec (omeprazole), Oxyfast (oxycodone), RisaQuad (lactobacillus acidophilus), and vitamin D_3.

■ CASE STUDY QUESTIONS

1. What is the prevalence and incidence of osteoporosis?
2. What is the gender difference for osteoporosis?
3. What is unique to the female pelvis versus male? Why does this make women more susceptible to pelvic fractures than men?
4. What imaging is needed for diagnosis of osteoporosis? Why is it important? How often should an individual have the imaging?
5. What is a FRAX Risk Assessment Tool, and what are its strengths and weaknesses? When is it an appropriate predictive tool?
6. What are the two types of skeletal bone structures? How do they differ, and how do they work together?
7. What are the risk factors for osteoporosis, physical and metabolic?
8. What is sarcopenia and how does it influence muscle strength and contribute to osteoporotic fractures?
9. What is the impact of osteoporosis-related kyphosis on falls?
10. What is the geriatric frailty syndrome and what impact does osteoporosis have?
11. How would the impact of a fall define the intervention and home exercise program to assist Doris in regaining function to prevent future falls and improve her functional status?

47

SPINAL STENOSIS: CASE 1

Meri Goehring, PT, PhD, GCS, CWS

Larry is a 73-year-old retired salesman who lives with his wife and two dogs. They live in a two-story home with the master bedroom and bathroom being upstairs. Larry enjoys playing golf with his fellow retired friends, watching his grandchildren play baseball, and working on his cars. He is very independent and has no underlying comorbidities with the exception of high cholesterol, which he is taking a statin for. His only complaint is low back pain with occasional "zingers"/shooting pain down his left leg. He notices that the pain is at its worst when he is walking or performing any activity that is overhead. Larry states that it does feel better when he sits in his recliner chair or when he sleeps on his side. He reports no change in bowel or bladder habits, no weight changes, or increased fatigue. Larry states that the only time he feels he can walk with limited to no pain in his back is when he is grocery shopping with his wife and he is able to drive the cart. His primary physician ordered an x-ray and found that his low back was unremarkable with the exception of osteoarthritis. You are seeing Larry in an outpatient sports medicine clinic.

You initiate the examination process with a systems review and you find BP: 132/85, HR: 74, RR: 16, SpO_2: 96%. You notice no integumentary issues nor do you notice any changes in skin temperature upon palpation. Larry has increased muscle guarding in the lumbar region compared to his thoracic spine and sacrum. No trigger points were found upon palpation. Upon sitting in a chair, light touch sensation appears intact. Upon standing for 3 minutes, light touch sensation appears intact with questionable sensation for the first digit (big toe) in the left foot. Larry demonstrates gross strength with 4+/5 bilaterally in his lower and upper extremities. Larry has 50% limited mobility in all directions except flexion when performing active range of motion with spinal movements. With repeated movement testing, Larry has no pain moving into a flexed position, stating he feels a slight stretch but no concordant symptoms. With repeated extension, Larry reports an increase in low back pain and pain in his left buttock. Repeated left side bending also increased his left buttock pain. Larry's goals are to be able to play nine holes of golf pain free, be able to watch his grandchildren play baseball, and work on his cars pain free if possible.

CASE STUDY QUESTIONS

1. What is the most likely diagnosis in this case?
2. What are some of the things thought to cause this problem?
3. What are some of the signs and symptoms of this problem?
4. At what age does this commonly occur?
5. What type of imaging is used to confirm the diagnosis?
6. What type of medical management might be included in Larry's treatment?
7. What might the patient demonstrate during the physical therapy examination?
8. What type of physical therapy treatments might be indicated?
9. Should modalities be routinely included in treatment?
10. Are braces/corsets used to treat spinal stenosis?
11. When might surgery be indicated?
12. Should a patient choose conservative or a surgical approach to treat spinal stenosis?
13. What is the minimally invasive lumbar decompression (MILD) surgical procedure?
14. What type of adverse events associated with spinal surgery for the treatment of lumbar spinal stenosis?
15. What are some standardized measures or functional outcomes tools that can be utilized by this population?

48

SPINAL STENOSIS: CASE 2

Meri Goehring, PT, PhD, GCS, CWS

Jane is a 77-year-old homemaker who lives with her 78-year-old husband. They live in a ranch-style home with the basement being the only level that requires navigation of stairs. Jane enjoys playing cards (bridge), reading, and babysitting her grandchildren. She is very independent in her daily activities and instrumental daily activities. She is considered overweight with a body mass index of 29.5, has type 2 diabetes mellitus, and osteoarthritis in both her knees and wrists. She comes to therapy today with a compliant of a 6-month history of low back pain that occasionally has shooting pain down into her posterior thigh and buttocks on the right side. She states that she has not noticed any changes in sensation in her

lower extremities or feelings of weakness in her legs. She reports no bowel/bladder changes including incontinence, no change in weight, and/or increases in fatigue. Jane states that the only position that she feels she is able to gain some relief is sitting on the couch and relaxing. She states that she does have some disrupted sleep from her back pain as she typically sleeps on her back. Jane went to her primary care physician and received an x-ray finding with no remarkable results other than "arthritis of the spine." Jane has come to see you in a general outpatient orthopedic clinic.

After taking a history, you begin the examination process with a systems review and you find: BP: 142/86, HR: 68, RR: 14, SpO_2: 97%. No noticeable integumentary abrasions or contusions were noted, nor were changes in skin temperature upon palpation. Jane has increased muscle guarding in her lumbar paraspinals and in her right buttocks, notably the gluteus medius and hamstring musculature. Light touch sensation and proprioception appear intact in both upper and lower extremities when she is upright sitting in a chair. When she sits with "good posture" she has increased pain in her low back, when she has "poor posture" she notices a relief of pain in her low back. Jane demonstrates a positive slump test bilaterally with right eliciting more pain at an earlier onset than left (30° of hip flexion vs 45° of hip flexion, respectively). Strength testing revealed lower extremity and abdominal muscle weakness. Jane graded at 4/5 in her lower extremities and 3/5 in her core stability. Reflex testing demonstrates 2+/5 in the upper extremities and left lower extremity. 1+ reflexes (patellar and Achilles) were noted in the right lower extremity. Straight leg raise is 80° bilaterally without pain. Jane scored a 58% on the Oswestry Disability Index. Jane's goals for physical therapy are to "get back to normal" and be able to play 2 hours of cards with no to minimal pain.

CASE STUDY QUESTIONS

1. What causes neurogenic claudication?
2. What are the symptoms of neurogenic claudication?
3. Why is a straight leg raise often pain free in individuals with lumbar spinal stenosis?
4. In individuals with spinal stenosis, where is this most commonly located?
5. Is there any potential reason why this is the most common location for stenosis?
6. What is the second most common location for stenosis?
7. Is this condition costly to our society?
8. If surgery is not performed, what other type of medical treatment might be incorporated?
9. What types of physical therapy treatment are indicated?
10. What standardized measures might be used during examination of this individual?

49

SPINAL STENOSIS: CASE 3

Sarah Dudley, MPT, GCS, CEEAA

Stacy Martin, PT, CEEAA

This case involves a 78-year-old male who is limited in his ADLs and IADLs by his spinal stenosis, weakness, and recurrent urinary tract infections (UTIs). He was referred to home health physical therapy with low back pain and lower extremity weakness following a hospitalization for *E coli* UTI. The patient's past medical history is significant for an L4-L5 microlaminectomy 2 years ago due to radicular lower extremity (LE) pain, which only minimally improved his pain. The patient experienced post-op saddle paresthesia, left foot drop, and neurogenic bladder that now requires a chronic Foley catheter and is the most likely cause of the resultant urinary tract infections. A recent lumbar MRI showed an L5-S1 spinal stenosis, multilevel degenerative disc disease, and osteophytes. He has no peripheral vascular disease. Additional past medical history includes dementia with behavioral disturbance, generalized osteoarthritis, diabetes mellitus type 2 with peripheral neuropathy, congestive heart failure, and macular degeneration. He lives alone and requires the increasing assistance from his sister-in-law who lives out of town and she reports she is unable to meet his growing demands. He does have a history of falls without overt injury, yet he has required multiple rehabilitative stays in the past 6 months and his home health physical therapy goal is to remain at home and return to his community level of mobility.

PHYSICAL THERAPY EXAMINATION

The patient lives alone in a second floor one level apartment with elevator access. He is anxious and highly distractible, but well groomed and dressed, alert, and oriented. His apartment is clean and free of clutter. He owns a rollator walker and single point cane, yet declines to use any assistive device while in the apartment. He uses the rollator for ambulation outside the apartment for community access.

The patient reports significant back pain that waxes and wanes. He initially reported he was having a good day with only a 1/10 pain report and then his pain increased throughout the session to a 6/10 in the lumbosacral region with bilateral (B) lower extremities (LE) radiculopathy, which caused him to require frequent seated rests. The pain limits standing tolerance to 60 seconds and a gait tolerance of 30 ft. His gait pattern is wide based and shuffling with high guard. He declines to use his rollator or cane while in the apartment today despite his elevated pain levels. His pain is relieved to a 0-2/10 in a seated position.

FUNCTIONAL ASSESSMENT

TUG scores: 19.5 with no AD (high fall risk)

Berg balance scores: 33 (high fall risk)

Postural assessment: Forward head, thoracic kyphosis, and decreased lumbar lordosis

Gait assessment: Forward lean with high guard gait pattern and wide base of support as well as absent heel strike B with foot drop R. Distance was limited to 30 ft without AD due to neck and back pain to 6-8/10.

Neurologic: Using Semmes-Weinstein filament testing, the patient had absent protective sensation from just below the knee to B toes. DTR to B Achilles are decreased. His proprioception is impaired to B great toe MTP joints and ankle.

Neuromuscular: The patient has right foot drop with DF at 3−/5, B hip extensors 3+5, B hip abductors 4/5, and B quadriceps 4/5.

Integumentary: The patient with decreased hair to BLE with cool distal LE.

Cardiopulmonary system: The patient has low BP at rest of 82/52 with an HR of 70, which increased to 100/50 and 72 beats per minute with activity. The patient was asymptomatic throughout and negative for orthostatics.

GI/GU: The patient has a chronic indwelling catheter due to his urinary retention after his lumbar surgery. He reports being constipated at this time with no bowel movement (BM) × 4 days, but has a history of nighttime bowel incontinence.

The patient presents to home PT with debilitating back pain with leg weakness and postural changes that places him as a high fall risk with low functional tolerance. This combination keeps him from his goal of being a community dwelling elder.

CASE STUDY QUESTIONS

1. What is the typical presentation (ie, signs and symptoms) associated with lumbar spinal stenosis (LSS)?

2. How is lumbar spinal stenosis diagnosed?

3. What are common impairments seen in patients with lumbar spinal stenosis?

4. Which questionnaires and functional tests should be utilized in this case?

5. What adaptive equipment can be helpful in treating those with lumbar spinal stenosis?

6. What physical therapy treatment interventions have been deemed effective for treating lumbar spinal stenosis?

7. How long should conservative management be trialed prior to surgical consult?

8. Are epidural steroid injections for lumbar spinal stenosis effective?

9. What are the types of surgical interventions performed for lumbar spinal stenosis?

10. Which is more effective surgical intervention or conservative management in treating symptomatic lumbar spinal stenosis?

11. What is the epidemiology of lumbar spinal stenosis?

12. What is the Semmes-Weinstein monofilament test for protective sensation?

50

SPINAL STENOSIS: L2-5 SURGICAL STABILIZATION

Lucy H. Jones, PT, DPT, MHA, GCS, CEEAA

Keith is a 53-year-old man presenting 2 weeks after surgery for home care physical therapy with spinal fusion of dorsal and dorsolumbar anterior and posterior columns at L2-5. A TENS was used for 1 month with only minimal amount of decrease in pain. An implanted muscle stimulator was then tried with this patient for 6 months prior to surgery but also had minimal effect on reducing pain. The patient had years of pain previously in his low back from several injuries as a youth. He smokes one pack of cigarettes a day, with past medical history of hypercholesterolemia, acid reflux, has 8/10 pain in low back, but no radicular symptoms. He wears a spinal brace while upright since surgery, with a metal upright descending from his spinal brace to his left knee with stabilizing cuff and hip lock mechanism to prevent left hip extension. Spinal surgery protocol includes no twisting, rotation, forward leaning, and no sitting longer than 30 minutes for the first 4 to 6 weeks. He is currently having systemic reactions of sweating and fatigue periodically in the day. He is also complaining of constipation.

Medications Keith was taking included:

Amitiza	24 mg	1–2× day
Colace	100 mg	1–2× day
Dilaudid (hydromorphone)	4 mg	PRN q4h
Lotrel	10–20 mg	1× daily
Lyrica (pregabalin)	75 mg	1–2× a day
Oxycodone	30 mg	1 q3h
Pravachol	20 mg	2 at bedtime
Prevacid	30 mg	1× day
Tenormin (atenolol)	50 mg	1× day
Valium	5 mg	q6h
Relistor (methylnaltrexone)	12 mg	Daily

Keith has several function-related goals. He wants to have reduced back pain during activities, do small jobs around his house, drive his car, and a golf cart to drive his friends around the golf course, as he had not been able to play golf for several years due to his back pain. He hopes he could return to work in the accounting business he had previously worked at before surgery.

■ CASE STUDY QUESTIONS

1. What is spinal stenosis?
2. What nonsurgical treatments could be utilized for spinal stenosis?
3. What is a muscle stimulator, and how does it function to decrease pain. What are indications and precautions?
4. What is the physical examination and differential diagnosis for spinal stenosis?
5. What is the difference in the presentation of pain between spinal stenosis and a herniated disc?
6. What are operative management options for spinal stenosis?
7. What are the surgical precautions for spinal surgery for spinal stenosis?
8. What are the medications Keith is taking for pain relief, the action of these pain medications, and their side effects?
9. Why would Keith be sweating periodically during the day with the systemic response?
10. How can constipation be managed in this case?
11. Describe the physiology of TENS and the gate control theory of pain. What would be a reason that TENS was not as successful as the patient would have liked as a pain relief mechanism?
12. What would the focus be for the home program for Keith, and the proposed discharge plan concerning his anticipated level of activity?
13. What is the purpose of the brace he is wearing?

51

BONE TUMORS: CASE 1

Meri Goehring, PT, PhD, GCS, CWS

Wilbur is an 84-year-old retired bricklayer. Wilbur lives with his 82-year-old wife in their one-story home with three steps to enter. They have one bathroom in their home with an elevated seat due to his wife having back surgery 3 months ago. His wife ambulates with a walker and needs assistance with car transfers only. Wilbur was independent in all ADLs and IADLs prior to his diagnosis of a bone tumor and states that he just performed "everything much slower than when he was 25 years old." Wilbur was diagnosed with a bone tumor 4 months ago and he recently had surgery (resection of the tumor with an iliac crest bone graft) to remove a chondrosarcoma in his left lower extremity, near the knee joint (distal femur). The surgery also included placement of an intramedullary rod in the femur. As of right now, it appears through imaging that the chondrosarcoma is fully removed and Wilbur is now in a state of remission. You are seeing Wilbur in the acute care hospital 1 day postoperatively, with a referral for evaluate and treat. His only restriction at this time is 50% weight bearing.

You begin the examination process with a review of systems and these are the findings that you find: HR: 77 beats per minute, BP: 136/84, RR: 19 breaths per minute, SpO_2: 95%. Sensation appears intact to light touch in the upper and lower extremities including around the surgical incision site. Light touch sensation is diminished on the surgical incision/scar. Reflexes are 2+ bilaterally.

The surgical incision site appears along the distal femur from lateral to medial with stitches, appearing healthy with no apparent signs of infection. The left knee joint is swollen. Wilbur demonstrates left lower extremity weakness and normal strength in the upper extremity with manual muscle test grades of 4+/5 grossly for the upper extremities and left lower extremity strengths of 3/5 hip flexion bilaterally, 2/5 for knee flexion and extension with severe pain of 7/10 with movement following surgery, 3/5 ankle dorsiflexion. Wilbur was able to complete three heel raises in standing position on his left leg and nine on his right leg. Wilbur demonstrates 4−/5 strength in his right lower extremity.

He is able to get out of bed with moderate assistance ×1, a standard walker, and an elevated bed height. Wilbur ambulated 43 ft partial non-weight bearing (NWB) with the standard walker and moderate assistance ×1 with 1 seated rest break for approximately 1 minute. He has a knee immobilizer that is to be worn when ambulating, but removed for active exercise while in the hospital. He is allowed to have 50% weight bearing but states it is too painful to put weight on the leg. Wilbur was able to complete the TUG test in 26.7 seconds and perform single leg stance on his right leg for 4 seconds.

■ CASE STUDY QUESTIONS

1. What are the different types of bone tumors?
2. What is another way (name) to describe multiple myeloma?
3. What is a chondrosarcoma?
4. At what age is chondrosarcoma most likely to develop?
5. How common are chondrosarcomas?
6. Where is a chondrosarcoma most likely to develop?
7. How are chondrosarcomas classified?
8. What are the clinical manifestations of a chondrosarcoma?
9. Why might this go undiagnosed?
10. Why might this be mistaken for another problem?
11. How is a diagnosis made?
12. What is the grading system for chondrosarcoma/tumors?
13. What is the staging system for these types of tumors?
14. What is the current treatment for chondrosarcoma?
15. What is the survival/prognosis for this disease?
16. What would be the physical therapy treatment for this patient at this time?

52

BONE TUMOR: CASE 2

Meri Goehring, PT, PhD, GCS, CWS

Wilbur is now out of the acute care hospital and was recently discharged home. He reports he is having difficulty ambulating with his walker, navigating stairs, getting in and out of the shower, donning/doffing shoes and socks, and getting in and out of the car to get to and from physical therapy. He has been out of the hospital for 7 days now and this is your initial examination of him in the outpatient setting since his discharge from the hospital following his cancer resection for chondrosarcoma of the distal femur and placement of a femoral intramedullary rod. His wife, Martha, accompanies Wilbur to the examination but has physical limitations of her own as she ambulates with a walker and requires car transfer assistance as well. Wilbur and Martha's daughter, Jane, was able to transport them to their physical therapy evaluation for today and possibly the next visit only as she had to take off work to do so. Wilbur lives in a one-story home with three steps to enter. They have one bathroom with an elevated seat that Wilbur is using now as he has a difficult time squatting so low on a normal toilet.

You begin your examination process with a systems review and these are your findings: HR: 74 beats per minute, BP: 128/82, RR: 16 breaths per minute, SpO2: 97%. Sensation appears intact to light touch in both the upper extremities and the lower extremities excluding the surgical site. The surgical site continues to have altered sensation with deficient light touch sensation and depressed sharp/dull sensation. Reflexes are 2+ bilaterally for upper and lower extremities with patellar reflexes withheld on the left lower extremity due to the large surgical incision site.

Wilbur continues to demonstrate normal strength in the upper extremities and right lower extremities with 4+/5 strength grossly in those two quadrants of the body. The left lower extremity displays moderate to severe weakness with manual muscle grades of 3+/5 for hip flexion, 2/5 knee flexion, 2−/5 knee extension, 2+/5 ankle dorsiflexion, and 4/5 ankle plantarflexion. Wilbur was able to complete three heel raises on his left leg and 11 heel raises on his right leg. Wilbur presents with moderate point tenderness and muscle tightness in his hip flexors bilaterally, left hamstring, left quadriceps, and left gastrocnemius/soleus. He has range of motion limitation of the left knee of 8° to 72° actively and 3° to 84° passively.

Wilbur states his pain at rest in the distal thigh and knee is 4/10 and with activity it climbs to 8/10 stating that partial weight bearing and fully bending his knee are the most painful of activities that he has tried. He currently ambulates with a walker and knee immobilizer and is toe touch weight bearing at this time (although his restrictions are 50% weight bearing). Upon demonstration of his ability to walk, he presents with increased hip hike for foot clearance during ambulation, non-weight bearing gait with exaggerated knee flexion throughout the gait phase to avoid his foot touching the ground. Wilbur is able to complete single leg stance on his right lower extremity for 7 seconds with notable increased sway and reliance on hip strategy. He is able to complete the TUG test in 25.4 seconds with notable difficulty turning his standard walker to the right.

■ CASE STUDY QUESTIONS

1. What is another name for a malignant fibrous histiocytoma?
2. Are chondrosarcomas typically slow- or fast-growing tumors?

3. What are the three classifications of bone tumors based on the location of the tumor?
4. What musculoskeletal disorders need to be ruled out when performing an examination?
5. What type of diagnostic imaging might be indicated?
6. What types of systems are available for grading or staging bone tumors?
7. What is the medical treatment of choice?
8. Based on a histological assessment, what is the prognosis for someone with a bone tumor?
9. Why was the intramedullary rod utilized in this case?
10. Is electrical stimulation indicated or contraindicated in this case? If indicated, what are the goals for this modality?
11. What standardized measures may be incorporated into the physical therapy examination?
12. The patient has progressed well and will need outpatient therapy. What interventions should now be added to the treatment?

53

RHEUMATOID ARTHRITIS: CASE 1

Meri Goehring, PT, PhD, GCS, CWS

Judy is a 73-year-old female who is a retired receptionist and has been widowed for 3 years. Judy enjoys spending time with her eight grandchildren and going to their extracurricular activities. Judy has been having pain in her upper extremities bilaterally that came on suddenly. Judy was unsure of the cause and thought maybe she overexerted herself gardening. Judy has been experiencing significant stiffness and pain in her arms and hands. Judy has some swelling in her upper extremity soft tissues. Judy was feeling very fatigued and when she went to the doctor she had a high *erythrocyte sedimentation rate* (ESR).

Judy was recently diagnosed with adult onset rheumatoid arthritis (RA) that is developed in persons 60 years old or older. Judy has been prescribed methotrexate and prednisone.

Judy's physician gave her a script for physical therapy and is presenting to an outpatient physical therapy clinic. Judy has a significant past medical history of osteoarthritis, a hysterectomy, chronic pain syndrome, and a heart arrhythmia. Judy does not participate in any formal exercise. A systems review reveals that her blood pressure is 135/70, heart rate is 70 beats per minute, respiration is 18 breaths per minute, and oxygen saturation is 96%. Neurologically, her light touch sensation is intact and DTRs are 2/4 throughout. Integument assessment reveals a rash that is present over elbows bilaterally, and her fingers are swollen. Judy's pain and stiffness in her upper extremities is 6/10 in the morning and improves to a 2/10 as the day progresses. Grip strength was equal bilaterally but weak and measured 60.4 lb on her left and 62.6 on her right. All upper extremity manual muscle tests were painful but Judy could resist against gravity. Shoulder flexion range of motion, abduction, internal rotation, and external rotation were limited by pain. Judy scored a 65 on the SF-36.

■ CASE STUDY QUESTIONS

1. What is the pathophysiology associated with rheumatoid arthritis?
2. What are the most common signs and symptoms of rheumatoid arthritis?

3. What are the common inflammatory markers of RA?

4. Do a positive rheumatoid factor and the presence of anti-CCP antibodies automatically indicate rheumatoid arthritis is present? Why or why not?

5. Is rheumatoid arthritis associated with any cardiac pathology?

6. What is the effect of rheumatoid arthritis on muscle?

7. What is the recommended medical treatment for RA?

8. What is the Disease Activity Score (DAS28)?

9. What are some lifestyle changes you would recommend for someone living with RA?

10. What are the objectives for physical therapy intervention?

11. Would you recommend high-intensity resistance exercise?

12. Is aquatic therapy (hydrotherapy) a viable option for this patient?

13. What patient education would you provide to this patient?

14. What modalities might you add to your intervention?

15. Should joint protection strategies be a part of your plan of care?

16. Would massage therapy assist this patient?

17. Where does therapeutic exercise and mobility training fit into the rehabilitation plan?

18. What are some standardized measures/functional outcomes tools that can be utilized in this population?

54

RHEUMATOID ARTHRITIS: CASE 2

Meri Goehring, PT, PhD, GCS, CWS

Maude is an 84-year-old retired waitress. Maude lives with her 87-year-old husband who has Alzheimer disease and is hard of hearing. She and her husband, Mervin, live in a one-story, ranch-style home with a walk-in shower, elevated toilet seat, and a ramp to enter her home in the front. She enjoys spending time with her three grandchildren and seven great grandchildren. Maude has been experiencing pain and stiffness in her hands and hips with moderate swelling noticeable in her hands. This pain exacerbation has been noticeable in the last two to three weeks. She complains of continual fatigue and that she has no energy to watch her great grandchildren. Upon further discussion, you learn that Maude was diagnosed with adult onset RA 3 years ago, but has no idea what that entails or what that even means. She has been taking methotrexate (Trexall) for the last 3 years and that seems to help, but otherwise no change in her symptoms has occurred. Maude is presenting to outpatient physical therapy.

Maude has a significant past medical history of cardiovascular disease, high cholesterol, fibromyalgia, and restless leg syndrome. She has a family history of heart disease as both her mother and father passed away of a myocardial infarction, and her brother passed away from a stroke thought to be caused from his atrial fibrillation. Maude recently started a senior fitness class, in which she attends once a week. She had been going for 2 months prior to her recent pain exacerbation. She has not gone since.

A systems review is performed and reveals that her blood pressure is 146/93 mm Hg, heart rate of 75 beats per minute, and respiratory rate of 14. Her reflexes present as 2+ bilaterally in her upper and lower extremities, light touch appears intact in both her upper and lower extremities. Both her hands are moderately swollen and appear red around the middle phalanx knuckles more notably on her right than her left hand. Grip strength was measured at 37 lb on the right and 49 lb on the left, both limited by pain. Manual muscle testing was performed and she demonstrates a gross upper extremity strength of 4−/5 and gross lower extremity strength of 4/5 with pain in her hips during resisted hip flexion. Maude rates her pain as 8/10 in the morning and by midday she reports that it decreases to a 4/10. With activity in the middle of the day, she reports 6/10 pain. Maude scored a 5.0 on the Disease Activity Score. She reports occasional flare-ups of the disease about four times per year.

■ CASE STUDY QUESTIONS

1. What medical treatment is common with rheumatoid arthritis?

2. What is the foremost reason that early diagnosis is important?

3. How does methotrexate work?

4. What are the side effects of methotrexate?

5. What are the possible complications of taking methotrexate?

6. What is the Disease Activity Score (DAS28)?

7. What factors influence prognosis?

8. Why is exercise important in individuals with rheumatoid arthritis?

9. What is the most critical benefit of exercise in individuals with rheumatoid arthritis?

10. What are the main objectives for physical therapy treatment in an individual with rheumatoid arthritis?

11. What are the minimal criteria to collect during the evaluation process?

12. What are the physical therapy treatment options for individuals with rheumatoid arthritis?

13. What modalities could be utilized?

14. What are joint protection strategies?

15. Should patients continue to exercise during acute flare-ups of the disease?

16. What are some of the functional measures that may be incorporated into the examination of an individual with rheumatoid arthritis?

17. What are some of the biologic agents being used to treat rheumatoid arthritis?

55

SARCOPENIA: CASE 1

Meri Goehring, PT, PhD, GCS, CWS

Longitudinal studies have demonstrated that muscle mass and size decreases by approximately 6% per decade in the average person beginning at approximately 45 years of age. This age-associated loss of skeletal mass and function is termed sarcopenia. The cause is multifactorial as disuse, change in endocrine function, chronic diseases, insulin resistance, nutritional deficiencies, and inflammation can lead to sarcopenias. Criterion has been set forth by the European Working Group on Sarcopenia in Older People (EWGSOP) to aid in the identification of sarcopenia. Gait speed is a performance level criterion and is used by both the EWGSOP and the International Working Group on Sarcopenia (IWGS). In addition, dual energy x-ray absorptiometry is used to determine the presence of sarcopenia; a low skeletal muscle mass greater than 2 standard deviations below a young adult is considered positive.

Josie has been referred to physical therapy by her primary care physician for lower extremity weakness. Josie is a 70-year-old woman who presents with difficulty walking that has slowly progressed over the last few years. Upon history, Josie reports that she has been having frequently falls secondary to fatigue. Activities of daily living (ADLs) have become challenging and she has been unable to play with her grandchildren when she cares for them two to three times per week. She has become limited in her activity level, and leaves her home only once or twice a week to shop for short periods of time. Prior medical history includes osteoporosis, hysterectomy, and obesity. Currently, Josie is taking Fosamax and Ambien as needed.

On evaluation, upper extremity strength was found to be 4/5 throughout and lower extremity 3+/5 via manual muscle testing. Using a handheld dynamometer, hand grip strength on her right, or dominant, side was 22 kg and her left side was 20 kg. Josie's neurological screen was unremarkable with no sensation loss. Josie performed a 6-m gait speed test, which revealed a walking speed of 0.8 m/s over level ground. Vitals for Josie's evaluation can be found in Table 55-1.

TABLE 55-1	Vital Signs		
	Before Examination	During Examination	After Examination
Blood Pressure	160/90	189/98	168/92
Heart rate (bpm)	87	130	95
Respiratory rate	20	25	23
Pulse oximetry	97%	94%	96%

■ CASE STUDY QUESTIONS

1. Is communication with Josie's primary care physician appropriate?
2. What specifically should be communicated?
3. What secondary health concern is worrisome?
4. How does obesity play a role in this case?
5. Why would handgrip strength be a useful measure?
6. Would you define/describe this patient as frail, why or why not?
7. Why would we be concerned with frailty?
8. Is there another functional test that may be utilized to test for frailty?
9. What physical therapy interventions should be included in Josie's plan of care?
10. What functional limitations should be addressed?
11. What education should be provided?
12. Would you make any other referrals? Why?

56

SARCOPENIA: CASE 2

Meri Goehring, PT, PhD, GCS, CWS

Ernie is an 82-year-old male who has just been diagnosed with sarcopenia based on the criterion set forth by the European Working Group on Sarcopenia in Older People (EWGSOP).[1] In addition, dual energy x-ray absorptiometry showed that his muscle mass is low and is greater than 2 standard deviations below a young adult. Ernie is now referred to physical therapy due to loss of muscle strength and the inability to perform basic activities of daily living (BADLs). Upon history taking, Ernie discloses that he is living alone in a semiassisted living center. His medications include a daily multivitamin, baby aspirin, Metolazone, and Captopril.

On examinations vitals were taken: blood pressure of 145/89, heart rate of 65, respiratory rate of 18, and pulse oximetry of 97%. Manual muscle testing for the upper extremities were graded 3+/5 throughout. Hip musculature 3+/5, knee 4/5, and ankle 3+/5. Sensation to upper extremities was intact but was altered within a stock-like pattern bilaterally throughout his lower extremities. Ernie performed a 6-m gait speed test, which revealed a decreased walking speed of 0.7 m/s over level ground with no abnormal vital response was noted.

■ CASE STUDY QUESTIONS

1. What could be the cause of Ernie's sarcopenia?
2. What additional questions could be asked to gain more insight into Ernie's history?
3. Has Earnie's fall risk increased over someone without sarcopenia?
4. Is Ernie at risk of having functional limitations?
5. Are there medical complications that can be associated with sarcopenia?
6. Are there personal and/or psychosocial factors that can be associated with sarcopenia?
7. What screening tools could be used during Ernie's evaluation?
8. What physical therapy interventions should be included in Ernie's plan of care?
9. Would you make any other referrals? Why?
10. Is prevention warranted for Ernie?

REFERENCE

1. Hernandez H, Harris-Love M. Ahead of the curve: preparing for the clinical diagnosis of sarcopenia. *GeriNotes*. 2014;21(2):5-9.

CHAPTER

3

Neuromuscular Cases

INTRODUCTION

AGE-RELATED CHANGES IN THE NEUROLOGIC SYSTEM

Deborah A. Kegelmeyer, PT, DPT, MS, GCS

The neuromuscular system undergoes many age-related changes that can negatively impact function. Normal age-related changes occur at a rate of 1% per year, starting at age 30.[1] Therapists need to understand the importance what constitutes a normal age-related change as opposed to pathologic changes as behaviors that fall outside of what is considered to be the range of normal function should be assessed and treated. Changes occur in the brain, spinal cord, and peripheral nervous system. These changes also lead to changes in the musculature. In addition, the sensory system declines with age and this impacts motor function. The cases in this chapter provide examples of both normal age-related and pathologic changes to the neuromuscular system.

It is necessary for therapists to have an understanding of the anatomy and physiology of the aging neurologic system to successfully treat their clients. Anatomic changes include a decline in brain volume overall with the greatest age-related differences in the prefrontal and orbitofrontal cortices. These areas are critical for executive function and memory.[2] The parietal cortex also shows more age-related differences in gray matter volume than either the temporal or occipital regions. Motor control is not only dependent on these areas but is also more dependent on these areas in the elderly than in young adults. Subcortical structures, including the cerebellum and basal ganglia, also exhibit reduced volume with aging. The cerebellum is important for movement timing and coordination, while the caudate nucleus of the basal ganglia is involved in skill acquisition, specifically motor planning. Declines in white matter volume begin later but continue at a more accelerated rate than gray matter changes. Changes in the corpus callosum, the largest white matter bundle, significantly impact interhemispheric communication that is critical for bimanual coordination. There is a decrease in myelin in the gracilis fasciculus and an associated decrement in vibration threshold, indicating that fibers conveying proprioception are most affected by aging, which may contribute to balance deficits due to the loss of long latency postural reactions.[2] Fortunately, some brain areas do not exhibit age-related changes, including the cingulate gyrus (influential in linking behavioral outcomes to motivation) and the occipital cortex (vision).[2]

In addition to the anatomic changes there are decreased levels of critical neurotransmitters in the aging brain. Acetylcholine declines are noted in the hippocampus and associated with changes in memory function.[3] Changes in dopamine are associated with declines in frontal lobe function, including executive function and working memory. In addition, the loss of dopamine is closely linked to impairments in gait, balance, and fine motor control.[3] Alterations

in serotonin with age correlate with declines in activity level and diminished balance in mice.[3] Norepinephrine levels decrease in the cerebellum and are related to diminished motor learning with age.

In the peripheral nervous system there is axonal degeneration and greater internodal length variability. The presence of shorter internodes suggests a process of denervation and then regeneration. The capacity for axonal regeneration and reinnervation is maintained throughout life but tends to be slower and less effective with aging.[4] This pattern of degeneration and reinnervation also leads to changes in the muscle. There is a decrease in the number of neurons per muscle fiber, leading to fiber grouping, a consequence of the above-mentioned process of denervation and subsequent reinnervation. The result of this pattern of changes is likely an increased recruitment of motor units for a given task in older adults. It takes more work to do any given task.

Normal age-related changes in the nervous system lead to small declines in the sensory and motor systems. This impacts all three systems related to balance visual, vestibular, and somatosensory systems. These age-related declines result in slowing of movement and difficulty in situations that require faster responses or a higher level of sensory-motor integration. Overall, individuals experiencing healthy aging remain able to engage in typical daily activities well into old age. In the old-old we would expect to see slowing of function and an inability to engage in high-level motor activities such as balancing on a moving surface or negotiating an unfamiliar area in low light. Any loss of function beyond this would potentially be beyond normal age-related changes and may be due to a treatable pathology.

Sensory changes related to normal aging include a reduction or alteration of sensations of pain, vibration, temperature, pressure, and touch. It is difficult to tell whether these changes are related to aging itself or to the disorders that occur more often in the elderly such as diabetic neuropathy. The ability of the eye to adapt to changes in lighting leads to difficulty seeing when moving from a light to a dark environment or vice versa as the pupil reacts more slowly to light with aging. In addition, the ability of the pupil to change focus quickly from far to near declines, this is presbyopia. Presbyopia is due to the lens becoming more dense and inelastic, leading to reduced accommodation. Far vision is easier because it is achieved by muscle relaxation. In addition, the aging eye has declines in its ability to detect contrast in objects that are close in color and has a decreased ability to adapt to glare. Visual acuity declines in situations with glare such as driving at night.

Changes in the visual system impact gait. We use vision to find obstacles and avoid them. Obstacle location and motor planning to avoid them happens long before the obstacle is "underfoot."[5] So, when vision is poor, the person is not able to locate the object until it is much closer or already underfoot. Knowing this they adapt by walking slower and walking with their head down. This adaptation leads to a slower gait and may contribute to postural changes such as kyphosis and forward head. While it helps locate objects and avoid trips it leads to many negative changes in other systems.

Cognition is another area that has taken on more importance for physical therapists as it has become evident that mobility relies

not only on motor and sensory function but also on the cognitive system. There is some change or decline in cognitive functioning, especially short-term memory, but if information is presented in a way to compensate for age-related changes in vision and hearing (slower) short-term memory is improved. Overall intelligence is not affected by normal aging. Nearly 30% of those over the age of 80 develop severe cognitive impairment or dementia which is not a normal part of the aging process. Cognitive disorders of all types account for two-thirds of nursing home admissions.

Pathologic changes in cognition fall into two categories: dementia or delirium. Dementia is a slow gradual onset of diminished ability to reason and make sound judgments, loss of social skills, and development of regressed or antisocial behavior. Alzheimer and multi-infarct dementia are the two most common forms of dementia. Cognitive problems can be reversible if they result from metabolic, toxic derangements or psychiatric illness. Delirium is a transient mental disorder with a relatively rapid onset, a course that typically fluctuates, and a brief duration of hours to 4 weeks. The essential features of delirium are reduced ability to maintain attention to external stimuli, and to appropriately shift attention to new external stimuli, and disorganized thinking as manifested by rambling, irrelevant, or incoherent speech. Physical activity in middle age can impact later cognitive function, the domain most likely to be influenced is executive function.[6] Studies support that physical activity is related to cognitive function with increased physical activity leading to better cognitive function and less dementia.[6,7]

The cases in this chapter also cover fall screening and prevention. The modality with the strongest evidence for efficacy in fall prevention or reduction is individualized exercise that includes balance training as a component.[8] Gait training by a physical therapist with prescription of an assistive device also has good evidence for efficacy.[9] There is also preliminary evidence that physical therapist-directed group exercise may help prevent falls.[9]

Neurologic disorders associated with aging that most commonly impact mobility and function are the neurodegenerative diseases such as Parkinson and Alzheimer diseases, stroke, dementia, and other cognitive disorders, traumatic brain injury, and spinal cord injury. Successful evaluation and intervention for each of these disorders rely on the therapist having an understanding of the aging process and incorporating this information in their treatment plan. Cases in this chapter provide the reader with the opportunity to explore the complex interaction of aging and each of these neurologic disorders.

The objectives of this chapter are to discuss age-related changes in the neurologic system and the primary neurologic disorders that affect the geriatric population. This chapter will also examine new research findings related to neurologic disorders examination and treatment and apply these findings to aged individuals with neurologic disorders.

REFERENCES

1. Mahncke HW, Bronstone A, Merzenich MM. Brain plasticity and functional losses in the aged: scientific bases for a novel intervention. *Prog Brain Res.* 2006;157:81-91.
2. Salat DH, Buckner RL, Snyder AZ, et al. Thinning of the cerebral cortex in aging. *Cereb Cortex.* 2004;14(7):721-730.
3. Li SC. Neuromodulation of behavioral and cognitive development across the life span. *Dev Psychol.* May 2012;48(3):810-814.
4. Peters A, Sethares C. Is there remyelination during aging of the primate central nervous system? *J Comp Neurol.* 2003;460:238-254.
5. Owsley C, McGwin GJ. Association between visual attention and mobility in older adults. *J Am Geriatr Soc.* 2004;52(11):1901-1906.
6. Kramer AF, Erickson KI, Colcombe SJ. Exercise, cognition, and the aging brain. *J Applied Physiol.* 2006;101(4):1237-1242.
7. Voss MW, Heo S, Prakash RS, Erickson KI, Alves H, Chaddock L, Szabo AN, Mailey EL, Wójcicki TR, White SM, Gothe N, McAuley E, Sutton BP, Kramer AF. The influence of aerobic fitness on cerebral white matter

integrity and cognitive function in older adults: results of a one-year exercise intervention. *Hum Brain Mapp.* 2013;34(11):2972-2985.
8. American Geriatrics Society, British Geriatrics Society. Clinical practice guidelines: prevention of falls in older persons. New York, NY: American Geriatrics Society; 2010. http://www.americangeriatrics.org/health_care_professionals/clinical_practice/clinical_guidelines_recommendations/2010/. Accessed June 22, 2010.
9. Panel on Prevention of Falls in Older Persons, American Geriatrics Society and British Geriatrics Society. Summary of the Updated American Geriatrics Society/British Geriatrics Society clinical practice guideline for prevention of falls in older persons. *J Am Geriatr Soc.* January 2011;59(1):148-157.

1

CVA: ACUTE STAGE

Deborah A. Kegelmeyer, PT, DPT, MS, GCS

Mr Stein is a 69-year-old male with a history of hypertension, lipidemia, and osteoarthritis. He does not smoke presently but has a 30-pack-year history. He quit smoking 7 years ago. He was admitted to the hospital through the emergency department (ED) last night with a diagnosis of embolic stroke. He noted that his right arm felt heavy when he woke up and as the day went on he began having trouble speaking and his arm became clumsy. He had no loss of consciousness and was continent of bowel and urine. On entering the ED he had been symptomatic for 12 hours. He was hypertensive (152/102) in the ED and tachycardic (96 beats per minute) with respiratory rate of 20.

At present he is mildly hypertensive (142/90), heart rate is 80 beats per minute, and respiratory rate is 18 breaths per minute. He is resting in his hospital bed.

Examination reveals mild aphasia and right-sided hemiplegia UE > LE. He is areflexic (0) on the right and DTRs on the left are 2+. Hoffman and Babinski reflexes are present on the right. Gross strength of the right upper extremity is 2/5 in the hand, 3/5 at the elbow, and 3+/5 in the shoulder girdle. Right lower extremity gross strength is 3/5 at the ankle, 3+/5 at the knee, and 4/5 at the hip. Sensation is intact in all four extremities.

Transfers: sit to/from supine requires minimal assist of one, and sit to/from stand requires contact guard assist (CGA). He is able to take several steps with moderate assist of one hand in hand and balance in standing requires assist when disturbed but able to maintain static balance. Sitting balance static is independent in a static pose but requires minimal assist for reaching out of the limit of stability to the right side.

Following these examination procedures his systolic BP rises by 10 mm Hg and his heart rate increases to 87 beats per minute on the monitor. ECG remains stable throughout the evaluation.

■ CASE STUDY QUESTIONS

1. Describe standard medical management for a patient fitting Mr Stein's description.

2. What are the precautions that should be followed in treating Mr Stein at this time?

3. What is the likely location of his stroke and what vessel is affected? (Be specific.)

4. What risk factors did Mr Stein have for stroke?

5. What further assessments should be done by the physical therapist at this time? Why?

6. What outcome measures would be appropriate at this time? Why? Be sure to include evidence for their validity in this situation.

7. What interventions should be initiated to improve lower extremity function by the therapist at this time?

8. What interventions should be initiated to improve upper extremity function by the therapist at this time?

9. What are the goals of these interventions?

10. What is Mr Stein's prognosis for returning home from the hospital rather than being admitted to long-term care? Is there any information the therapist could collect to further determine his prognosis for return to home?

2

CVA: SUBACUTE STAGE
Deborah A. Kegelmeyer, PT, DPT, MS, GCS

Mr Thomas is an 82-year-old male who suffered an ischemic stroke 5 days ago. He has just been admitted to a rehabilitation facility and is approved for up to 3 weeks of care. He has a history of hypertension, lipidemia, and COPD. In addition, he has lumbar spinal stenosis. Mr Thomas is retired and lives in a two-story single family home with his wife. Bedroom and full bath are on the second floor.

He had a left CVA with right-sided hemiplegia and moderate aphasia. The right arm is spastic with no active movement in the hand or elbow and isolated strength in the shoulder girdle is 2/5. When asked to raise his arm he shrugs his shoulder and then elevates at the shoulder to 45°. His right leg strength is 1/5 in the dorsiflexors, 2/5 in the plantar flexors, 3−/5 at the knee, and 3+/5 at the hip. He is hypertonic in the right upper extremity and lower extremity with Ashworth scores of 2 to 3 in the shoulder adductors and internal rotators, elbow flexors, and wrist and finger flexors. Modified Ashworth scores of 2 to 3 are present in the hip adductors, knee flexors, and ankle plantar flexors. Unsustained clonus is noted in the right wrist and ankle.

He has a right visual field cut and exhibits no signs of hemineglect. Transfers require one person moderate assist. Gait in the parallel bars requires moderate assist of one to maintain balance and assist in advancing the right leg. He tolerates being up in a chair for >3 hours and blood pressure has been stable in hospital.

When walking in the parallel bars he keeps his weight on his left leg and attempts to drag the right leg with the foot in plantar flexion and inversion. All transfers are made with all of his weight on his left side.

■ CASE STUDY QUESTIONS

1. What is the Modified Ashworth Scale?

2. What outcome measures would be appropriate for this setting and Mr Thomas' condition?

3. Describe a task-oriented intervention to promote equal weight bearing in sitting.

4. Describe a task-oriented intervention to promote:

   a. Equal weight bearing during sit-to-stand transfer

   b. Transferring stand to sit with controlled lowering and forward flexion of the trunk

   c. Initiating swing cycle on the right with hip flexion and not hip hike or circumduction

   d. Increasing stance time on the right leg during left swing phase

5. Describe appropriate gait activities for Mr Thomas at this stage of his rehabilitation.

6. Describe appropriate gait activities when Mr Thomas is able to improve swing initiation and weight bearing on the right in isolation but not during gait.

7. Describe the pros and cons of using a cane or quad cane during gait while in the rehabilitation facility. What are alternative devices to use during rehabilitation in the facility?

8. Describe treatment approaches for decreasing tone in Mr Thomas' UE and LE and provide evidence of the effectiveness of each one.

9. Describe methods to strengthen Mr Thomas' UE and LE and provide evidence of their potential benefit and safety.

10. Describe methods to improve Mr Thomas' balance in standing and gait and provide evidence for their efficacy in this situation.

11. What are the treatments for his right visual field cut? (By both other providers and the physical therapist.)

3

CVA: CHRONIC STAGE REHABILITATION IN THE HOME SETTING
Deborah A. Kegelmeyer, PT, DPT, MS, GCS

Mr Thomas, an 82-year-old male, suffered an ischemic stroke 4 weeks ago. He is beginning home health rehabilitation. He has a history of hypertension, lipidemia, and COPD. In addition he has lumbar spinal stenosis. Mr Thomas is retired and lives in a two-story single family home with his wife. His bedroom and a full bath are on the second floor.

He had a Left CVA with right-sided hemiplegia and moderate aphasia. The right arm is spastic with no active movement in the hand and synergistic movement in the elbow and isolated strength in the shoulder girdle is 3/5. When asked to raise his arm he shrugs his shoulder and then elevates at the shoulder to 105°. His right leg strength is 2/5 in the dorsiflexors, 3/5 in the plantar flexors, 4/5 at the knee, and 4/5 at the hip. He is hypertonic in the right upper extremity and lower extremity with Ashworth scores of 2 to 3 in the shoulder adductors and internal rotators, elbow flexors, and wrist and finger flexors. Ashworth scores of 2 to 3 in the hip adductors, knee flexors, and ankle plantar flexors. Positive clonus, unsustained in the right wrist and ankle.

He has a right visual field cut and exhibits no signs of hemineglect. Transfers require one person minimal assist in bed and CGA from firm surfaces. Gait with quad cane requires CGA on level uncluttered surfaces with minimal weight shift to the right leg.

When walking he keeps greater weight on his left leg and hip hikes to initiate swing with the right leg with the foot in plantarflexion and inversion. All transfers are made with greater weight on his left side.

Mr Thomas is unable to climb stairs and is in a hospital bed in the dining room with a bedside commode.

■ CASE STUDY QUESTIONS

1. What are the rules for qualification for home health coverage from Medicare?

2. What are the factors related to the characteristics of the stroke lesion that determine prognosis after CVA? Apply them to Mr Thomas.

3. What are other factors that impact an individual's prognosis after CVA? Apply to Mr Thomas.

4. What would be the primary goal for rehabilitation at this time for Mr Thomas?

5. What therapeutic interventions will be effective to improve Mr Thomas' stair climbing independence?

6. What type of transfer training would be appropriate?

7. In what way will his lumbar stenosis impact therapy and how will you modify therapy due to this comorbidity?

8. How will his COPD potentially impact therapy sessions? What red flags should the therapist watch for while working with a client who has COPD?

9. Describe appropriate exercises for the shoulder girdle at this point in his rehabilitation.

10. At what point in his rehabilitation should Mr Thomas be transferred to outpatient rehabilitation?

4

CVA: WITH HEMINEGLECT

Deborah A. Kegelmeyer, PT, DPT, MS, GCS

Mr Urse is a 72-year-old male who is recovering from a right CVA that has left him with left hemiplegia. He has mild spasticity in the left arm and leg and weakness and sensory impairment. He has been admitted to a skilled nursing facility for rehabilitation. On examination the therapist notes that he has fixed gaze deviation to the right and his left arm is hanging down by the wheel of the wheelchair and the left foot has fallen off of the footrest and is dragging on the floor while he is wheeling himself in circles using his right arm to propel the chair. When the therapist approaches him from the left he does not respond to her until she is directly in front of him and cues him by touching his right shoulder.

■ CASE STUDY QUESTIONS

1. What condition do Mr Urse's symptoms indicate? (gaze deviation, dragging left leg, not notice therapist when on his left side) Describe this condition. Which area of the brain leads to this condition?

2. What examination techniques and outcome measures are used to assess for hemineglect? —*Behavioural Inattention test*

3. What are treatment techniques to improve spatial awareness? (awareness of objects and external space) *Figure ground dis, form discrim, spatial rel'n, topographic*

4. Describe how to perform mirror training to improve awareness of self and body parts.

5. Describe how transcutaneous electrical nerve stimulation (TENS) is used to treat unilateral neglect.

6. Describe how visual imagery and movement imagery are used to treat unilateral neglect.

7. Describe how vibration is used to treat unilateral neglect.

8. Describe what optokinetic stimulation is and how it is used to treat unilateral neglect.

9. What is Mr Urse's prognosis for recovery from unilateral neglect?

10. What are the payment policies of Medicare for receiving rehabilitation in a skilled nursing facility (SNF)?

↳ 60 days of Wellness
3 nights in Hospital
> 65 yrs
significant medical...

5

CVA WITH PUSHER SYNDROME → MCA

Deborah A. Kegelmeyer, PT, DPT, MS, GCS

Mrs Epley is a 76-year-old female who has a history of smoking and hypertension. She has had stents placed into two coronary arteries in the past and was admitted to the hospital 3 days ago for a right CVA. She exhibits neglect on the left side, hemianopsia, and hemiparesis of the left arm and leg. While in the hospital it was noted that during transfers she leans posteriorly and to the left and does not support her weight on the left leg. Due to the severity of her stroke and the signs of neglect she has been admitted to a skilled nursing facility under Medicare Part A for rehabilitation.

On examination, Mrs Epley does not notice people and objects on her left side but is very friendly and conversational when people stand in front of her or to the right side. She talks a great deal and when asked why she is there she states, "I'm your supervisor and I'm here to make sure you do right." When her left arm or leg is moved passively she knows that they are her limbs. She tries to stand up without help and when told she should not do that as she has had a stroke and is weak she denies having any weakness on the left side.

Anosognosia → Denial & lack of awareness.

■ CASE STUDY QUESTIONS

1. What condition related to body perception is being described in this case?

2. What area of the brain is impacted that leads to this syndrome? Describe what the patient is experiencing that leads to the pushing behavior.

3. What evaluation methods are valid and reliable for measuring contraversive pushing? → *Posterolateral thalamic damage*

4. Describe visual feedback treatment techniques that evidence shows work to resolve "pushing" in Mrs Epley.

5. Describe the sequence of recovery that is necessary for clients with Pusher syndrome.

6. Describe the potential benefits of designing therapy to have the Mrs Epley move out of pushing rather than the therapist resisting the "pushing" behavior.

7. Describe some activities that could be used to treat Mrs Epley in supine and sitting to encourage weight shift to an upright alignment.

8. Describe therapeutic activities that can be done during standing to promote active weight bearing on uninvolved lower extremity and upright posture with reduced pushing behavior.

9. Describe therapeutic activities that can be done during gait to promote active weight bearing on the involved lower extremity.

10. Describe therapeutic activities that can be done during gait to promote active weight shift onto the uninvolved side and out of pushing.

6

PARKINSON DISEASE, EARLY TO LATE STAGES: PART 1

Deborah A. Kegelmeyer, PT, DPT, MS, GCS

Mrs Wykowski is a 67-year-old female who just received a diagnosis of Parkinson disease. She is considered to be in Hoehn and Yahr (H&Y) stage 1 and scored a 10 on the MDS-UPDRS (Unified Parkinson Disease Rating Scale). Her neurologist has sent her to physical therapy for a consultation on exercise and Parkinson disease. She states that she noticed she was walking slower when she could not keep up with her husband on their evening walks. Additionally her husband remarked that she did not swing her left arm when walking. She is a retired administrative assistant and she and her husband enjoy reading, going to the movies and evening walks. She keeps a tissue in her right hand and tabs her lips every 2 to 3 minutes.

Medical history: para ×2 and gravida ×2; lipedema controlled with statins. Gallbladder removal at age 42 and is postmenopausal.

Medications: Lipitor, multivitamins, and occasional use of ibuprofen for "arthritis" in her knees.

Physical therapy examination results:

- TUG score of 10.0 seconds
- Gait is safe and independent with a time of 1.1 m/s on the 10-Meter Walk Test
- Strength and range of motion are WNLs throughout.
- MoCA (Montreal Cognitive Assessment) score of 30
- Nine-Hole Peg Test time is 21 seconds on the right and 23 seconds on the left. She is right handed.
- Integument is intact.
- Vital signs at rest: HR 72 beats per minute, regular; RR 16 breaths per minute; BP 126/78; SpO$_2$ 98%; temp 98.7°F.
- Neurological: slight tremor, DTRs 2/4, light touch, proprioception, 2-point discrimination is intact.

■ CASE STUDY QUESTIONS

1. What are the defining characteristics of the Hoehn and Yahr stages?
2. What does the UPDRS measure? Is this a diagnostic, screening, or outcome measure?
3. Define rigidity and discuss how it is best measured.
4. Define bradykinesia and discuss ways to measure it.
5. What type of tremor is common in Parkinson disease? Describe this tremor and common areas of the body impacted by tremor.
6. Describe the area of the brain impacted by Parkinson disease. What pathways are impacted?
7. At the time of diagnosis how much of this area of the brain is usually already absent on imaging?
8. What do the results of her examination by the physical therapist tell you? Discuss age normed scores for each outcome measure and how her scores relate to age normed scores.
9. Based on her history and examination what would you prescribe for her in an exercise program?
10. Would an exercise program be beneficial for her? If yes, what evidence is there that exercise at this stage in her disease would be beneficial?

7

PARKINSON DISEASE, EARLY TO LATE STAGES: PART 2

Deborah A. Kegelmeyer, PT, DPT, MS, GCS

Mrs Wykowski who has Parkinson disease (see Part 1) and was just diagnosed was assessed using the following measures:

- MDS-Unified Parkinson Disease Rating Scale (MDS-UPDRS)
- Timed Up and Go (TUG)
- Montreal Cognitive Assessment (MoCA)
- Nine-Hole Peg Test
- 10-Meter Walk Test

You completed your examination and evaluation yesterday. You have a new student who you want to work with this new patient. As a clinical instructor your student is very curious as to why you chose these measures and has several questions for you.

■ CASE STUDY QUESTIONS

1. Which of these measures is recommended for use by the PD EDGE task force for the Neurology Section of the APTA?
2. What are the other core outcome measures recommended by the PD EDGE task force and describe what constructs each one measures?
3. What is the best measure for assessing freezing of gait according to the PD EDGE task force?
4. What is the best measure for assessing fear of falling in those with PD according to the PD EDGE task force?
5. Discuss the benefits of performing an initial assessment of every individual with PD at the time of diagnosis using a core set of measures that are also used by other clinics across the country.
6. What are the benefits of using a core set of measures for every individual with PD from time of diagnosis and throughout all stages of the disease?
7. What is the incidence of Parkinson disease?
8. What causes Parkinson disease?
9. What is dysphagia and is it common in Parkinson disease?
10. Why is it important to determine if the patient has dysphagia?

8

PARKINSON DISEASE, EARLY TO LATE STAGES: PART 3

Deborah A. Kegelmeyer, PT, DPT, MS, GCS

Mrs Wykowski is now 70 years old and her neurologist recently modified her medications to include Sinemet (carbidopa and levodopa). She has again been referred to physical therapy for gait and balance issues. Mrs Wykowski reports that she is stiff on both sides of her body with the left being more affected than the right. She is having trouble keeping up with her friends and her husband and finds shopping difficult as it just takes too long. Additionally it now takes her an hour to get dressed and groomed in the morning. States she has had no falls but has had many "near falls" where she stumbles and catches herself on furniture or the wall or her husband catches her.

Physical therapy examination results:

- TUG score of 14 seconds.

- She states that she has trouble getting up from her couch and sometimes from the toilet. It often takes several attempts and lots of rocking back and forth. She is able to rise from the firm chair in the clinic independently with no arms.

- Gait is slow and shuffling with no device with a time of 0.9 m/s on the 10-Meter Walk Test.

- Strength is WNLs throughout.

- Range of motion is limited in the knees, hips, and spine: lacks 5° of knee extension and hip extension bilateral and is in a kyphotic posture with a forward head and is unable to lay flat on the plinth.

- MoCA (Montreal Cognitive Assessment) score of 30.

- The Nine-Hole Peg Test time is 25 seconds on the right and 28 seconds on the left. She is right handed.

- She is complaining of difficulty with her handwriting stating it is getting smaller and as she writes it gets smaller and smaller. She is having trouble writing checks and thank you notes.

- Vital signs at rest: HR 70 beats per minute, regular; RR 17 breaths per minute; BP 122/76; SpO$_2$ 98%; temp 98.7°F.

- Neurological: increased tremor, DTRs 2/4, light touch, proprioception, 2-point discrimination is intact.

■ CASE STUDY QUESTIONS

1. Based on her description what Hoehn and Yahr (H&Y) stage is she now in? Why?

2. What does her Timed Up and Go (TUG) score mean? How sensitive, specific, reliable, and valid is this score in Parkinson disease?

3. What does her Nine-Hole Peg Test score mean?

4. What intervention would you prescribe for her loss of range of motion? Is this pattern of loss typical for PD?

5. Should she be placed on a strengthening program? If yes, what muscle groups should she focus on?

6. Mrs Wykowski has not been doing any exercise programs though she does continue to try to take evening walks with her husband. What barriers to exercise are common in individuals with PD? How may these have played a role in Mrs Wykowski's noncompliance with her home exercise program?

7. What interventions have been shown to be effective in increasing gait speed and balance?

8. What intervention would you use to improve her sit to and from stand transfer?

9. Is motor learning changed by Parkinson disease? How?

10. Mrs Wykowski would like to work on her handwriting as she finds it difficult to write checks and thank you notes, given this and her Nine-Hole Peg Test score what intervention(s) would you implement that have been shown to improve micrographia?

11. Describe the evidence behind the following interventions for Parkinson disease and briefly describe the parameters for using each as an intervention:
    a. Treadmill training
    b. Dance
    c. Bicycle
    d. Tai Chi
    e. LSVT BIG

PARKINSON DISEASE, EARLY TO LATE STAGES: PART 4

Deborah A. Kegelmeyer, PT, DPT, MS, GCS

Mrs Wykowski is now 75 years old and returns to physical therapy following a wrist fracture from a fall. At her most recent visit with the neurologist they increased her Sinemet (carbidopa and levodopa) dose. She states that the Sinemet generally works but she has "off" periods when she has great difficulty walking and transferring between doses of Sinemet. These periods are most common in the late afternoon. She requires help from her husband with dressing. She states this is because she is so slow and cannot balance to put on her socks and shoes. She reports having four falls in the last 3 months, the last one of which resulted in a Colles fracture.

Physical therapy examination results:

- TUG score of 25 seconds.

- She states that she has trouble getting up from all chairs and tends to "plop" when sitting down. She requires assistance to get off of the toilet about 50% of the time. She is unable to rise from the clinic chair without using her arms. Tends to lean backward.

- Gait is slow and shuffling with no device with a time of 0.5 m/s on the 10-Meter Walk Test.

- Strength is grossly 4/5 throughout except hip extension, back extension, and knee extension are 3+ to 4− out of 5.

- Range of motion is limited in the knees, hips, and spine: lacks 15° of knee extension and hip extension bilateral and is in a kyphotic posture with a forward head and is unable to lay flat on the plinth.

- MoCA (Montreal Cognitive Assessment) score of 24.

- Nine-Hole Peg Test time is 45 seconds on the right and 58 seconds on the left. She is right handed.

- History of falls, two occurred immediately after standing up and two occurred while walking to the bathroom.

- She reports increased difficulty swallowing and occasionally chokes when drinking water.

- Vital signs at rest: HR 68 beats per minute, regular; RR 20 breaths per minute; BP 116/70; SpO$_2$ 98%; temp 98.7°F.

- Neurological: significant resting tremor bilaterally, DTRs 2/4, light touch, proprioception, 2-point discrimination is intact.

■ CASE STUDY QUESTIONS

1. What does her TUG score indicate?

2. Her gait velocity of 0.5 m/s makes her which type of ambulatory? Community, limited community, or household?

3. Does a gait speed of 0.5 m/s indicate any increased risk of negative health status such as increased probability of hospitalization or of death? If yes, how does gait speed correlate with health status?

4. She has decreased range of motion into extension in her spine, hips, and knees. Describe a treatment plan for these issues.

5. Describe a treatment plan to improve her gait stability and safety and make her a community ambulatory.

6. How will you address her inability to independently transfer when she is having "off" periods with her Sinemet?

7. Would you prescribe an assistive device for her to use when walking? Why or why not? If you do prescribe a device, which one would you prescribe? Is there evidence for the efficacy of this device?

8. Is dual task ability impacted by PD? How?

9. How would you measure Mrs Wykowski's ability to dual task while walking? Give evidence for the efficacy of the method you have chosen.

10. Would impairment in dual task skill impact the ability to use an assistive device? If so, which device would be least impacted by declines in dual task ability?

11. Describe a physical therapy intervention program to improve dual task ability during walking.

12. Do auditory or visual cues aid in improving size or speed of movement in PD? Describe research findings to date regarding the use of cueing for increasing size and speed of movement.

13. What can be done for her swallowing problem?

PHYSICAL THERAPY EXAMINATION

- 10-Meter Walk Test—0.8 m/s
- Sit-to-stand transfer can be done independently with no hands but he has to rock back and forth 10 times and is unstable on initial standing.
- Gait is shuffling with very short step lengths. After about 10 ft of gait he begins to walk faster and faster with a rapid cadence and small shuffling steps. His weight is on the balls of his feet and he is in increasing trunk flexion. He is unable to stop and runs into a chair to stop.

■ CASE STUDY QUESTIONS

1. What is "freezing" of gait? What causes this?

2. He is also exhibiting "propulsive" gait, what is this? Are freezing of gait and propulsive gait related?

3. Is he a candidate for an assistive device? If he is, would reverse brakes be helpful to his gait problems?

4. Name at least three strategies to teach him to utilize when he experiences "freezing."

5. How are freezing of gait and falls related?

6. What strategies can he use to improve his transfers and minimize the need for rocking?

7. What strategies can he use to improve his step length?

8. What is Sinemet?

9. When is the best time for the patient to take Sinemet?

10. Are there any long-term side effects to taking Sinemet?

11. What are dopamine agonists?

10

FREEZING IN PARKINSON DISEASE

Deborah A. Kegelmeyer, PT, DPT, MS, GCS

Your 2:00 PM patient comes in 15 minutes late and appears quite distressed. He states that he became "frozen" in place after exiting his car in the parking garage and that is why he is late for his appointment. He is a 74-year-old male in good health with a diagnosis of Parkinson disease (PD) that he states he has had for 5 years. In the last year he has started falling, as often as three times a week and is experiencing freezing episodes. He describes these as times when he cannot move and it feels like his feet are "stuck in cement." He believes these occur most often when he has to turn such as when doing a transfer in and out of a car or from a chair at a table or when he is walking in a restaurant or theater and has to turn and walk in a small, cramped space. He has begun to limit his activities outside of the home due to these episodes. He is still driving and is not using an assistive device. He has purchased knee pads and is wearing one on each knee.

Vital signs: HR 62; RR 18; BP 112/68; SpO$_2$ 96%, temp 98.4°F

Medications: Sinemet (carbidopa and levodopa). He is also taking a dopamine agonist for the last 4 years. The Sinemet was added last year when his resting tremors became worse and decreased his hand function to perform IADLs.

11

MEDICAL MANAGEMENT OF PARKINSON DISEASE

Deborah A. Kegelmeyer, PT, DPT, MS, GCS

You are seeing a client with Parkinson disease in clinic today for shuffling gait and difficulty with transfers. Your client states that they love the new casino and have started spending a lot of time there even though this person never gambled before. In addition, his wife is concerned because he was talking about seeing spiders on the walls and she did not see any bugs but he was quite insistent.

In addition, his wife wonders if his medications should be changed. She states that she heard that Mirapex (pramipexole) or Requip (ropinirole) or Comtan (entacapone) would be good for him to use since her friend's cousin was prescribed these medications.

You review his medication list and find he is on the following medications:

Entacapone 200 mg tab 1 tab by mouth two times daily—Oral

Benztropine 1 mg tab take 1 tab by mouth three times daily—Oral

Carbidopa-levodopa 25-100 mg tab CR take two tabs by mouth three times daily—Oral

Propranolol 80 mg PO cap XR take 80 mg by mouth daily—Oral

Garlic supplements

■ CASE STUDY QUESTIONS

1. What is Sinemet or carbidopa-levodopa? What is its mechanism of action of this medication in treating PD?

2. What are the possible side effects of Sinemet or carbidopa-levodopa?

3. What is entacapone and what is its mechanism of action for treating PD?

4. What may be the underlying cause of this patient's gambling behavior?

5. What may be the underlying cause of this patient's visual hallucinations?

6. Which medications that the wife is asking about are typically used early in the disease for management of the symptoms of PD?

7. Give the mechanism of action for pramipexole, ropinirole, and entacapone?

8. How do MAO-B inhibitors work in PD?

9. Why would an anticholinergic medication be prescribed to someone with PD?

10. What are some common side effects of anticholinergic medications?

11. Define the abnormal tone commonly found in Parkinson disease.

12. What is the known efficacy of garlic supplements in PD?

12

CAMPTOCORMIA

William H. Staples, PT, DHSc, DPT, GCS, CEEAA

You are evaluating a patient with Parkinson disease who has a newly diagnosed postural disorder called camptocormia. He is currently being treated with Sinemet (levodopa). This patient is able to achieve upright posture in standing against a wall with great effort but quickly succumbs to the pull of the flexor musculature. He ambulates with a hyperflexed posture without an assistive device. Upon palpation the abdominals are quite taught and perhaps spastic in standing but relaxed in supine. The patient has had a diagnosis of Parkinson disease for 5 years and the symptoms of camptocormia that have been worsening for the last 2 years. This condition has become socially disabling for the patient and interferes with community participation. Remarkably the patient is not falling and functions reasonably well in the home. Rigidity in the limbs is not present and the patient has a small resting, unilateral tremor in the right hand, and the patient states that it worsens at the end of his medication cycle.

After your evaluation you determine that you need to do more research for this rare disorder to determine your treatment approach. Please answer the following questions based on your research.

■ CASE STUDY QUESTIONS

1. What is camptocormia?

2. What is the prevalence of camptocormia for people with Parkinson disease?

3. What functional test(s) would be beneficial to conduct on this patient?

4. Has camptocormia been found to be responsive to sensory cues (as this is helpful in other forms of dystonia)?

5. Has camptocormia been found to be responsive to core (extension) exercises?

6. Are there any other exercises that would be important for this patient?

7. Would you prescribe an assistive device for ambulation? Why or why not? What type?

8. Would you consider bracing for this patient? What type?

9. Would any modalities be helpful?

10. Are there other types of medications that might assist this patient's problem?

11. Deep brain stimulation has been used to help treat Parkinson disease, might it help with this condition?

12. Have any other medical interventions been attempted to alleviate this problem?

13

ESSENTIAL TREMOR

William H. Staples, PT, DHSc, DPT, GCS, CEEAA

A 67-year-old widowed male comes into your outpatient practice and you observe severe tremors in both hands when trying to complete his intake form. The tremors disappear when he stops writing. You also observe some difficulty when the patient ambulates due to tremors in the lower extremities that were not noticed when sitting. On examination, the patient states that his physician told him that he had essential tremors. The physician suggested that physical therapy might be able to help. He has been placed on two medications to control the tremors which are propranolol (Inderal) 40 mg orally twice a day and gabapentin (Neurontin) 300 mg three times daily 3 days ago. The patient states that he thinks the medications are helping. The patient is upset and anxious to start therapy because the physician told him that if the therapy and medications do not work that deep brain stimulation surgery is the only other option.

He also complains of mild right shoulder pain on a 3/10 verbal pain scale. The patient states that performing routine tasks (ADLs) like drinking, eating, handwriting, dressing, and grooming has become very difficult. He has had to wear a bib when eating because of the difficulty getting food to his mouth, and has therefore stopped dining out with his friends. He has had trouble paying his bills because he can no longer write a legible check. Otherwise this patient is in general good health. The patient does state he saw a medication on the Internet containing valerian root that might stop the tremors and asks you if he should try it.

■ CASE STUDY QUESTIONS

1. What is an essential tremor?

2. What functional tests/measures would you include in your examination?

3. What would your treatment plan consist of?

4. What would be your goals for this patient?

5. What might be the cause of the shoulder pain?

6. What might make the symptoms worse?

7. Would you order any specialized equipment to make ADLs easier for this patient?

8. Are there any dietary restrictions or other suggestions you would make for this patient?

9. Would any other services be beneficial?

10. What are the side effects of the medications to watch for?

11. Would these medications affect the therapy?

12. What would you tell your patient about valerian root?

13. What do you know about the brain surgery the patient mentioned?

14

PARKINSON DISEASE VERSUS PROGRESSIVE SUPRANUCLEAR PALSY

William H. Staples, PT, DHSc, DPT, GCS, CEEAA

A 64-year-old male with a recent diagnosis of Parkinson disease is evaluated in your clinic. He visited a neurologist following a number of falls at home and in the community. He was put on Sinemet 25 to 100 (carbidopa-levodopa) one tablet by mouth three times a day, 3 weeks ago by his physician. The patient states that he does not feel the medication has improved his walking ability. He is taking no other medication.

The patient's chief complaint is frequent loss of balance, and "stiffness" of his gait. He cannot remember the mechanism of the falls, but he states he usually ends up "on my buttock." He works as an accountant which does not require much walking during the day. He states that he is able to drive a car without difficulty. Lately he has been having difficulty working on his computer and describes the screen as blurry. During the subjective interview you notice slight slurring of the speech and that the patient rarely makes eye contact with you. Objective findings include: normal muscle strength throughout; slight loss of range of motion in bilateral shoulder abduction and flexion; bradykinesia when initiating movement, slow gait pattern; absence of resting or intention tremor. He ambulates with a "swaggering"-type pattern with a straight cane that he bought at a local drug store. When walking with him using a gait belt and doing balance testing, you find that the loss of balance reactions is primarily posteriorly. Posture during gait is upright.

You perform the following functional tests with resultant scores.

Unified Parkinson Rating Scale (UPDRS): Motor Experience of Daily Living (Part II) self-administered and Motor Examination (Part III). Part II score is 12 and Part III score is 20.

Hoehn and Yahr Classification of Disability is stage III.

10-Meter Walk Test (10MWT): 1.2 m/s with cane
STEADI: Four-Stage Balance Test

1. Stand with your feet side by side: 10 seconds

2. Place the instep of one foot so it is touching the big toe of the other foot: 10 seconds

3. Place one foot in front of the other, heel touching toe: 5 seconds

4. Stand on one foot: 3 seconds

Timed Up and Go (TUG): 12.5 seconds with a cane
30-Second Chair Stand Test: 10 times
MMSE: 27/30
Depression screening using Geriatric Depression Scale: 5/30

■ CASE STUDY QUESTIONS

1. What is progressive supranuclear palsy?

2. What is the most frequent first symptom of progressive supranuclear palsy?

3. What are some other common symptoms of progressive supranuclear palsy?

4. What is the normal progression of the disease?

5. What is the relationship to Parkinson disease?

6. When is the diagnosis of progressive supranuclear palsy absolutely confirmed?

7. What is the importance of a therapist knowing the clinical difference between Parkinson disease and progressive supranuclear palsy?

8. What is the STEADI tool and what do the scores on the tests mean?

9. What does the score on the Geriatric Depression Score indicate?

10. What are some treatment strategies for progressive supranuclear palsy?

11. What do the two measures of Parkinson disease tell you? (Unified Parkinson Rating Scale and Hoehn and Yahr Classification of Disability)

15

TBI IN AN ELDERLY CLIENT—COMA: PART 1

Deborah A. Kegelmeyer, PT, DPT, MS, GCS

George and Maura Smith were involved in a motor vehicle accident and both suffered traumatic brain injuries (TBI), with bruising and lacerations to the front and side of their heads. In addition, George has a fracture to his right distal femur and Maura has two rib fractures on her right side. George is 77 years old and Maura is 69 years old. Both have a history of hypertension and Maura has a history of atrial fibrillation and takes anticoagulants due to this condition. Both were unconscious when the driver in the truck that struck their vehicle approached their car. Both regained consciousness before the EMTs arrived. George was taken to surgery to repair his femur fracture and then placed in a drug-induced coma immediately following surgery. Glasgow coma scale (GCS) as rated on entry to the emergency room for George was 11 = E3 V3 M5, and Maura was 13 = E4 V4 M5.

■ CASE STUDY QUESTIONS

1. Both George and Maura are considered to be in the elderly age group. What is their prognosis compared to individuals aged 25 to 50 years old? Is the prognosis the same for those 60 to 75 as those over 75 years old?

2. What is the most common mechanism of TBI in those over 60 years old? What is it in those younger than 60 years old?

3. What type of brain injury are the Smiths most likely to have based on their age? Extradural hematoma or subdural hematoma? Is this different than what is seen in young and middle-aged adults?

4. Maura was discharged home after 36 hours in the hospital. The following day her daughter noted that she was having trouble speaking and her answers to questions did not make sense. She also noted that her coordination seemed "off." What is likely happening with Maura?

5. What are the underlying anatomical and pathological conditions in the elderly that lead to poorer outcomes after TBI in this population?

6. Maura eventually undergoes surgical evacuation of a brain bleed. Discuss the prognosis for Maura compared to younger individuals now that she has had a subdural hematoma and surgery.

7. Discuss response to rehabilitation for individuals over age 60. Consider potential benefit and recommended intensity.

8. What is the relationship between TBI and cognition and depression in the elderly?

9. George is in a drug-induced coma. Why is this done? What is the appropriate physical therapy intervention during this time?

10. What is the appropriate physical therapy for individuals who are in a coma or vegetative state?

3. As Maura progresses she is no longer agitated and now is impulsive and demonstrates perseveration. She follows simple instructions. What Ranchos stage is she in and why?

4. What is the recommended method to manage impulsive behavior? What are the unique dangers of impulsivity in an elderly individual?

5. Describe perseveration and how it may impede physical therapy. How is perseveration managed?

6. Give an example of physical therapy goals for gait and transfers incorporating behaviors of impulsivity and perseveration. Assume that she starts to rock back and forth to go sit to stand and continues rocking, perseverating on this motion. In addition, she climbs steps without using the handrail and goes too fast.

7. What does Ranchos stage VI look like? How is it different from Ranchos stage V?

8. George also fractured his femur and is now in rehabilitation with a long leg cast and weight bearing as tolerated. He is considered to be in Ranchos LOC VI. How will this impact gait and transfer training for George?

9. What is a netbed and why is it used?

10. What is the recommended method for managing individuals who are highly agitated? Are restraints appropriate?

16

EARLY RANCHOS STAGES: TBI PART 2

Deborah A. Kegelmeyer, PT, DPT, MS, GCS

George and Maura Smith were involved in a motor vehicle accident and both suffered traumatic brain injuries (TBI), with bruising and lacerations to the front and side of their heads. In addition, George has a fracture to his right distal femur and Maura has two rib fractures on her right side. George is 77 years old and Maura is 69 years old. Both have a history of hypertension and Maura has a history of atrial fibrillation and takes anticoagulants due to this condition. Both were unconscious when the driver in the truck that struck their vehicle approached their car. Both regained consciousness before the EMTs arrived. George was taken to surgery to repair his femur fracture and then placed in a drug-induced coma immediately following surgery. Glasgow coma scale (GCS) as rated on entry to the emergency room for George was 11 = E3 V3 M5, and Maura was 13 = E4 V4 M5.

Maura was discharged home after 36 hours in the hospital. The following day her daughter noted that she was having trouble speaking and her answers to questions did not make sense. She also noted that her coordination seemed "off."

Maura eventually undergoes surgical evacuation of a brain bleed. When Maura Smith awakens after surgery she is agitated and pulling at her lines and tubes. When she is given an injection she tries to slap the nurse's arm away. When asked her name or other questions she gives nonsensical responses such as the dog ate a purple cow. She is in a netbed as she fell out of bed when trying to get up by herself during the night.

■ CASE STUDY QUESTIONS

1. What Ranchos Los Amigos Levels of Cognitive Functioning Scale (LOCF) best fits the description of Maura?

2. What is the key to treatment when a person status post TBI is agitated? (Ranchos LOCF IV)

17

LATE RANCHOS STAGES: TBI PART 3

Deborah A. Kegelmeyer, PT, DPT, MS, GCS

George and Maura Smith were involved in a motor vehicle accident and both suffered traumatic brain injuries (TBI), with bruising and lacerations to the front and side of their heads. In addition, George has a fracture to his right distal femur and Maura has two rib fractures on her right side. George is 77 years old and Maura is 69 years old. Both have a history of hypertension and Maura has a history of atrial fibrillation and takes anticoagulants due to this condition. Both were unconscious when the driver in the truck that struck their vehicle approached their car. Both regained consciousness before the EMTs arrived. George was taken to surgery to repair his femur fracture and then placed in a drug-induced coma immediately following surgery. Glasgow coma scale (GCS) as rated on entry to the emergency room for George was 11 = E3 V3 M5, and Maura was 13 = E4 V4 M5.

George Smith has returned home and receives home health nursing and physical therapy with an aide coming to the house to assist with bathing. Maura is in a skilled nursing facility and is now in Ranchos LOC VII but continues to exhibit impulsivity and when frustrated she becomes agitated. She often wanders at night and nursing feels that she is exhibiting signs of early dementia and sundowning.

■ CASE STUDY QUESTIONS

1. Describe the features of Ranchos LOCF VII.

2. Is it unusual that Maura continues to have periods of agitation? If not, explain why she would still have agitation.

3. At this stage how will therapy address impulsivity?

4. What are the safety concerns regarding impulsivity in an elderly individual like Maura and how would these impact her returning to home?

5. What is Maura's prognosis for full recovery to her previous status? Explain your answer.

6. What is George's prognosis for full recovery to his previous status? Explain your answer.

7. What is the link between cognitive impairment (ie, delirium and dementia) and TBI?

8. There are now Ranchos LOC stages beyond VII, what are they? Briefly describe each one.

9. What would be the criteria for Maura to be discharged from the SNF to home? Consider all variables and not just her physical condition.

10. How will Medicare coverage impact discharge plans for Maura?

18

AGING WITH SPINAL CORD INJURY

Deborah A. Kegelmeyer, PT, DPT, MS, GCS

Mr Lynch is a 63-year-old male who has tetraplegia due to a gunshot wound which left him an ASIA level A at C7-8. He has full use of the elbow and limited use of the wrist and hands due to this spinal cord injury (SCI) from a gunshot wound that occurred 22 years ago. He had a cervical fusion from C6-T1. He was a police officer and is on disability due to the SCI. Mr Lynch's wife is 61-year-old who works full time as an accountant. She assists Mr Lynch with bathing and dressing. Their home is wheelchair accessible and Mr Lynch has been independent in transfers and wheelchair mobility. Mr Lynch has come to outpatient physical therapy due to a partial tear in the right rotator cuff that has left him dependent in transfers and is limiting his wheelchair mobility.

His vital signs are HR: 72 beats per minute, BP: 126/80, RR: 16 breaths per minute, SpO$_2$: 98%. He has 3/5 strength in right active shoulder abduction, and has pain with resistance into abduction and external rotation. He also complains of a burning pain and numbness extending down his right arm anteriorly to the palm. When actively abducting the arm there is a slight shoulder hike and an Empty Can Test is positive. He has no weakness or pain in the left shoulder. Bilaterally, sensation to light touch is intact and deep tendon reflexes are 2+ throughout.

■ CASE STUDY QUESTIONS

1. When taking his vitals you note that Mr Lynch does not have hypertension. Does this mean that he is at equal or lower risk for cardiovascular disease than his age-matched peers?

2. What are the potential impacts of aging with a spinal cord injury on Mr Lynch's gastrointestinal and genitourinary systems?

3. Discuss whether Mr Lynch's shoulder problems are likely due to normal aging, his SCI, or both. How common is this problem in those s/p SCI?

4. When having Mr Lynch perform exercises what precautions should be taken with his skin based on the changes related to an individual with SCI aging?

5. Which musculature of the shoulder is likely to be underdeveloped secondary to the types of activities Mr Lynch engages in?

6. Mr Lynch has pain complaints that appear to be partially neuropathic. Is this common after SCI? Is this pain likely to respond to therapy?

7. Mr Lynch's wife is 61 years old and works full time. What are the implications for her that Mr Lynch is having these difficulties?

8. With aging individuals report some degree of activity limitation. How does aging with an SCI impact this?

9. Mr Lynch comes to therapy and reports that while transferring the day before he missed the edge of the bed and fell to the floor landing on his buttocks. He reports no pain but you note that he has increased spasticity in his legs. What might be causing his spasticity worse?

10. What underlying condition that is common in individuals' aging with SCI would put Mr Lynch at increased risk of fracture from this fall? Discuss management and prevention of this condition in those with SCI.

11. What does ASIA level A at C7-8 mean?

19

SPINAL CORD INJURY IN AN ELDERLY CLIENT: CERVICAL INCOMPLETE

Deborah A. Kegelmeyer, PT, DPT, MS, GCS

Mrs Tedesky is a widower aged 77 and lives in a two ranch home with three steps to enter the home. She has a history of hypertension, osteoarthritis, and hypothyroidism. Two days ago she was brought to the ED via ambulance after a fall down her stairs while exiting her home. She has a laceration with 16 sutures on her forehead and a diagnosis of a spinal cord contusion. She has just been moved to a standard unit in the hospital from the ICU and is to begin therapy for mobilization.

At evaluation at her bedside the therapist finds that Mrs Tedesky has 4/5 strength in bilateral dorsiflexors and 5/5 strength throughout her other lower extremity musculature; bilaterally she has 3/5 shoulder strength, 2/5 in the elbows, and only trace movement in her hands. Trunk muscles are 3/5. She also has periodic episodes of incontinence.

■ CASE STUDY QUESTIONS

1. Given her age and mechanism of injury what type of spinal cord injury is Mrs Tedesky at high risk for? (Consider that she landed face first and likely hyperextended her neck.)

2. What are the factors that make Mrs Tedesky at high risk for this kind of an injury, and at risk for sustaining this injury from a low impact fall in the home?

3. Which cervical level is more prone to injury in the elderly than in younger adults? Why?

4. Initial nursing and therapy care should focus on prevention of what common sequelae of spinal cord injury (SCI) and immobility?

5. Reviewing the findings on evaluation, which spinal cord syndrome does this fit? In what pattern will she recover and is she likely to regain full function of all four extremities?

6. Briefly describe rehabilitation for Mrs Tedesky to regain function in transfers and gait.

7. Describe an assessment tool to measure trunk control after spinal cord injury.

8. What challenges will she have that are unique due to her age?

9. Mortality after SCI is high in the elderly. What are the reasons for higher mortality in this group?

10. What type of damage is typical when the mechanism of injury is hyperflexion of the cervical spine?

20

SPINAL TUMOR

Deborah A. Kegelmeyer, PT, DPT, MS, GCS

Bella LaRue is a 77-year-old female who fell while walking in her yard and fractured her tibia. While being treated it was noted that she had decreased sensation in her bilateral feet and spasticity in bilateral lower extremities. She reports that her feet have felt funny for years. She did not notice the spasticity but did notice that she felt stiffer and clumsier in the past few months. During her medical workup and evaluation a meningioma was discovered in the T5-6 area of the spine with a CT scan. She has now been released to a skilled nursing facility for rehabilitation.

Mrs LaRue is currently non-weight bearing with a plaster cast on the right leg due to her tibial fracture. She continues to have significant spasticity in bilateral hip adductor muscles and mild spasticity in the quadriceps and gastrocnemius bilateral. On entry to the rehabilitation facility she requires one person max assist to do a sliding board transfer from chair to mat, one person moderate assist to go sit to stand, and one person minimal assist to go stand to sit. She has not ambulated.

■ CASE STUDY QUESTIONS

1. What is a meningioma and which tissues does it involve?

2. Are meningiomas usually benign or malignant?

3. What is the prognosis for recovery?

4. Which area of the spine is most often involved and what are the typical symptoms along with their time of onset?

5. What complications could occur postoperatively? How will these potentially impact therapy?

6. In the hospital the therapists tried sliding board transfers. Given the level of assist required for the sliding board transfer as compared to going sit to stand should she continue with a sliding board transfer or work on stand pivot transfer? Explain your logic.

7. Discuss options for assistive devices for gait for Mrs LaRue.

8. Mrs LaRue continues to have spasticity. Describe the functional implications of her spasticity and how to manage it therapeutically.

9. Mrs LaRue is now (6 weeks after onset) in a removable hard splint on her right ankle and is permitted full weight bearing. She scissors with gait and tends to keep the right leg in extension throughout the gait pattern. Describe some task-oriented activities that could be done to encourage an appropriate gait pattern.

10. Biofeedback is a treatment method that can be used during gait training. What types of biofeedback could be used during gait training with Mrs LaRue and is there evidence to support their use?

11. Discuss balance activities that could be done with Mrs LaRue to improve balance and lower her risk of future falls.

21

DIFFERENTIAL DIAGNOSIS OF DEMENTIA

Deborah A. Kegelmeyer, PT, DPT, MS, GCS

Mrs Delaney scores a 21 on both the Montreal Cognitive Assessment (MoCA) and on the Mini-Mental Status Exam (MMSE). Her neurologist has informed the family that she has cognitive impairment that is pathological and not a part of normal aging. The neurologist is performing tests and working up Mrs Delaney to determine the underlying cause of her cognitive impairment. The physical therapist communicates with the neurologist regarding behaviors observed in therapy and is awaiting final word as the type of dementia and how it could impact how best to work with Mrs Delaney in therapy.

■ CASE STUDY QUESTIONS

1. List potential causes of dementia for Mrs Delaney.

2. List causes of dementia that are potentially reversible or can be treated.

3. Discuss ways to assess Mrs Delaney to determine whether or not she has any treatable medical conditions that could be causing or contributing to her cognitive decline.

4. If Mrs Delaney has a B_{12} deficiency, what would her symptoms be?

5. If Mrs Delaney has normal pressure hydrocephalus, what would her symptoms be?

6. If Mrs Delaney has vascular dementia, what would she present like in therapy?

7. There is a suspicion that Mrs Delaney has dementia with Lewy bodies (DLB), what symptoms would be present to cause the physician to suspect DLB?

8. If Mrs Delaney had dementia with Lewy bodies, what would her motor and balance tests look like?

9. Mrs Delaney has been told that she does not have Pick disease or any form of frontotemporal dementia (FTD). What factors would indicate that she does not fit the profile for FTD? What are the signs and symptoms of FTD?

10. Mrs Delaney is diagnosed with vascular dementia and depression. Discuss the role of physical therapy in treating her cognitive symptoms and overall care.

22

A POSTSURGICAL CASE IN AN ELDERLY CLIENT

Deborah A. Kegelmeyer, PT, DPT, MS, GCS

Mrs. McConnell, a 75-year-old female, has been admitted to a skilled nursing facility following colorectal surgery. She had the surgery 6 days ago. She is admitted for skilled care for deconditioning, gait and transfer training. She lives alone in a two-bedroom apartment that is one story. She is a retired nurse and volunteers at the reception desk of the local hospital 1 day a month. She also plays bridge and belongs to two bridge groups. She played bridge and did her volunteer work the week prior to her surgery with no difficulty. When she is evaluated by physical therapy she is unable to tell you what month it is but does know where she is and why she is in the facility. When asked about her surgery she is able to tell you that she had abdominal surgery but rambles and appears to get some facts confused. She seems overly happy and laughs a lot but says she is tired and does not feel up to doing therapy.

Gait without an assistive device and transfers require one person minimal assist. Her strength is grossly 4+/5, ROM is within normal limits throughout, and sensation to light touch is intact. Her reflexes are 2+ throughout and the cranial nerves are intact. Her vital signs are: HR 74, RR 18, BP 136/84, SpO$_2$ 96%, temp 98.7°F.

During her second day of therapy she does not remember meeting you but is able to tell you the month and year. She is given a Montreal Cognitive Assessment (MoCA) and scores a 21. During the interdisciplinary team meeting nursing states that her cognitive status is at times very good and at other times she is confused and unsafe in daily tasks without supervision.

■ CASE STUDY QUESTIONS

1. Does the description of Mrs. McConnell's cognitive status best fit delirium or dementia? Explain your answer.

2. What are the essential features of delirium? Explain how it affects attention, thought processes, and level of consciousness.

3. Who is at risk for delirium and in what situations is it likely to occur?

4. What is the cause of delirium?

5. What are the guidelines for managing delirium?

6. Describe how to implement these guidelines in PT for Mrs. McConnell who is now going to undergo PT and OT with PT including therapeutic exercise, balance exercise, transfer, and gait training.

7. Cognitive reserve has been noted to mitigate the impact of dementia. Given the same amount of brain atrophy and plaque formation individuals who have higher education and more cognitively challenging jobs will perform better than those with lower cognitive reserve (lower level of education and less demanding jobs). Does cognitive reserve protect against postsurgical delirium?

8. How long will Mrs. McConnell's delirium last?

9. How does delirium impact prognosis for recovery?

10. Mrs. McConnell is now 4.5 weeks postsurgery and is still at the skilled nursing facility. She continues to demonstrate poor safety awareness, poor problem solving, and impaired short-term memory. Her level of consciousness has stabilized and she is consistently oriented to person, time, and place. What is likely the cause of her impaired judgment and short-term memory? Delirium or dementia?

Her children have noted bruising on her knees and abrasions on her legs and elbows. They believe that she is falling. When visiting they have noticed that her apartment is messier than usual and have found objects in strange locations such as finding a hair brush in the silverware drawer. In addition, when her daughter came to pick her up to take her to a grandchild's wedding shower she had no memory of being invited to the event or that her granddaughter was due to be married.

Later that month Mrs Delaney was taken to a memory clinic for a complete medical workup, and also referred to physical therapy to assess and treat for balance and falls. The physical therapist evaluation found the following: vital signs: HR 74 beats per minute, RR 16 breaths per minute, BP 128/78, SpO$_2$ 97%. Strength was grossly 4+/5 except hip extensors, back extensors, abdominal, dorsiflexors, and plantar flexors, which are 3/5. ROM is functionally intact with 15° to 20° loss of terminal shoulder abduction and flexion bilaterally. Bilateral hips have only 5° of extension and she has 5° of dorsiflexion bilaterally. She ambulates independently without an assistive device with a slight forward posture, for greater than 100 ft before stopping without being asked to stop. Deep tendon reflexes 2+ throughout, and sensation to light touch is intact. She has glasses that are used for reading and her hearing is intact. The therapist chose a balance measure based on the results of the other tests.

■ CASE STUDY QUESTIONS

1. Describe normal changes in intelligence and memory and compare/contrast with the changes Mrs Delaney is experiencing.

2. If Mrs Delaney has cognitive impairment, what are the possible reversible and irreversible causes of her impairment?

3. What are some screening tools that PTs can use to screen for possible dementia/cognitive impairment?

4. Describe brain plasticity and how the negative plasticity theory applies to cognitive function.

5. What are the key components of a program aimed at inducing plasticity in the brain?

6. Can exercise play a role in improving Mrs Delaney's cognitive function?

7. Could cognitive decline contribute to declines in ambulation status? Explain how these interact.

8. What method is typically used to assess for the impact of attention on gait?

9. Does administering the TUG Cognitive Test improve fall screening accuracy over the TUG?

10. What functional test could be utilized to test cognition and balance simultaneously for community ambulators?

11. Describe possible gait interventions for improving Mrs Delaney's balance and safety.

23

COGNITION AND DEMENTIA

Deborah A. Kegelmeyer, PT, DPT, MS, GCS

Mrs Delaney is a 73-year-old female who lives alone with her pet poodle. She lives in an apartment that she has rented for the past 10 years. She is a retired secretary and has three grown-up children.

24

ALZHEIMER DISEASE AND PHYSICAL THERAPY

Deborah A. Kegelmeyer, PT, DPT, MS, GCS

Parker Davis, your patient, is an 80-year-old male with a diagnosis of Alzheimer disease. He lives in a split level home with his wife. He wanders at night and sleeps during the day. His wife is 78 years old and has been overwhelmed in recent months with his care and her lack of sleep. Three days ago she fell while struggling to bring him back into the house and fractured her hip. She underwent open reduction internal fixation (ORIF) and both she and Mr Davis have been admitted to the skilled nursing facility. She for rehabilitation and he for care during her stay. He has been admitted to the Alzheimer unit in a different wing of the facility.

Patient history: hypertension (HTN), hyperlipidemia, and a myocardial infarction (MI) 5 years ago. His wife states that he has a history of bilateral knee pain secondary to osteoarthritis. Physical therapy assessment finds that he responds to greetings with "hello" and "how are you" but when asked where he is he does not know the answer. When asked the date he says 1950 and he believes that the woman across the hall from him is his mother. Transfers are independent but at times he is impulsive and off balance; he has a shuffling gait with a forward head posture. He does not follow directions consistently for MMT but overall tests are good to normal in all major muscle groups. He wears glasses and one hearing aide. His vital signs at rest are: HR 78, RR 16, BP 134/84, SpO$_2$ 97%, temp 98.6°F.

■ CASE STUDY QUESTIONS

1. Mr Davis has Alzheimer disease (AD), is this a common or rare form of dementia? Discuss the epidemiology of AD.

2. Alzheimer disease goes through stages; some sources break it down into as many as six stages and others three stages. Using the three-stage system (early, intermediate, and late stage), describe which stage you believe Mr Davis is in and defend your answer.

3. Is there any medication that can be used to improve cognitive function in those with AD? If so, what is it and can it help slow the disease? Would it be beneficial for Mr Davis at this time?

4. In the evening when attempting to get Mr Davis ready for bed the staff report that Mr Davis becomes agitated and can be aggressive. This occurs while trying to remove his clothing and put on a hospital gown. His wife reports that he wore pajama bottoms to bed at home. Discuss possible causes of his behavior and ways to address this behavior.

5. In the previous question we identified that the change in bedtime clothing could be an agitating factor for Mr Davis. Describe a method or ways to determine what might be causing agitation in a client like Mr Davis during therapy.

6. Mr Davis is in PT and has just completed a sit-to-stand transfer from a soft chair followed by walking from his room into the hallway. While in the hallway he begins to say "the road goes to the East" over and over getting faster and louder each time. Describe possible causes and how you would approach managing his agitation within this therapy scenario.

7. Mr Davis is having falls and balance problems and the PT determines he needs a walking device. Discuss the pros and cons of different devices and can he be taught to use a device at this stage in his disease?

8. Is motor learning possible in individuals with AD? Is it impaired?

9. Why can individuals with Alzheimer disease and other dementias motor learn?

10. How do the changes in motor learning impact physical therapy?

11. Do therapists generally enjoy working with people with Alzheimer disease?

25

CERVICAL MYELOPATHY

Deborah A. Kegelmeyer, PT, DPT, MS, GCS

Mrs Kimble is a 74-year-old female who reports a history of neck and arm pain going back at least 10 years. She tends to have burning pain and intermittent numbness in her left arm. She has managed it with ibuprofen, heating pads, and physical therapy. On this visit she complains that her hands are clumsy and she is having trouble knitting. She also reports three falls in the last 6 months.

On evaluation she presents with bilateral hand weakness (3/5) and diminished sensation on the right of light touch and vibration. The right lower extremity is grossly 4−/5 strength. Except for the hand weakness strength is grossly intact on the left side.

■ CASE STUDY QUESTIONS

1. Describe the epidemiology of cervical stenosis?

2. Which signs/symptoms are due to radiculopathy?

3. What signs/symptoms indicate that an individual with cervical stenosis has developed myelopathy?

4. How are the upper motor signs of myelopathy managed?

5. What are the indications for surgical management of myelopathy?

6. What is the common surgical management of myelopathy?

7. Describe Brown-Sequard syndrome.

8. Myelopathy and motor neuron disease can present very similarly. How are they differentiated?

9. Mrs Kimble reports recent onset of decreased coordination in the hands and balance problems including three falls in the past 6 months. Based on these findings is she a candidate for surgery? What factors would predict whether her symptoms remain the same or improve after surgery?

10. What physical therapy treatment is known to lead to spinal cord plasticity after traumatic injury? Would there be any basis to believe it could be beneficial in cases of myelopathy?

11. After surgery will Mrs Kimble still be at risk for falls? Should she have a fall risk assessment?

26

CHARCOT-MARIE-TOOTH DISEASE

William H. Staples, PT, DHSc, DPT, GCS, CEEAA

A 57-year-old male with a 5-year diagnosis of Charcot-Marie-Tooth (CMT) disease comes to your outpatient clinic due to difficulty walking. He presents with bilateral gastrocnemius and soleus atrophy, hammer toes, and high foot arches. He is 5 ft 9 in and weighs 215 lb. Vital signs are: heart rate 70, respiratory rate 16, blood pressure 124/78, and pulse oximetry 97%. He has a primary complaint of recent "stumbling" and falls. Balance testing utilizing the Berg Balance Scale (38/56) and Dynamic Gait Index (18/24) reveal static and dynamic problems. Deep tendon reflexes (DTRs) are 1/4 bilateral ankle, but normal 2/4 for the quadriceps and upper extremities. Sensation to light touch is diminished to light touch in a stocking-like pattern, but he complains of pain 2-3/10 (verbal analog scale) in both feet during weight bearing. Muscle strength of the dorsiflexors and plantar flexors is 3/5 to 3−/5 bilaterally with visible atrophy of the triceps surae. All other major muscle groups are 5/5. He exhibits a slight steppage gait pattern. A 6-Minute Walk Test is measured at 653 ft. The patient states he was never athletic and always considered himself a little clumsy. He states that his neurologist had suggested starting an exercise program 5 years ago, but he was busy with family and work issues.

■ CASE STUDY QUESTIONS

1. Describe the pathology of Charcot-Marie-Tooth disease.
2. Is a diagnosis of CMT disease usually made at this age?
3. How common is this disease?
4. Are the neurological changes exhibited here to be expected?
5. What do you need to know about Charcot-Marie-Tooth disease to complete a thorough evaluation and examination of this patient?
6. Are the tests and measures utilized for this patient appropriate? Are there other tests you would utilize?
7. What do the functional tests tell you?
8. What do you need to know about Charcot-Marie-Tooth disease to design an exercise program for this patient?
9. What can be done to improve the patient's gait pattern?
10. What can be done for the pain?
11. Would you want to measure and document grip strength with a dynamometer? Why or why not?
12. How might this patient be better motivated to continue a home exercise program?
13. Are there any other suggestions you would make to this patient?
14. Are there any medications or food supplements that should be prescribed for this patient?
15. What is the expected long-term outcome for this patient?

27

CEREBRAL VASCULAR ACCIDENT—OT AND PT

Jana Grant, OT/L, MS

Katie Houghtaling, MSPT, GCS, CEEAA

The patient is a 70-year-old female with 10-year history of diabetes mellitus type 2 and Charcot foot deformity for the past 2 years that is progressively worsening. The patient is seen for home health care following hospitalization for 5 days, and 2 weeks in a skilled nursing home, with new left middle cerebral artery (MCA) cerebral vascular accident (CVA) with resultant right-sided weakness, affecting her right upper extremity more so than her right lower extremity. The patient was referred to physical and occupational therapy.

She is right-hand dominant and the primary caregiver of her elderly mother. The patient lives with her husband; however, he works during the day, so he needs to leave the patient home to function independently and take care of her elderly mother with dementia. The patient's husband is unable to take any more time off from work as he took time off when the patient was hospitalized. He is the only source of income for the family. The patient is now presenting with complaints of fatigue, inability to successfully perform her IADLs, and great difficulty with her ADLs. The patient's medications consist of the following:

5 mg of Coumadin with weekly INRs
10 mg of simvastatin daily
Extra strength Tylenol 500 mg one to two tabs every 8 hours as needed for pain in her feet
glipizide 5 mg three times daily before meals

The patient's home is two stories with no stairs to enter except one large step up from the garage into kitchen, which is the most used method of entry to home. She has a half bath on the first floor with the only shower being on the second floor. First floor is uncluttered with open floor plan and free of scatter rugs. The patient has 12 stairs with right-sided rail only, to get to second floor where bedroom and main bath are located. She has a tub-shower with high sides and glass sliding doors. No grab bars are present. She has a high toilet with which she has no trouble getting on and off independently. The bed is neutral height and the patient is able to transfer in/out without difficulty.

PHYSICAL THERAPY EVALUATION

On examination, the patient presents with generalized weakness throughout the right upper extremity (UE), more so distally than proximally, with shoulder grossly 4−/5, elbow grossly 3/5, and wrist and grip grossly 2/5. Right lower extremity (LE) strength is grossly 4+/5 at hip, 4/5 at knee, and 3−/5 at ankle within limited ROM from chronic changes with Charcot deformity in both feet. The left-sided extremities are grossly within functional limits (WFL) for strength. ROM is WFL throughout all extremities except bilateral ankles which have AROM to 0° dorsiflexion (DF) and 10° plantar flexion (PF), with PROM at 5° DF and 12° PF. The patient has varying pain from 2 to 4/10 in bilateral feet depending on her level of activity and if she is wearing her supportive diabetic shoes. Sensation is intact throughout the left UE and LE, with sensation only intact to deep pressure on the right UE and LE with good localization, and protective sensation on bilateral feet with Semmes Weinstein monofilament (5.07) tested 8/10 correctly.

A Postural Assessment Scale for Stroke Patients (PASS) was performed. Gait is abnormal, with a steppage-type pattern, due to right LE weakness and decreased coordination, as well as decreased ankle ROM. The patient is using a single-point cane and was able to ambulate 200 ft before fatiguing. Her gait speed is 0.6 m/s, indicating limited community ambulation. Vitals at rest were as follows: BP 112/64 mm Hg, HR 64 beats per minute, O_2 sat 99% on room air, RR 18, temp 98.7°F. After activity there was no change in BP or O_2 sat; however, HR increased to 88 beats per minute and RR increased to 24 breaths per minute.

OCCUPATIONAL THERAPY EVALUATION

The patient presents with flat effect but with good recall of current and past events. She does appear confused at times when asked about her medications. She is able to verbalize when to take them, and that she uses a pill box which she fills herself. However, she becomes confused when asked about specific medications she is taking and the method she uses to fill the pill box.

The patient is able to demonstrate moderate independence for upper body (UB) dressing using compensation techniques for donning a bra, which she previously did not need to do. She is able to don pants and underwear using a reacher, but relies on her husband to don shoes and socks due to fatigue and decreased functional reach. Her husband leaves for work early in the morning, which is inconvenient for the patient, but is currently their only way to get her shoes and socks on for the day. She is able to stand at sink level in the bathroom to demonstrate grooming tasks; however, she becomes fatigued easily and needs rest breaks during this task. She has been doing only sponge baths due to poor setup of shower and low endurance level. A Medi-Cog Assessment was also performed.

The patient is able to move around her kitchen with a straight cane, and make meals for herself and family, but has resorted to cooking preprepared meals or frozen meals in the microwave. This has led to discouragement and frustration for her as she always enjoyed cooking and serving her family meals. Her husband is currently doing the laundry as the washer and dryer are in the basement level. He has also taken on the heavy home cleaning. The patient does assist with folding laundry, but often gets extremely fatigued by this task.

The patient has an elderly mother with a diagnosis of dementia who lives down the street from her. Her mother has hired help, but the patient is responsible for coordination of this and filling the gaps when hired caregivers are not there.

■ CASE STUDY QUESTIONS

1. What considerations should be made for treatment with a patient on Coumadin?

2. What considerations should be made for the Charcot foot deformity with increasing activity?

3. What is the importance of monitoring vitals before, during, and after activity?

4. What is the Postural Assessment Scale for Stroke Patients (PASS)?

5. What is the Medi-Cog Assessment and why would it be beneficial in this case?

6. How can the patient's blood sugar affect her participation in therapy?

7. What are common medical concerns poststroke to be aware of during treatment?

8. Describe the typical effects of an MCA CVA?

9. How have the patient's life roles now changed, and what emotional impact can that have on her recovery process?

10. What is the occupational therapy framework and how can a clinician use it for this case?

CHAPTER 4

Cardiovascular and Pulmonary Cases

INTRODUCTION

CARDIOVASCULAR AND PULMONARY ISSUES RELATED TO REHABILITATION OF THE GERIATRIC PATIENT

William H. Staples, PT, DHSc, DPT, GCS, CEEAA

The aging cardiopulmonary and respiratory systems are important to understand in relation to rehabilitation. Understanding the normal cardiovascular and pulmonary changes can assist therapists when judging the functional capacities of aging adults either with or without other comorbidities.

There are minimal changes in resting heart rate, plasma volume, or hematocrit readings as people age normally without pathology. Several decreases occur, however. There is an overall reduction in distensibility, contractility, and elasticity. The decreases include loss of maximal aerobic capacity, maximal heart rate, maximal cardiac output, stroke volume, peak heart rate, maximum O_2 consumption, endothelial reactivity, maximal skeletal muscle blood flow, capillary density, vascular insulin sensitivity, heart size, end-diastolic filling, compliance of large arteries, and secretion and release of catecholamines. A decrease in pacemaker cells in the S-A node can lead to slightly slower heart rate, and tonic modulation of the cardiac period. Decreased sensitivity of the baroreceptors can lead to postural hypotension in response to stress. There is diminished speed of red blood cell production in response to stress of illness, along with decreased levels of HDL (good) cholesterol, and lipoprotein lipase activity, which may then promote obesity and atherosclerosis.[1-3]

There are increases in the cardiovascular function as well, but increases are not necessarily a good thing. There is an increase in fat (noncontractile) and fibrous (nondistensible) tissue. The left ventricular mass and wall thickness amount of blood the chamber can hold may actually decrease, leading to heart filling more slowly. There is thickening of valvular structures and addition to the epicardial fat. Heart rate and blood pressure response to submaximal exercise increase as do peripheral vascular resistance, total cholesterol, and LDL (bad) cholesterol.[1-3]

The functional implications of these cardiovascular changes is significant and leads to lower HRmax, lower stroke volume and cardiac output, and increased blood pressure. An increased threat of cardiovascular disease may lead to premature death and/or function. A reduced blood flow and therefore reduced oxygen to the skeletal muscles will also limit function as we age. Decreased VO_2 max and reduced skeletal muscle oxidative capacity will lead to reduced exercise capacity and blunted exercise response that will also limit function.[1-3]

Pulmonary changes as we age will also affect us as we age. There is little to no change in total lung capacity, but there are many decreases. Decreases include vital capacity, tidal volume, vascular insulin sensitivity, maximal air flow rates, respiratory muscle strength, lung expansion, and elastic recoil. Decreases also accompany the aging process and including loss of alveolar surface area, up to 20%, which leads to decrease in maximum O_2 uptake. Alveolar vascularity and the number of cilia/function also decrease. Alveoli tend to collapse sooner on expiration due to the loss of elasticity.[3-5]

Increases to the aging pulmonary system include loss of residual volume (between 30% and 50%), stiffness of chest wall, the number of mucus producing cells, functional residual capacity, and respiratory rate. The functional implications of pulmonary changes will also affect function in older adults. Vital capacity is reduced as is the maximal ventilatory capacity and the ability of forced expiratory volume in 1 second (FEVsec-1). Up to 20% increase in work of respiratory muscles is required. A ventilation/perfusion mismatch decreases the ability to oxygenate the blood. These changes make older adults more vulnerable to respiratory infections, and the body becomes less efficient in monitoring and controlling breathing, and there is a lower threshold for shortness of breath.[3-5]

Aging affects many aspects of respiratory system by increasing the work of breathing due to the loss of elasticity and recoil of lung tissue, increased rigidity in rib cage, and increased anterior-posterior diameter of chest. Postural changes may lead to restrictive lung dysfunction. Osteoporosis can lead to increased thoracic curvature, making the tidal volume of oxygen less. The loss of alveoli surface area can decrease by 4% each decade. Additionally, decreased respiratory muscle strength, combined with the collapse of smaller airways, increases air flow resistance, which in turn increases the physical effort of breathing by 29% from the age of 20 to 70. Other respiratory effects include diminished gag and cough reflexes, which may lead to aspiration pneumonia. Medications such as sedatives, pain relievers, and alcohol can further depress the respiratory system, leading to hypoxia or aspiration. Overall, an increased amount of unoxygenated blood will decrease the functional reserve, and may even cause cognitive impairment. Aerobic capacity decreases with age ($\approx 1\%$ /year) because there is a decrease in size and number of mitochondria, which produce energy, and a decreased capillary/fiber ratio also leads to decreased blood flow, leading to a decreased work capacity of 20% to 30% from age 30 to 70 years.[3-5]

Due to a decrease in vascularity there is a reduced capacity for O_2 transport. Oxygen uptake, or the ability to extract and utilize O_2 on a cellular level, demonstrates a decrease in the VO_2 difference due to less effective O_2 extraction from the bloodstream. Sedentary individuals have a twofold decrease in VO_2 max compared to active individuals.[3-5]

According to Spirduso et al, 25% of older adults are frail and dependent, requiring assistance with basic ADLs and IADLs.[6] Seventy percent are independent and fully functional now, but low activity levels may cause physical declines, leading to frailty in the future and only 5% are in the fit/elite category, which are highly active people who should remain mobile into late life barring injury/illness.[6]

Older adults and physical activity appear to be odds with each other despite the propensity of evidence that reports the need to keep active. Coleman et al studied nearly 1.8 million individuals (18+) to see if exercise vital sign (EVS) included in electronic medical record provides estimate of physical activity (PA) levels.[7] The authors categorized EVS into completely inactive (0 minute of exercise/week), insufficiently active (more than 0, less than 150 minutes/week), and sufficiently active (150 minutes or more/week). The authors found that 36.3% were completely inactive; 33.3% were insufficiently active; and only 30.4% were sufficiently active. Being physically inactive was found to be more common if older, obese, of a racial/ethnic minority, and had higher disease burden.[7]

Cardiovascular dysfunction attributed to the aging process closely mimics the decline in cardiac function seen with inactivity. Inadequate physical activity is responsible for 30% of deaths due to heart disease and other systemic diseases.[8]

Cardiovascular-pulmonary endurance or cardiac reserve is important for community engagement. Some important signs and symptoms of reduced cardiac reserve for clinicians to understand include a marked need for rest even after mild exercise, an extensive time to recover from exercise, shortness of breath, dyspnea, and an increased heart rate with slow or incomplete recovery during rest. Some people may develop an irregular heart rhythm, a decrease in heart rate or systolic blood pressure with an increased workload, which would indicate the need for a medical workup before advancing exercise. A bluish hue to skin, lips, or fingertips may indicate pulmonary system involvement.

Benefits of exercise for older adults include improvements to both the cardiovascular and pulmonary systems. Benefits include decreased blood pressure, increased HDL (good cholesterol), decreased incidence of coronary artery disease, decrease in platelet aggregatibility ("stickiness"), decreased angina/ischemia, decreased O_2 requirement, decreased respiratory disease and complications, and less hospitalization. Incidence for angioplasty is decreased by 19%, for CABG 13%, and fatal MI by 21%.

Other benefits of increased activity include that ADLs can be performed better and below anginal threshold, an increased glucose utilization, improved weight management, and increased exercise tolerance. Improved psychological status, quality of life, ability to return to work, and decreased mortality have also been noted.

Previous health factors add to stress on the cardiovascular system including smoking, weight gain, stress, and depression. The most common cause of death in the United States is cardiovascular disease with men at 47% and women at 53%.[9,10] It is important to note that 45% of US women do not know that they are at risk.[9] Of people who died from sudden cardiac death, 50% of men and 63% of women had no previous symptoms. As therapists we need to do more to both educate and exercise our patients to reduce these numbers.[10]

REFERENCES

1. Smirnova IV. The cardiovascular system. In: Goodman CC, Fuller KS, eds. *Pathology Implications for the Physical Therapist*. 4th ed. St Louis, MO: Elsevier; 2015:538-665.
2. Cohen M. Cardiac considerations in the older patient. In: Kauffman T, Scott R, Barr JO, Moran ML, eds. *A Comprehensive Guide to Geriatric Rehabilitation*. 3rd ed. China: Churchill Livingston; 2014:34-39.
3. Watchie J. *Cardiovascular and Pulmonary Physical Therapy: A Clinical Manual*. 2nd ed. St Louis, MO: Saunders-Elsevier; 2010.
4. Cohen M. Pulmonary considerations in the older patient. In: Kauffman T, Kauffman T, Scott R, Barr JO, Moran ML, eds. *A Comprehensive Guide to Geriatric Rehabilitation*. 3rd ed. China: Churchill Livingston; 2014:40-44.
5. Packel L. The respiratory system. In: Goodman CC, Fuller KS, eds. *Pathology Implications for the Physical Therapist*. 4th ed. St Louis, MO: Elsevier; 2015:772-861.
6. Spirduso WW, Francis KL, MacRae PG. *Physical Dimensions of Aging*. 2nd ed. Champaign, IL: Human Kinetics; 2005.
7. Coleman KJ, Ngor E, Reynolds K, et al. Initial validation of an exercise "vital sign" in electronic medical records. *Med Sci Sports Exerc*. 2012;44(11):2071-2076.
8. Stewart KJ, Ouyang P, Bacher AC, Lima S, Shapiro EP. Exercise effects on cardiac size and left ventricular diastolic function: relationships to changes in fitness, fatness, blood pressure and insulin resistance. *Heart*. 2006;92:893-898.
9. CDC, NCHS. Underlying Cause of Death 1999-2013 on CDC WONDER Online Database, released 2015. Data are from the Multiple Cause of Death Files, 1999-2013, as compiled from data provided by the 57 vital statistics jurisdictions through the Vital Statistics Cooperative Program. Accessed February 3, 2015. http://wonder.cdc.gov/ucd-icd10.html
10. CDC. Million hearts: strategies to reduce the prevalence of leading cardiovascular disease risk factors. United States, 2011. *MMWR*. 2011;60(36):1248-1251. http://www.cdc.gov/mmwr/preview/mmwrhtml/mm6036a4.htm?s_cid=mm6036a4_w.

1

ABDOMINAL AORTIC ANEURYSM

Stacey Brickson, PT, PhD, ATC

James S. Carlson, MPT, CCS

PT CONSULT: BACK PAIN

The patient is a 71-year-old male referred to physical therapy for back pain. Onset of symptoms began 6 weeks ago without any specific mechanism of injury. The patient presented to local emergency department (ED) about 2 weeks ago for chest pain (CP), midback pain, and shortness of breath. Workup in the ED showed normal troponin and B-type natriuretic peptide (BNP) levels. Lungs were clear and no abnormal heart sounds appreciated. Electrocardiograph (ECG) demonstrated no ischemic changes. Chest radiograph was negative for acute pulmonary pathology. Chest pain and dyspnea felt to be related to anxiety associated with spinal muscle spasms. The patient was discharged with a prescription for lorazepam and Flexeril (see the medication list). The patient was referred to a cardiopulmonary physical therapy specialist (CCS) for his back pain due to his comorbidities of COPD and cardiac disease.

PAST MEDICAL HISTORY (PMH)

Coronary artery bypass graft (CABG) × 3 15 years ago
Hypertension (HTN)
Hyperlipidemia
Tobacco (1 pack per day for 43 years. Has now stopped for 10 years)
Enlarged prostate
Chronic obstructive pulmonary disease (COPD)

MEDICATIONS

Metoprolol (Lopressor) 100 mg once per day — β blocker
Lisinopril (Prinivil) 10 mg once per day — ACE Inhibit

Simvastatin (Zocor) 20 mg once per day

Aspirin (ASA) 81 mg once per day

Fish oil 1000 mg

Lorazepam (Ativan) 1 mg two times a day

Cyclobenzaprine (Flexeril) 5 mg three times a day

Tamsulosin (Flomax) 0.4 mg once daily one-half hour following the same meal each day

Albuterol (ProAir HFA) metered-dose inhaler: two puffs every 4 to 6 hours as needed.

Budesonide/formoterol (Symbicort) two inhalations twice daily.

Pulmonary Function Test (PFT): 2012

Value	Actual	%Predicted	Predicted
FVC (L)	3.10	80	3.84
FEV$_1$ (L)	2.01	65	3.10
FEV$_1$/FVC	0.67		
TLC (L)	6.31	100	6.37
RV (L)	2.23	110	2.03
DLCO	20.75	75	27.61

PATIENT PRESENTATION IN CLINIC

Pulse: 100-110 beats per minute, irregular

BP: 90/60 mm Hg with subjective complaint of dizziness

RR: 18

Pulse oximetry (SpO$_2$): 93% on room air

Temp: 98.7°F

Pain: 7/10 (verbal analog scale) in midback with referral to left lower quadrant as well as radiating pain (5/10) into left lower extremity

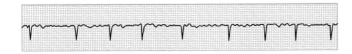

ECG (telemetry)

Auscultation

Breath sounds: decreased breath sounds with atelectasis in bilateral lower lobes

Heart sounds: normal S1/S2, no murmur, S3 or S4

Abdominal clearing: tenderness left lower quadrant, which exacerbates low pain, pulsatile abdominal mass to palpation

Neurological and musculoskeletal screen: Sensation and reflexes of LE normal. SI joint cleared. AROM for lumbar flexion, extension, side bending, and rotation WFL. No pain with overpressure at end range PROM. Palpation of the paraspinals are nontender and do not exacerbate the pain. Gross strength of LE muscles WNL. Spring passive intervertebral motion (PIVM) testing for thoracic and lumbar vertebrae normal. Slump test and Lasègue sign (straight leg raise) negative.

■ CASE STUDY QUESTIONS

1. What is B-type natriuretic peptide (BNP)?

2. What is the likelihood of low back pain due to mechanical versus visceral causes?

3. Based on the information provided in the case, which signs and symptoms are consistent or inconsistent with a musculoskeletal etiology for midback pain? Identify and describe the specific tests that were administered during the examination to assist with diagnostic classification of low back pain.

4. What questions might you ask during the patient interview to more specifically probe for the likelihood of underlying musculoskeletal etiology?

5. Describe the stages of COPD. Which stage does this patient present with? Are any of the patient's symptoms consistent with a COPD exacerbation?

6. The referral to a cardiopulmonary specialist was issued for a patient with back pain due to his comorbidities of COPD and prior CABG. How would COPD impact rehabilitation in a patient with back pain of musculoskeletal etiology?

7. Does long-term use of inhaled steroids pose a risk for osteoporosis?

8. Identify the cardiac rhythm the patient is presenting. What two major ECG changes would you anticipate in the event of ischemia?

9. Given his prior CABG, one might suspect occlusion and acute coronary syndrome. Discuss the likelihood of ACS based on the incidence of occlusion with a left internal mammary artery (LIMA) versus saphenous vein graft (SVG).

10. What evidence rules in the possibility of an abdominal aortic aneurysm?

11. How is an abdominal aortic aneurysm diagnosed?

12. What are the signs and symptoms of a ruptured aneurysm? What is the risk of rupture for an abdominal aortic aneurysm?

13. What is your next clinical decision?

2

ACQUIRED COAGULATION DISORDER

Eric Shamus, PT, DPT, PhD

Wendy Song, DO

Family Medicine Resident, Mount Sinai Beth Israel Residency in Urban Family Medicine, New York City, New York

A 70-year-old male presents with a left thigh bruise and knee pain from a fall 1 week ago. He has been taking Ibuprofen four times a day for his knee pain. The patient has a history of celiac disease and has noticed increased bruising and prolonged gum bleeding after brushing his teeth for the last week. He has not adhered to his gluten-free diet due to hectic work hours as a police chief.

Vital signs are temperature: 98.2°F, heart rate: 84, respirations: 16, blood pressure: 130/86, and SpO$_2$: 98%. Physical exam shows diffuse small ecchymosis on his upper and lower extremities, left thigh with deep ecchymosis, and gingival petechiae. Lab tests show low hemoglobin of 11.0, normal platelet count with a prolonged prothrombin time and mildly elevated partial prothrombin time.

After your evaluation you determine that you need to do more research for this disorder to determine what your treatment approach should be. Please answer the following questions based on your research.

■ CASE STUDY QUESTIONS

1. What is a coagulation disorder?

2. What are the possible contributing causes of a coagulation disorder?

3. What are the common symptoms of a coagulation disorder?

4. What are the common laboratory tests for this disorder?

5. Can the bleeding occur spontaneously?

6. What types of medications may mimic a coagulation disorder?

Prim Hemostasis.
asc .

7. How does blood clotting occur?

8. Are there any exercises that would be precautionary for this patient? → *High Intensity Exercis*

9. Are there any modalities that would be precautionary for this patient? ↓ *All*

10. What is the prognosis for a patient with a coagulation disorder?

3

AORTIC REGURGITATION (AR)

Eric Shamus, PT, DPT, PhD

Natalie V. Wessel, DO, MPH

A 68-year-old male presents knee pain as a direct access patient. He reports intermittent chest pain that does not seem to be correlated with exercise and frequent episodes of palpitations. He also complains of a "pounding" heartbeat when lying down, particularly on his left side.

Vitals are pulse: 96, respirations: 18, blood pressure: 140/50, and SpO$_2$%: 98%. On physical examination, the patient has a "water hammer" pulse in the brachial and radial arteries bilaterally. You notice a head bob occurring with each heart beat and audible systolic and diastolic sounds over the femoral arteries. On auscultation, there is a diastolic murmur in the second right intercostal space.

After your evaluation you determine that you need to do more research for this disorder to determine what your treatment approach should be. Please answer the following questions based on your research.

■ CASE STUDY QUESTIONS

1. What should the physical therapist do first?

2. What vitals should be taken?

3. If a patient complains of a heavy heart beat, where should auscultation occur?

4. What is aortic regurgitation?

5. What are the possible contributing causes of aortic regurgitation?

6. What are the common symptoms of aortic regurgitation?

7. What are the common tests if aortic regurgitation is suspected?

8. What happens to the stroke volume?

9. What types of medications may the patient be taking?

10. What are the appropriate functional tests and measures?

11. What are the common impairments?

12. What is the prognosis for a patient with aortic regurgitation?

13. Can a person with aortic regurgitation exercise?

4

AORTIC STENOSIS: CASE 1

William H. Staples, PT, DHSc, DPT, GCS, CEEAA

You are seeing a 64-year-old male patient who has undergone mechanical aortic valve replacement secondary to severe aortic stenosis (AS) 14 weeks ago. He has undergone cardiac rehabilitation and now wants to continue exercise under some supervision. His vital signs are heart rate 60, blood pressure 114/72, respiratory rate 16, and oxygen saturation of 98%. He is taking Coumadin at an INR of 1.5 to 2.0, plus 81 mg aspirin, and lisinopril (Zestril) 10 mg daily. Before treating the patient you decide to research this condition.

■ CASE STUDY QUESTIONS

1. What are the typical symptoms of aortic stenosis?

2. What is the surgical procedure to replace the aortic valve?

3. How common is aortic stenosis?

4. How is the diagnosis of aortic stenosis made?

5. What is aortic regurgitation?

6. What is the medical management for a patient with aortic stenosis?

7. Are there medications that can slow the progression of the disease?

8. What is the typical prognosis for aortic stenosis?

9. What is the difference between a mechanical and biological heart valve?

10. Is exercise recommended prior to valve replacement?

11. Can people exercise after a valve replacement surgery?

12. What is the purpose of the medications he is taking?

5

AORTIC STENOSIS: CASE 2

Eric Shamus, PT, DPT, PhD

Jennifer Shamus, PT, DPT, PhD

An 80-year-old male is being treated for lateral elbow pain from playing golf. While the patient is performing arm exercises, he becomes short of breath. The patient states that he is dizzy and has chest pain. Vitals are: pulse: 98, respirations: 22, blood pressure: 142/86, and SpO$_2$: 96%. On physical examination, the patient has a slow rate of rise in the carotid pulse, a systolic ejection murmur at the right second intercostal space, and a reduced intensity of the second heart sound. You work in a multidisciplinary sports medicine clinic with physical therapists, physicians, nutritionists, and psychologists.

After this has occurred you determine that you need to do more research for this disorder to determine what your treatment approach should be. Please answer the following questions based on your research.

■ CASE STUDY QUESTIONS

1. What should the physical therapist do first?

2. What vitals should be taken?

3. What would an ECG present with for a patient with aortic stenosis?

4. What is aortic stenosis?

5. What are the possible contributing causes of aortic stenosis?

6. What are the common symptoms of aortic stenosis?

7. What are the common tests for aortic stenosis?

8. What happens to the blood flow?

9. What types of medications may the patient be taking?

10. What are the appropriate functional tests and measures?

11. What are the common impairments?

12. What is the prognosis for a patient with aortic stenosis?

ASTHMA

Eric Shamus, PT, DPT, PhD

Ingrid Quartarol, PT, MS

A 67-year-old nonsmoking male complains of a 3-month history of a nonproductive cough that is worse at night and with exercise. He has a history of smoking. He has just moved to the area by the beach 3 months ago from living in the mountains for the last 20 years. He was evaluated by his physician and his blood markers were negative for cancer cells. A chest radiograph was read as normal. Auscultation of his lungs presents a wheeze on forced expiration. On the posture evaluation, he has increased tone in the accessory breathing muscles, postural disorders with rounded shoulders, and increased thoracic kyphosis. His capillary refill is slow bilaterally and O_2 saturation 95%. Functionally, he is having difficulty with stairs in his new house and feels tightness in his chest with activity.

After your evaluation you determine that you need to do more research for this disorder to determine what your treatment approach should be. Please answer the following questions based on your research.

■ CASE STUDY QUESTIONS

1. What is asthma?

2. What does moving to a new area have anything to do with asthma?

3. What are the possible contributing causes of asthma?

4. What are the common symptoms of asthma?

5. What are the common heart and lung/breathing sounds for asthma?

6. What causes the lung sound?

7. What are the appropriate functional tests?

8. What muscles are used for accessory breathing?

9. What are the appropriate diagnostic procedures?

10. What types of medications are used for treatment?

11. Are there any exercises that would be important for precautionary or this patient?

12. What are the functional implications of asthma?

13. What is the prognosis for a patient with asthma?

14. What postural changes are seen in asthmatic patients?

ATRIAL FIBRILLATION

William H. Staples, PT, DHSc, DPT, GCS, CEEAA

A 69-year-old female patient who had taken up playing tennis 6 weeks ago and suddenly felt her heart pounding and began to feel dizzy 3 weeks ago after an hour of tennis. At first she thought it was just the heat, but her friend convinced her to see a physician. She is newly diagnosed with atrial fibrillation after having a stress test by a cardiologist and comes to you because she wants to exercise safely. She comes to your hospital outpatient clinic because you are equipped to provide ECG monitoring during exercise. Her current vital signs are heart rate 62 regular, respiratory rate 16, blood pressure 128/84, and pulse oximetry 98%. She began regularly taking ibuprofen following her tennis because of some mild knee pain. She is anxious about exercising but would like to increase her activity level.

■ CASE STUDY QUESTIONS

1. What is atrial fibrillation?

2. Is atrial fibrillation common in older adults?

3. What are the signs and symptoms of atrial fibrillation?

4. Is atrial fibrillation a dangerous problem?

5. What is the treatment for atrial fibrillation?

6. Do people with atrial fibrillation require medication?

7. What are some of the anticoagulant medications that may be prescribed?

8. What are the pluses and minus of the medications to control blood clots?

9. What are some of the antiarrhythmic medications that may be prescribed?

10. What does atrial fibrillation look like on ECG?

11. How is atrial fibrillation classified (are there different types)?

12. Are nonsteroidal anti-inflammatory medications linked to a higher risk for atrial fibrillation?

13. Can people with atrial fibrillation exercise?

BRONCHITIS

Eric Shamus, PT, DPT, PhD

Marangela Prysiazny Obispo, PT, DPT, GCS

A 69-year-old female arrives to the clinic with a complaint of recent onset of thoracic/rib pain. She reports difficulty performing ADLs like vacuuming and shopping due to symptoms of pain and fatigue. She has been a second-hand smoker for 25 years due to her past job setting as a waitress. The patient revealed that she had a mild fever 3 days ago, which went away after taking acetaminophen (Tylenol)

500 mg four times a day, which she continues to take due to her back pain. She also reports onset of a cold approximately 1 week ago with current symptoms of sore throat, productive cough, and chest pain after coughing. She reports presence of sputum when coughing, which turned from clear to yellowish in the last 2 days. Upon examination, the patient presents with normal vital signs with an SpO_2 saturation of 94% at rest. She has normal range of motion (ROM) of all extremities and lumbar and cervical spine but limited (due to pain) in side-bending to the left. Tenderness to palpation is present on the right paraspinal muscles from T10 to T12. She has normal strength of all extremities. Functional mobility (walking) was normal with increased time (self-reported) required mainly due to fatigue. Her breath sounds were abnormal with wheezing present after coughing.

After your evaluation you determine that you need to do more research for this disorder to determine what your treatment approach should be. Please answer the following questions based on your research.

■ CASE STUDY QUESTIONS

1. What might be the cause of this patient's thoracic/rib pain?
2. What are the two types of bronchitis?
3. What are the demographics of bronchitis?
4. What are the common symptoms of bronchitis?
5. What are the common lung/breathing sounds for bronchitis?
6. What functional test(s) would be beneficial to conduct on this patient?
7. What is the normal SpO_2 saturation rate?
8. What are the appropriate diagnostic procedures?
9. What is an appropriate treatment for her pulmonary condition?
10. What would you do about the thoracic back pain?
11. Are there any exercises that would be important for this patient?
12. What are the functional implications of bronchitis?
13. What are the possible contributing causes of bronchitis?
14. What differentiates an acute episode from a chronic bronchitis?

9

CAROTID ARTERY DISEASE

Eric Shamus, PT, DPT, PhD

Natalie V. Wessel, DO, MPH

A 78-year-old male presents for a vestibular examination with complaints of dizziness. He is on aspirin, lovastatin, and hydrochlorothiazide. Vitals are pulse: 82, respirations: 17, blood pressure: 130/86, temperature: 98.6°F, and SpO_2%: 98. On physical examination with auscultation there is a bruit in the left side of the neck. The patient is sent back to their primary physician. The physician orders a carotid ultrasound, which reveals 70% blockage of the left carotid and 35% blockage of the right carotid.

After your evaluation you determine that you need to do more research for this disorder to determine what your treatment approach should be. Please answer the following questions based on your research.

■ CASE STUDY QUESTIONS

1. Did the therapist make the correct decision in referring back to the physician?
2. What vitals should be taken?
3. If a patient complains of dizziness, where should auscultation occur?
4. What are the possible contributing causes of carotid artery disease?
5. What are the common symptoms of carotid artery disease?
6. What medical tests are used to diagnose carotid artery disease?
7. What are the common physical therapy differential tests?
8. What happens to the circulation to the brain with carotid artery disease?
9. What types of medications may the patient be taking?
10. What are the common laboratory tests for carotid artery disease?
11. What are the common functional tests performed for carotid artery disease?
12. What are the common impairments found in carotid artery disease?
13. What is the prognosis for a patient with carotid artery disease?
14. What medical procedures may be used in severe carotid artery disease?

10

CONGESTIVE HEART FAILURE

William H. Staples, PT, DHSc, DPT, GCS, CEEAA

PART 1

You are evaluating a new home health referral who was released from the hospital yesterday, following a 5-day stay with a diagnosis of acute congestive heart failure. He has comorbidities of hypertension, coronary artery disease, diabetes mellitus, and obesity. He lives alone in a small single-story home and works as an accountant and wants to return to work as soon as possible. He does not smoke or drink alcohol. His physician wants him started on an exercise program.

On examination the 60-year-old Caucasian male is pleasant, alert, and oriented. At rest his heart rate (HR) is 92 regular and strong, respiratory rate (RR) is 16, blood pressure (BP) is 132/84, oxygen saturation (SpO_2) is 96%, rate of perceived exertion (RPE) is 2/10, and temperature is 98.6°F. The therapist is unable to use your standard blood pressure cuff on his upper arm so the cuff is placed on the forearm proximal to the wrist to obtain a reading. His blood sugar taken this morning was 120 mg/dL. He has no complaint of pain. He is 5 ft 11 in and weighs 351 lb. You are able to measure his weight using one scale the patient has and one you keep in your car as an experienced home care therapist. He stands with one foot on each scale and you add up the weight.

You ask him if he has any dietary restrictions and states that "the nurse at the hospital told me I need to eat better and to improve my diet to lose weight." His eyesight and hearing are intact.

Medications include Lasix (furosemide), Altace (ramipril), Aldactone (spironolactone), Glucophage (metformin), and baby aspirin.

On auscultation, lung sounds are clear. Heart auscultation reveals normal first and second heart sound. All four areas are auscultated, aortic, pulmonic, tricuspid, and mitral with no murmur.

Range of motion and strength are normal. The patient has mild 2+ pitting edema proximal to both ankles. Integument is clear of any open areas. Sensation is intact to light touch.

Functional test performed were the Timed Up and Go: 8.6 seconds, and 2-Minute Step Test for endurance: 48 steps. Vital signs taken after endurance test reveal a change in vital signs from rest as: HR 98, BP 148/86, RR 28, SpO_2 98%, RPE 8/10.

PART 2

The therapist returns in 3 days for a second visit and reassesses the patient and hears wheezing even before auscultation and the patient is short of breath at rest.

■ CASE STUDY QUESTIONS: PART 1

1. What is congestive heart failure?
2. What is the goal of medical treatment for heart failure?
3. What type of medication is Altace?
4. What type of medication is Aldactone and are there any risks?
5. What are the signs of hyperkalemia?
6. Why did the therapist choose the 2-Minute Step Test to measure endurance, and how is it performed?
7. What do the results of the 2-Minute Step Test tell you?
8. Is taking the blood pressure at the wrist acceptable?
9. How is pitting edema measured and scaled?
10. What type of exercise program would you begin with?
11. What recommendations would you make today?

■ CASE STUDY QUESTIONS: PART 2

12. What might that wheezing breath sound mean?
13. What other measures would you want to take now?
14. What findings would lead you to call 911?
15. What was the outcome?

11

CHRONIC OBSTRUCTIVE PULMONARY DISEASE (COPD): CASE 1

William H. Staples, PT, DHSc, DPT, GCS, CEEAA

A new 82-year-old female resident in the continuing care community (CCC) in which you work is having difficulty making it to meals. She complains of getting "winded" easily. She has a 62 year history of smoking cigarettes. On examination, she is alert and oriented and decided to come live in the CCC because she was fatiguing at home just trying to complete simple tasks around her home.

She tells you that she has not been to a physician in 10 years because "the only thing they tell me is to quit smoking."

She is currently not taking any prescription medication. Vital signs at rest are: HR 84 steady, RR 24, BP 146/88, SpO_2 92%. Lung auscultation reveals wheezing on exhalation. Range of motion is normal for all joints. Muscle strength is grossly 4/5 throughout. A 10-Meter Walk Test results in a 1.0 m/s gait speed. A 6-Minute Walk Test following Senior Fitness Test guidelines results in a distance of 380 yd (1140 ft or 347.5 m) during which she stopped to take two short rest breaks and has dyspnea by the finish, rating it a 3 on ACSM's Dyspnea Scale.

■ CASE STUDY QUESTIONS

1. What are the signs and symptoms of COPD?
2. As a physical therapist, how can you screen for COPD?
3. How many people are affected by COPD?
4. What are red flags that may require hospitalization for someone with COPD?
5. What causes COPD?
6. How is COPD diagnosed?
7. What types of medications are usually prescribed to people with COPD?
8. What is the target (purpose) of the medications used by patients with stable COPD?
9. What are some possible adverse effects of long-term use of corticosteroids?
10. What else should treatment consist of?
11. Can people with COPD exercise?
12. Where does this patient compare to others in her age group performing the 6-Minute Walk Test?
13. How is dyspnea measured?

12

CHRONIC OBSTRUCTIVE PULMONARY DISEASE (COPD): CASE 2

Stacey Brickson, PT, PhD, ATC

James S. Carlson, MPT, CCS

A 70-year-old man is referred to physical therapy for falls risk reduction after a fall at home. He presents in the clinic complaining of shortness of breath for the past 2 weeks. Prior to the onset of symptoms 2 weeks ago he could walk to all his community destinations without limitations, but now he becomes fatigued after a short walk through the grocery store. He also notes that he has felt his heart racing even when he is at rest. In addition, he reports night sweats and a worsened morning cough of clear to yellow/green-tinged sputum. Extremity range of motion and strength are within normal limits. His past medical history includes hypertension, hypercholesterolemia, a 40 pack per year tobacco history, chronic obstructive pulmonary disease (COPD), type 2 diabetes mellitus (DM), and peripheral neuropathies in both feet.

PULMONARY FUNCTION TESTS: 2013

Value	Actual	%Predicted	Predicted
FVC (L)	2.67	70	3.84
FEV$_1$ (L)	1.40	45 %	3.10
FEV$_1$/FVC	52	64	
TLC (L)	6.69	105	6.37
RV (L)	3.55	175	2.03
DLCO (units)	18.5	67	27.61

6-MINUTE WALK TEST (2013): 270 M (886 FT)

Rest	HR 89	SpO$_2$ 94%	FiO$_2$: room air
Exertion (walk)	HR 104	SpO$_2$ 90%	FiO$_2$: room air
Recovery (2 minutes)	HR 92	SpO$_2$ 94%	FiO$_2$: room air

MEDICATIONS

Hydrochlorothiazide 25 mg daily
Amlodipine 10 mg daily
Metformin 1000 mg once daily at night
Simvastatin 20 mg once daily
Albuterol 200 µg 2 puffs every 4 to 6 hours
Tiotropium 18 µg powder once daily
Budesonide/formoterol 160/4.5, two inhalations twice daily

VITALS

Pulse: 107 beats per minute, irregular
BP: 130/90 mm Hg
RR: 18 breaths/min
SpO$_2$: 94% on room air
Temp: 37°C (98.6°F)

PHYSICAL EXAMINATION

Observation: Appears comfortable and speaks in full sentences without difficulty.
Head and neck: No jugular venous distension (JVD), normal thyroid.
Auscultation: Decreased breath sounds in both lung bases, inspiratory and expiratory wheezing in the right middle lung fields. Heartbeat irregular and rapid, without murmurs, rubs, or gallops.
Extremities: No edema.
Abdomen: Soft and nontender.
Telemetry ECG is shown below.

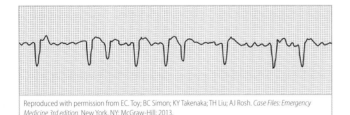

Reproduced with permission from EC. Toy; BC Simon; KY Takenaka; TH Liu; AJ Rosh. *Case Files: Emergency Medicine 3rd edition.* New York, NY: McGraw-Hill; 2013.

■ CASE STUDY QUESTIONS

1. What stage of COPD does this patient have according to the GOLD classification? *stage III*

2. Identify the inhaled medications. Are these medications consistent with an appropriate regimen based on his stage of disease? Identify other components of optimal medical management for this stage of COPD. →

3. Are there any side effects of these inhaled medications that would impact PT, either directly or indirectly?
→ Cough, headache, runny nose, muscle pain, dizzy

4. Identify the rhythm seen on telemetry. How might this rhythm impact a PT session? *BBB*

5. What are the most common arrhythmias associated with COPD? *Supraventricular arrhythmias*

6. What are the signs and symptoms of a COPD exacerbation? Discuss the classification of COPD exacerbations. What are the most common etiologies for a COPD exacerbation?

7. What signs and symptoms does this patient demonstrate that would support a diagnosis of respiratory infection? How does early recognition of these signs and symptoms by the PT impact the course of medical treatment and outcome for the patient?

8. What additional tests and measures might a physical therapist choose for this patient?

9. What is FiO$_2$?

10. What is amlodipine? *→ CCB NORVASC*

13

CHRONIC OBSTRUCTIVE PULMONARY DISEASE (COPD): CASE 3

Eric Shamus, PT, DPT, PhD

Arie J. van Duijn, PT, EdD, OCS

A 65-year-old female presents to your office with a referral diagnosis of functional decline. The patient complains of shortness of breath (SOB) with exertion. She has a cough that is not productive. She has a 30-year history of smoking, but quit 5 years ago for her 60th birthday. She is having difficulty with breathing when performing overhead activities as a component of ADLs. The patient reports decreased ability to walk inside her home and has difficulty with all ADLs due to fatigue and shortness of breath (SOB). The patient requires increased time for bed mobility, transfers, and gait with multiple rest breaks due to SOB.

On examination, the patient's blood pressure is 115/70 mm Hg, her pulse is 94 beats per minute, and her respiratory rate is 20 breaths per minute with shallow breathing. There is increased activity of the accessory musculature during respiration. Resting oxygen saturation (SpO$_2$) is 90%. The patient has forward head posture with rounded shoulders. There is decreased muscle length of the upper trapezius, levator scapulae, and pectoralis minor bilaterally. The 6-Minute Walk Test (6MWT) demonstrates 200 ft with frequent rest stops as a result of shortness of breath. The patient's modified Borg Dyspnea Scale increased from 3/10 (moderate breathing difficulty) before the 6MWT to 9/10 (very, very severe breathing difficulty) post 6MWT. Her SpO$_2$ saturation during the 6MWT drops to 86%. The patient has a decreased forced expiratory volume (FEV$_1$). The patient also has a decreased forced vital capacity (FVC) and an FEV$_1$/FVC ratio of 60%.

■ CASE STUDY QUESTIONS

1. What is chronic obstructive pulmonary disease?

2. What are the demographics of chronic obstructive pulmonary disease?

3. What are the common symptoms of chronic obstructive pulmonary disease?

4. What are the common lung/breathing sounds for chronic obstructive pulmonary disease?

5. What is paradoxical inspiration?

6. What functional test(s) would be beneficial to conduct on this patient?

7. What are the normal O_2 saturation rate and FEV_1/FVC ratio?

8. What is the most appropriate diagnostic procedure?

9. What is an appropriate treatment for her pulmonary condition?

10. How and why would you address the abnormal posture?

11. What are the functional implications of chronic obstructive pulmonary disease?

12. What are the possible contributing causes of chronic obstructive pulmonary disease?

13. What medications might she be taking for this condition?

14. Would you recommend the use of supplemental oxygen for this patient?

14

LOWER LEG PAIN

Eric Shamus, PT, DPT, PhD

Oseas Florencio de Moura Filho, PT (Brazil), MSc

A 70-year-old patient presents following abdominal surgery 3 days ago for a large abdominal cyst. The patient is being seen at home to begin general mobilization. Following your evaluation yesterday you began gait training with a straight cane for support. Today she complains of soreness in the left lower leg. The patient states when she was up walking her calf felt tight and had some "aching" pain. On examination, she has swelling in the left lower leg and some tenderness of the calf. She has a positive Homans sign that increases when the calf is gently squeezed. There is no redness of the leg, but she has point tenderness and warmth in the posterior lower leg/calf muscles. The student physical therapist working with you wants to know if he can do some massage on the leg to loosen the muscle cramp up. The patient is anxious to get back to her normal daily routine and is concerned about her calf pain interfering with this.

■ CASE STUDY QUESTIONS

1. What is a deep vein thrombosis (DVT)?

2. What are the possible contributing causes or risk factors for developing a DVT?

3. What are the common symptoms of a deep vein thrombosis?

4. Is a Homans sign diagnostic for a DVT?

5. What are the differential diagnoses of a DVT?

6. What should a physical therapist do if a DVT is thought to be present?

7. What is the physiology behind the formation of a thrombus?

8. What are the appropriate diagnostic tests for a DVT?

9. What types of medications are used for treatment?

10. What can be done to help prevent a DVT after surgery?

11. What can affect the prognosis for a patient with a DVT?

12. What are the systemic implications of a deep vein thrombosis?

13. Should you allow the student PT to perform a massage to the calf muscle?

15

HIP FRACTURE WITH COMPLICATIONS

Stacey Brickson, PT, PhD, ATC

James S. Carlson, MPT, CCS

The patient is an 82-year-old male who had an open reduction internal fixation (ORIF) of the right hip subtrochanteric fracture due to a fall in the kitchen. The patient developed chest pain and shortness of breath (SOB) in the recovery room. Cardiac labs were drawn and patient had a + troponin (Tn) bump to 4.5 ng/mL with a brain natriuretic peptide (BNP) of 800 pg/mL. A 12-lead ECG demonstrated no ST-segment changes or T-wave inversion. The patient was subsequently transferred to the cardiac care unit for monitoring. On post-op day (POD) 1, the patient developed worsening renal function with a creatinine spike to 1.8 mg/dL. It is now POD 2 and the physician has requested that mobilization be initiated at this time with touchdown weight bearing (TDWB) on the right lower extremity.

His past medical history includes coronary artery disease (CAD), drug-eluting stents (DES) to left anterior descending (LAD) and oblique marginal 1 (OM1) arteries in 2003, hypertension (HTN), congestive heart failure (CHF), and gastroesophageal reflux disease (GERD).

PRIOR LEVEL OF FUNCTION

Lives alone on the second floor of a two-story elderly occupied apartment building. Nearest support person is the patient's son who lives 200 miles away. Was previously very sedentary, left his apartment only to go to his physician's office and the pharmacy. His housekeeper performs most of his daily chores, including grocery shopping.

MEDICATIONS

Metoprolol (metoprolol tartrate) 100 mg bid.
Lisinopril (Zestril) 40 mg daily.
Aspirin 81 mg daily.
Simvastatin (Zocor) 20 mg daily.
Omeprazole (Prilosec) 20 mg daily.
Percocet (acetaminophen and oxycodone 5/325) two tablets qid.
Examination reveals an elderly, cachectic male who is noted to be mildly confused. He is oriented to time and place, but thinks the year is 1974.
Auscultation heart: S1, S2, +S3, no S4, no murmurs.
Auscultation lungs: Diminished breath sounds throughout, crackles in the upper lung fields.
Extremities: Bilateral upper and left lower extremities are within normal limits for strength and range of motion.
Circulation/integument: Normal capillary refill, 2+ pitting edema right lower extremity, 1+ on the left lower extremity. Bruising and ecchymosis right lateral and anterior upper thigh. Wound dressing intact without soak through drainage.
Vital signs: HR: 105 beats per minute; BP: 135/67 mm Hg; SpO_2: 99%; FiO_2: room air; respirations: 16 breaths per minute.

TELEMETRY

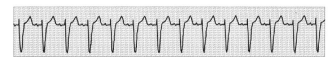

V_3

Current Labs					
RBC	3.1	Creatinine	1.4	Troponin	0.005
WBC	10.2	BUN	32	BNP	800
Hgb	9.8	Na$^+$	138	INR	1.4
Hct	28	K$^+$	3.6	Albumin	3.1
Glucose	98	Mg^{2+}	2.4	Amylase	50

BEDSIDE CHEST X-RAY

Mild cardiomegaly, no evidence of infiltrate, pleural effusion, or pulmonary edema.

BEDSIDE TRANSTHORACIC ECHO

Left ventricle: Mild to moderate LV dilation, EF 50%, mild reduced left ventricular wall motion anterior and anterolateral. Wall motion score of 1.1. Grade 2 diastolic dysfunction.

Left atrium: Mild dilation.

Aortic valve: No evidence of stenosis or regurgitation.

Mitral valve: Mild regurgitation. No evidence of stenosis.

Right ventricle: Normal chamber size. No evidence of concentric hypertrophy.

Estimated right ventricle systolic pressure of 18 mm Hg. No evidence of pulmonary hypertension.

Right atrium: Normal chamber size.

Tricuspid valve: No evidence of regurgitation or stenosis.

RIGHT HIP FILM

Stable alignment of internal fixation.

■ CASE STUDY QUESTIONS

1. How is capillary refill time measured?
2. What is the scale used for edema measurement?
3. What evidence supports the development of congestive heart failure postoperatively for this patient?
4. What is the relevance of developing congestive heart failure for the treating physical therapist?
5. What is the significance of crackles on lung auscultation findings?
6. How might this finding impact this patient's rehabilitation potential and clinical decision making for treatment?
7. Identify the rhythm on telemetry. Does this rhythm have any clinical implications for this patient's rehab care?
8. Differentiate systolic and diastolic heart failure and determine which type of CHF this patient presents with. What are the similarities or differences in clinical presentation and overall mortality?
9. What prognostic value does wall motion score and grading of diastolic dysfunction on echocardiogram have?
10. What are the common postoperative complications following surgical fixation of a hip fracture? What complications, if any, is this patient at risk for?
11. What functional tests and measures have prognostic implication for this patient's successful discharge to home and prevention of repeat hospitalization?
12. What gait speed would be an appropriate expectation for the treating outpatient clinician to reduce morbidity and mortality?

16

HEMATOMA

William H. Staples, PT, DHSc, DPT, GCS, CEEAA

Your patient is a 75-year-old white male with a medical history of hypertension, knee osteoarthritis, chronic atrial fibrillation, congestive heart failure, and peripheral vascular disease. You are seeing her as an outpatient because she wants to initiate an exercise program. Current medications include aspirin (81 mg, daily), prazosin (1 mg tid), hydrochlorothiazide (HCTZ) (25 mg bid), lisinopril (40 mg daily), warfarin (2 mg M, W, F; 1 mg Sa, Su, Tu, Th), salsalate (two 750 mg tablets, bid), and a potassium supplement. Physical examination reveals mild erythema on the posterior aspect of the left calf, which is warm to touch, slight swelling that is 2.5 cm larger than the right, diffuse superficial tenderness, ecchymosis distally at level of the malleoli, and a positive Homans sign.

The patient denies any trauma or recent surgery. Her gait pattern is slightly antalgic with decreased plantar flexion at terminal stance. You are concerned that she may have a medical problem requiring physician's care.

TREATMENT

She saw her physician and was started on a course of oral erythromycin for presumed cellulitis and instructed to curtail physical activity until seen again. Laboratory data: WBC 8.2, PT/INR 3.3, and an erythrocyte sedimentation rate (ESR) of 35 mm/h. There was no improvement in symptoms after 3 days; in fact there was worsening of the pain and swelling and she returned to her physician for follow-up.

■ CASE STUDY QUESTIONS

1. What is salsalate?
2. What is hydrochlorothiazide?
3. What is prazosin?
4. Does this patient need to take a potassium supplement?
5. What would be the differential diagnosis for this problem?
6. Why would you or would you not suspect a deep vein thrombosis?
7. What is "coup-de-fouet" syndrome?
8. What is a hematoma?
9. Are there any risks for hematoma with this patient?
10. What are the signs and symptoms of a hematoma?
11. What is the medical workup for this problem?
12. What is the PT/INR and what does it mean?
13. What is the common medical treatment for this problem?
14. What complications may occur with this problem?
15. What are some common comorbidities seen in this condition?
16. What are some drug interactions that may increase the risk for bleeding?
17. How was this case handled medically?

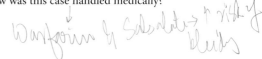

17

UNMOTIVATED PATIENT

William H. Staples, PT, DHSc, DPT, GCS, CEEAA

An 88-year-old woman admitted to subacute rehab after a three night stay in an acute care hospital following a fall at home with resultant multiple areas of bruising/trauma but no fractures. At the hospital she was found to have moderate hypertension of 168/100 for which she had already been taking furosemide (Lasix) 20 mg daily. The dose of furosemide was increased to 40 mg daily and she was also started on lisinopril (Zestril) 10 mg daily. She was also started on ibuprofen 400 mg q6 hours for the pain, which was 5/10 in her left shoulder and hip on which she landed when she fell. She did not receive therapy at the hospital due to pain complaints. The only other pertinent medical history was for anxiety for which she was taking sertraline (Zoloft) 50 mg daily. Previous to her fall she was living independently in an apartment in a continuing care community.

The day after admission to the subacute rehab section of the nursing home, the therapist attempts to get the woman to therapy but the patient refuses on multiple attempts, giving one- to three-word answers and refusing to look the therapist in the eyes. She asked to be left alone. She refused therapy for the first 2 days. The therapist attempted to give her the two-question depression test, but the patient told the therapist to "go away" and to "leave me alone." Discussion began between nursing and the physician to increase her sertraline because of her lack of motivation. The physician ordered lab work, with results below. Her vital signs in bed are HR 88, RR 18; BP 110/68; SpO$_2$ 96%.

Laboratory studies showed the following:

- Sodium level—126 mEq/L
- Potassium level—3.9 mEq/L
- Chloride level—94 mEq/L
- Total CO$_2$—23
- Blood urea nitrogen (BUN) level—10 mg/dL
- Creatinine level—0.6 mg/dL
- Glucose level—93 mg/dL
- Uric acid level—1.6 mg/dL
- Plasma osmolality—260 mOsm/kg

Urine studies revealed the following:

- Sodium level—173 mEq/L
- Potassium level—45 mEq/L
- Creatinine level—168 mg/dL
- Uric acid level—52 mg/dL
- Urine osmolality—565 mOsm/kg

Complete blood count findings were normal, and nonfasting lipid profile found the following:

- Total cholesterol—223 mg/dL
- Triglyceride level—188 mg/dL
- Low-density lipoprotein level—170 mg/dL
- High-density lipoprotein level—46 mg/dL

CASE STUDY QUESTIONS

1. What is homeostasis?
2. What happens to homeostasis as a person ages?
3. What is lisinopril? ACE Inhibitor
4. What is sertraline? Antidepressant, SSRI
5. What is the normal range for serum sodium? 135-145
6. What diagnoses would you consider at this point? ↓ HTN
7. What is hyponatremia? < 135
8. Is hyponatremia common in the older population? Yes
9. What are the signs and symptoms of hyponatremia? headache, confusion, stupor, seizures.
10. What effect does aging have on water metabolism?
11. Is there more than one type of hyponatremia?
12. What can cause salt depletion in older adults? ↑
13. What is the first thing to consider whenever there is an acute change in condition of an older adult?
14. What is SIADH? furosemide & Zoloft
15. Are there any drug interactions that may be of concern? both ↑ concochn
16. What is the medical treatment for hyponatremia?
17. Do you think that this patient was able to recover from this problem? — NO

Common causes of Hyponatremia:
- Diuretic use, diarrhea, heart failure, liver disease.

18

MYOCARDIAL INFARCTION OR URINARY TRACT INFECTION

William H. Staples, PT, DHSc, DPT, GCS, CEEAA

An 82-year-old woman residing in a skilled nursing facility has been referred for physical therapy evaluation due to worsening of her "Alzheimer symptoms" with "increased confusion and loss of independent gait status" in the last 2 days with a fall yesterday. No injuries are reported from the fall. She had no complaints of chest or urinary pain. She also has diagnoses of type 2 diabetes mellitus and atherosclerotic heart disease. On admission 6 months ago an MMSE was 23/30. Vital signs are HR 92 beats per minute, RR 18 breaths per minute, BP 118/74, SpO$_2$ 94%, temp 98.8°F, and 2+ dyspnea when transferring with moderate assist from the bed to a bedside chair.

At the time of the therapy evaluation, she had difficulty following simple commands or responding verbally to questioning. The therapist decided to curtail the evaluation and request that the physician order blood and urine labs before continuing the evaluation. The labs returned were as follows:

10-40 → liver damage

Blood Labs (Cardiac Biomarkers)		Urinalysis	
AST (aspartate transaminase)	63 U/L	Specific gravity	1.010
Troponin I	30 µg/L	Glucose (mg/dL)	50
Glucose	110 mg/dL	pH	6.9
LDH (lactic dehydrogenase)	982 U/L	Leucocytes	Trace

100-190

Blood Labs (Cardiac Biomarkers)		Urinalysis	
Creatine kinase	1.3 mg/dL	Nitrite	Negative
WBC	6.3 k/mm³	Protein (mg/dL)	++/100
RBC	4.2 m/mm³	Ketones	+Small
Myoglobin	120 (ng/mL)	Bilirubin	Negative
		Blood (ery/μ)	Negative
		Color	Yellow
		Appearance	Clear

■ CASE STUDY QUESTIONS

1. What are the typical signs and symptoms of a myocardial infarction?
2. Are symptoms in older adults the same for men and women?
3. What is a "silent heart attack?"
4. Why are blood tests performed?
5. What is troponin?
6. What is creatine kinase and why is it measured?
7. What does the myoglobin level indicate?
8. What is AST (aspartate transaminase)?
9. What is LDH (lactic dehydrogenase) and what does it indicate?
10. Is the glucose level normal?
11. What does the overall blood work for this patient indicate?
12. Does it appear that this patient has a UTI or MI? Why or why not?
13. Do people with diabetes have a higher risk for MIs? Why or why not?

19

MITRAL VALVE PROLAPSE (MVP)

Eric Shamus, PT, DPT, PhD

Ahmed Elokda, PT, PhD, CLT, CEEAA, FAACVPR

A 68-year-old woman presents for a vestibular examination for complaints of dizziness. Upon further questioning, it is revealed that she also has palpitations and anxiety. She states that nothing in particular has been causing her stress lately, but she feels her "heart racing." Vitals are pulse: 84, respirations: 18, blood pressure: 110/70, and SpO$_2$%: 99%. On examination, there is an audible nonejection click and a faint, late systolic murmur. On the musculoskeletal exam, there is a narrow anteroposterior chest diameter and a mild scoliosis.

The patient is sent back to their primary physician for a cardiac workup. The physician orders an echocardiogram; there is a 2.5-mm displacement of the mitral valve leaflet.

After your evaluation, you determine that you need to do more research for this disorder to determine what your treatment approach should be. Please answer the following questions based on your research.

■ CASE STUDY QUESTIONS

1. Did the therapist make the correct decision in referring back to the physician?
2. What vitals should be taken?

3. If a patient complains of dizziness, where should auscultation occur?
4. What are the possible contributing causes of mitral valve prolapse?
5. What are the common symptoms of mitral valve prolapse?
6. What are the common physical therapy differential tests?
7. What types of medications may the patient be taking?
8. What are the common laboratory tests for mitral valve problems?
9. What are the common functional tests for mitral valve problems?
10. What are the common impairments for mitral valve problems?
11. What is the prognosis for a patient with mitral valve prolapse?

20

MITRAL STENOSIS

Eric Shamus, PT, DPT, PhD

Jennifer Shamus, PT, DPT, PhD

A 60-year-old female, originally from Guatemala, is preparing to run her first 5K. On history, she stated that she had rheumatic fever as a child, but has been very healthy ever since. Vitals are pulse: 80, respirations: 16, blood Pressure: 126/80, and SpO$_2$: 99%. On physical examination, there is an opening snap and a faint diastolic murmur over the cardiac apex. Her strength and range of motion are normal. After 5 minutes on the treadmill, her heart was racing and she coughed up a little bit of blood.

The patient is sent back to their primary physician for a cardiac workup. The physician orders a chest x-ray. The ECG is within normal limits and the cardiac echo reveals a narrowing of the mitral valve.

After your evaluation, you determine that you need to do more research for this disorder to determine what your treatment approach should be. Please answer the following questions based on your research.

■ CASE STUDY QUESTIONS

1. Did the therapist make the correct decision in referring the patient back to the physician?
2. What vitals should be taken?
3. Where should auscultation occur?
4. What are the possible contributing causes of mitral valve stenosis?
5. What are the common symptoms of mitral valve stenosis?
6. What are the common differential tests?
7. What types of medications may the patient be taking after diagnosis?
8. What are the common laboratory tests for mitral stenosis?
9. What are the common functional tests for mitral stenosis?
10. What are the common impairments for mitral stenosis?
11. What is the prognosis for a patient with mitral valve prolapse?

21

PERICARDITIS

Eric Shamus, PT, DPT, PhD

Christopher C. Felton, DO, ATC

A 60-year-old male presents with a recent onset of substernal chest pain. The pain is sharp and stabbing and has started to radiate to the left trapezius muscle. Inspiration causes the pain to become more severe, but sitting up and leaning forward helps relieve it. The patient states the pain is limiting his functional ability. This patient's review of systems reveals a recent viral illness, including "flu-like" symptoms and low-grade fever for 1 week. His past medical history is otherwise unremarkable.

His current temperature is 100.9°F, BP is 130/84, HR is 95 beats per minute, RR is 24 breaths per minute, and O_2 sat is 99% on room air. Heart auscultation reveals a scratchy, rubbing sound at the lower left sternal border. Lungs are clear, but breathing is shallow.

After your evaluation, you determine that you need to do more research for this disorder to determine what your treatment approach should be. Please answer the following questions based on your research.

■ CASE STUDY QUESTIONS

1. What should the therapist do?
2. What is pericarditis?
3. What are the common symptoms of pericarditis?
4. What are the common lung/breathing sounds for pericarditis?
5. What is the most common classification of functional status for objective assessment of heart disease?
6. What are the functional implications?
7. What are the appropriate diagnostic procedures?
8. What is an appropriate treatment for her pulmonary condition?
9. Are there any exercises that would be important for this patient?
10. What type of medications may be appropriate?
11. What are the possible contributing causes of pericarditis?

22

PULMONARY EDEMA

Eric Shamus, PT, DPT, PhD

Greg Hartley, PT, DPT, GCS, CEEAA

A 77-year-old male in a telemetry unit of an acute care facility for exacerbation of congestive heart failure (CHF) presents to the physical therapist during the second day of treatment with a sudden (new) onset of shortness of breath (respiration rate is 24, a pulse oximetry reading of 92% saturation of peripheral oxygen [SpO_2] while on 2 L of O_2 via nasal cannula); crackles without wheezing are heard upon lung auscultation. The patient has an elevated blood pressure (177/109), anxiety, profuse diaphoresis, frothy pink sputum, and 3+ pitting edema is present in both feet. The patient's current relevant

medications include furosemide (Lasix) as a diuretic 40 mg two times per day and enalapril (Vasotec) for an angiotensin-converting enzyme (ACE) inhibitor 20 mg twice a day. He is in some distress and is unable to respond to questions reliably or without further anxiety. Upon cardiac auscultation you hear an "extra" beat that sounds like a horse galloping. The physical therapist notified the nurse and the physician who obtained the following stat test results: a standard chest radiograph revealed fluid in the alveolar walls and upper lobe diversion; an echocardiogram confirmed impaired left ventricular function; a complete blood count (CBC) with differential revealed a mildly elevated white count (10,800 cells/μL/mm³); the blood urea nitrogen (BUN) was 30 mg/dL; creatinine was 1.5 mg/dL; B-type natriuretic peptide (BNP) was 600 pg/mL; and arterial blood gases revealed elevated carbon dioxide and low oxygen concentration.

After your evaluation, you determine that you need to do more research for this disorder to determine what your treatment approach should be. Please answer the following questions based on your research.

■ CASE STUDY QUESTIONS

1. What is pulmonary edema?
2. What are the demographics of pulmonary edema?
3. What are the common symptoms of pulmonary edema?
4. What are the common heart and lung/breath sounds for pulmonary edema?
5. Where and how would you auscultate to hear the "gallop?"
6. What functional test(s) would be beneficial to conduct on this patient?
7. What are the normal results/ranges for the diagnostic procedures ordered by the physician?
8. What is an appropriate treatment?
9. Are there any exercises that would be important for this patient?
10. What are the functional implications of pulmonary edema?
11. What are the possible contributing causes of pulmonary edema?
12. What is hypercapnia?

23

PULMONARY EMBOLUS (PE): CASE 1

Stacey Brickson, PT, PhD, ATC

James S. Carlson, MPT, CCS

A 70-year-old male is referred to outpatient physical therapy 7 days status post right total knee arthroplasty (TKA) secondary to severe osteoarthritis (OA). The patient was discharged from the hospital's orthopedic nursing unit 3 days ago with a prescription for enoxaparin for deep vein thrombosis (DVT) prophylaxis. The patient has been inactive at home with the exception of completing activities of daily living (ADLs) with the assistance of his wife. This morning, the patient noted some mild chest pain and shortness of breath while watching television. The breathlessness has persisted all morning.

On examination, he appears slightly short of breath, anxious, and uncomfortable. The patient denies headache, fever, nausea, vomiting, cough, and chills. Vital signs at rest were a blood pressure of 110/78 mm Hg, heart rate of 101 beats per minute, pulse oximetry

SpO$_2$ of 92% on room air, and respiratory rate of 26 breaths per minute. The entire right lower extremity has limited ROM with slight redness, warmth, and gross edema from knee distal. The patient complains of pain 7/10 in the right knee and 8/10 in the right calf on a verbal analog scale. The patient transfers very slowly with a standard walker and appears very short of breath.

Cough is nonproductive, but the patient reports mild left-sided chest pain with coughing. The pain does not radiate and is not reproducible by touch. The lungs are clear to auscultation with no evidence of wheezing/crackles. Heart sounds with a strong S1, S2, no S3/S4 or murmur. The abdomen is soft, nontender, and nondistended. Bowel sounds present on auscultation.

PAST MEDICAL HISTORY (PMH)

Hypertension (HTN) × 30 years
Dyslipidemia × 25 years
Chronic stable angina × 2 years (negative adenosine stress test 2 months ago)
Chronic kidney disease (CKD) secondary to previously uncontrolled HTN, stage 4 (baseline creatinine 1.8-2.0 mg/dL)
Osteoarthritis (OA)
Obesity with a BMI of 32
S/P TKR right leg (postoperative day #7)

SOCIAL HISTORY

The patient is retired. He lives at home with his wife. Prior to surgery, he avoided most physical activity due to severe osteoarthritis. He has no history of tobacco abuse. He also denies alcohol use.

MEDICATIONS

- Aspirin 81 mg PO once daily
- Metoprolol (Toprol-XL) 50 mg PO bid
- Amlodipine (Norvasc) 10 mg PO once daily
- Hydralazine 25 mg PO tid
- Atorvastatin (Lipitor) 20 mg PO once daily
- Nitroglycerin (Nitrostat) 0.4 mg sublingually PRN chest pain
- Calcium acetate (PhosLo) 667 mg PO tid with meals
- Enoxaparin (Lovenox) 30 mg SC q 24 hours
- Oxycodone SR (OxyContin) sustained release 20 mg PO q 12 hours
- Oxycodone (Roxicodone) immediate release 5 mg PO q 6 hours PRN pain
- Docusate (Doculase) 100 mg PO qhs

VITAL SIGNS

BP 110/78, P 101, RR 26, T 36.9°C, wt 85 kg, ht 5 ft 4 in, O$_2$ saturation 88% on room air

ECG

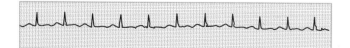

■ CASE STUDY QUESTIONS

1. What subjective and objective information is consistent with a diagnosis of pulmonary embolus?

2. During the differential diagnosis procedure, what other etiologies might manifest with shortness of breath and mild chest pain? What are alternative diagnoses for right calf pain and swelling?

3. Identify the rhythm this patient is presenting with. Is this rhythm typical for a patient presenting with pulmonary embolus?

4. What are risk factors for developing a deep vein thrombosis and pulmonary embolus? Which ones are present in this case?

5. The Wells score is a clinical prediction rule for PE. What clinical characteristics are listed in the Wells score? Is this patient low, intermediate, or high risk for pulmonary embolus?

6. How is the diagnosis of a pulmonary embolus confirmed? What tests are ordered when the patient is high risk versus low risk for pulmonary embolus?

7. What are the differences between acute and chronic pulmonary emboli?

8. What is the common medical treatment algorithm for a pulmonary embolus?

9. Is the patient stable for physical therapy intervention? Defend your answer.

10. Are there special precautions/contraindications or monitoring that need to be taken for someone following treatment for pulmonary embolus during therapy?

11. What interventions would be useful for this patient?

12. What is the risk for a future pulmonary embolus in this patient?

24

PULMONARY EMBOLUS (PE): CASE 2

Eric Shamus, PT, DPT, PhD

Elysa Roberts, OTR, PhD

A 77-year-old male is being seen in an inpatient rehabilitation facility 1 week post-right total hip replacement. The patient is being cotreated by occupational therapy (OT) and physical therapy (PT). The patient just finished with occupational therapy and the physical therapist has come to work on weight shifting and gait training. The patient states that he is fatigued and is having shortness of breath. After walking about 10 ft the patient is complaining of being light-headed, right calf pain, and is having increased difficulty with breathing. The patient is seated and vital signs are taken. Heart rate is 106 beats per minute (at rest was 72), respiratory rate is 28 (rest was 18), blood pressure is 132/82 (128/78 at rest), and oxygen saturation (SpO$_2$) is 90% (98% at rest). He is showing signs of cyanosis with his increased heart rate. You call a code and the patient is taken to the hospital via ambulance where the physician orders a cardiopulmonary workup and ultrasound of his lower leg.

After your evaluation, you determine that you need to do more research for this disorder to determine what your treatment approach should be. Please answer the following questions based on your research.

■ CASE STUDY QUESTIONS

1. What is a pulmonary embolism?

2. What are the demographics of the patient with a pulmonary embolism?

Handwritten note at top: signs of DVT, Chest pain, diff breathing, Pulse

3. What are the possible contributing causes and/or risk factors of a pulmonary embolism? *77 Y/ M, imm, rect Sx*

4. What are the common signs and symptoms of a pulmonary embolism? *lgt headed, Cl chest pain, diff breathi, ↑ HR, signs of cyanosis*

5. What are essentials of the diagnosis?

6. The patient returns to your facility in 1 week. What functional test(s) would be beneficial to conduct on this patient? *– Endurance testg → 2 MWT*

7. What are the normal results/ranges for the diagnostic procedures ordered by the physician?

8. What is the appropriate medical and/or pharmacological treatment? *Anticoaglns → Heparn/Wafarn*

9. What are the functional implications following a pulmonary embolism? *↓ mobility*

10. What is the appropriate PT/OT treatment when the patient returns from the hospital? *→ ambul CM out & leg exercises*

11. What do research studies or clinical practice guidelines offer to inform your clinical reasoning and treatment planning?

25

PULMONARY TUBERCULOSIS (TB)

Eric Shamus, PT, DPT, PhD

A 65-year-old female presents to your office with a referral diagnosis of functional decline. The patient complains of shortness of breath (SOB) with exertion. Over the last month she has lost about 5 lbs. She states her appetite has decreased. She does have a productive cough with green sputum. On examination, she has a heart rate of 82 beats per minute, blood pressure of 132/82, temperature of 100.2°F, and respiratory rate of 16 breaths per minute. Lung sounds are clear with a few rales in the right lobes. When asked about recent sickness or travels, she reports she went on a cruise to the Caribbean about 2 months ago and was able to walk all around the ship.

After your evaluation, you determine that you need to do more research for this disorder to determine what your treatment approach should be. Please answer the following questions based on your research.

■ CASE STUDY QUESTIONS

1. What is pulmonary tuberculosis (TB)?

2. Is TB contagious?

3. What are the common symptoms of TB?

4. What are the common lung/breathing sounds for TB?

5. What is extrapulmonary TB?

6. What functional test(s) would be beneficial to conduct on this patient?

7. What are the normal O_2 saturation rate and FEV_1/FVC ratio?

8. What is the most appropriate diagnostic procedure?

9. What is an appropriate treatment for her pulmonary condition?

10. What are the functional implications of TB?

26

RESPIRATORY FAILURE

Stacey Brickson, PT, PhD, ATC

James S. Carlson, MPT, CCS

PART 1

The patient is a 61-year-old female librarian admitted to the ICU following a syncopal episode. The patient was carrying a box of books across the school library when she became severely short of breath, light-headed, and lost consciousness. A coworker witnessed the event and emergency medical services (EMS) was called. Upon arrival of the paramedics, the patient was alert and oriented ×3 and in severe respiratory distress. The patient was transported to emergency department (ED) where vital signs, labs, electrocardiograph (ECG), blood gases, and chest radiograph were completed.

Vital Signs	ABG	Lab Results
Pulse: 110 beats per minute, regular	PaO_2: 45 mm Hg	RBC: 4.4
ECG: Sinus tachycardia, no ST or T-wave changes	$PaCO_2$: 70 mm Hg	WBC: 9.9
	SaO_2: 78%	Hct: 50%
BP: 100/60 mm Hg		Hgb: 12 g/dL
RR: 32 breaths per minute		Troponin: 0.04 mg/mL
Temp: 37.8°C (100°F)		BNP: 1000 pg/mL
SpO_2: 75%		
FiO_2: 44% (6 L) nasal cannula		

PMH

Coronary heart disease (CAD): Angina with 40% blockage in left anterior descending (LAD), treated with medical management, no percutaneous intervention (PCI).

HTN

Family history: Mother died of pulmonary fibrosis in her 50s.

Social history: Social: married and live in a two-story home. House is 100 years old and only has an upstairs bathroom with a shower. There is no downstairs bathroom. Nonsmoker.

Prior function: Employed part-time as a librarian. Was having worsening dyspnea with exertion and sleeping propped up on two pillows the past 3 weeks, according to her husband. She was also experiencing a frequent cough

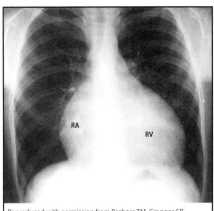

Reproduced with permission from Bashore TM, Granger CB, Jackson K, Patel MR. Heart Disease. In: Papadakis MA, McPhee SJ, Rabow MW. eds. *Current Medical Diagnosis & Treatment 2015.* New York, NY: McGraw-Hill; 2014.

Admission medications: Multivitamin, lisinopril (Zestril) 20 mg once per day, and metoprolol (Toprol-XL) 100 mg once per day.

Chest radiograph: Cardiomegaly. No evidence of consolidation or infiltrates.

Right heart catheterization

Right atrial pressure: 10 mm Hg

Right ventricle pressure: 40/20 mm Hg

Pulmonary artery pressure: 55 mm Hg

PCWP: 8 mm Hg

Echocardiogram

Left ventricle: EF 55%, normal chamber size, no hypertrophy

Mild anterior wall hypokinesis: wall motion score of 1.1

Mitral valve: no stenosis or regurgitation

Left atrium: mild dilation

Aortic valve: no evidence of stenosis/regurgitation

Right ventricle: moderately dilated, moderate concentric hypertrophy

Tricuspid valve: moderate regurgitation

Right atrium: moderate to severe dilation

Pulmonary artery pressure: 40 mm Hg

The patient was admitted to the ICU in respiratory failure and intubated. The patient has been intubated for 3 days and is now weaning toward extubation. The patient is conscious and fully alert and oriented. PT has been consulted to initiate early ICU mobility. The patient's current status is as follows:

Vitals	ABG
HR: 78 beats per minute	PaO_2: 70 mm Hg
BP: 114/64 mm Hg	PCO_2: 45 mm Hg
RR: 16 breaths per minute	SaO_2: 96%
Temp: 37.6°C	
FiO_2: Pressure support	

ECG

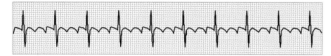

Auscultation: Diffuse crackles throughout all lung fields. S1 murmur, S2, soft S3.

Physical examination: Mild JVD, 2+ pitting edema in lower extremities from knee distal.

Mobility/strength/function: Strength is mildly decreased at 3+ to −4/5 throughout upper and lower extremities via bedside myotomal screen.

PART 2

The patient completes bed mobility and transitions to standing with the following hemodynamic changes:

HR: ↑ to 117 beats per minute

BP: ↓100/50 mm Hg

SpO_2: 88%

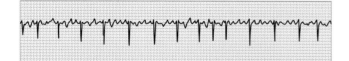

■ CASE STUDY QUESTIONS: PART 1

1. What are the functions of the prescription medications she is taking?

2. Define the types of respiratory failure by PaO_2 and $PaCO_2$ levels and give possible reasons or underlying etiology for each type of failure.

3. Based on the preintubation arterial blood gas, what type of respiratory failure does this patient have?

4. What rhythm is demonstrated in the ECG? What are the risks associated with this rhythm?

5. What information in the case supports a diagnosis of congestive heart failure?

6. Based on the right heart catheterization results, identify which values are elevated. Which value is used to differentiate between right and left heart failure? Determine the type of heart failure (right sided or left sided) in this patient.

7. What are the most common etiologies for right- and left-sided heart failure?

8. Is this patient appropriate to begin early mobilization in the ICU? Defend your answer.

9. What are the demonstrated benefits of early mobility in the ICU?

■ CASE STUDY QUESTIONS: PART 2

10. What rhythm is the patient in now?

11. What is your next clinical decision?

12. What factors need to be considered in disposition planning for home?

27

TRICUSPID VALVE REGURGITATION

Eric Shamus, PT, DPT, PhD

Jennifer Shamus, PT, DPT, PhD

A 67-year-old male presents to physical therapy for weakness, cold skin, sensation of blood vessel pulsations in the neck, and fatigue. The fatigue and weakness have progressed to the point where he is not comfortable going out grocery shopping and driving around town. He has a history of mild hypertension that is well controlled on lisinopril (Zestril) 40 mg orally once a day. Vitals are pulse: 70, respirations: 14, blood pressure: 124/84, temperature: 97.9°F, and SpO2%: 96.

On physical examination, there is mild distension of the jugular veins on the right side of the neck and a palpable right ventricular heave. On auscultation, there is a holosystolic murmur at the right midsternal border. With leg raising, the murmur gets louder. The patient was referred to the cardiologist. ECG and chest x-ray show signs of right atrial and ventricular enlargement. Echocardiography reveals a vena contracta of 0.8 cm and a dilated tricuspid annulus.

After your evaluation, you determine that you need to do more research to determine what your treatment approach should be. Please answer the following questions based on your research.

■ CASE STUDY QUESTIONS

1. What is ventricular heave?

2. What is a holosystolic murmur?

3. What is tricuspid valve regurgitation?

4. What are the demographics of tricuspid valve regurgitation?

5. Where would the placement of the stethoscope be appropriate for auscultation of a pansystolic heart murmur?

6. What do the ECG results of a vena contracta of 0.8 cm and a dilated tricuspid annulus indicate?

7. What would you look for on a chest x-ray?

8. What would be an appropriate diagnostic procedure?

9. What functional test(s) would be beneficial to conduct on this patient?

10. What are common signs and symptoms?

11. Has exercise been found to be beneficial for tricuspid valve regurgitation?

12. Are there any other exercises that would be important for this patient?

13. What are common impairments?

14. What are the common medications for heart failure induced by tricuspid regurgitation?

15. What would be an appropriate treatment goal?

28

UPPER RESPIRATORY TRACT INFECTION (URI OR URTI)

Eric Shamus, PT, DPT, PhD

Mitchell L. Cordova, ATC, PhD, FNATA, FACSM

A 72-year-old female arrives to the clinic with a complaint of recent right shoulder pain. The patient states that she had a cold that started 5 days ago. The patient states that 2 days prior to her cold, she went outside to do some yard work when her right shoulder began to hurt. She states that her shoulder bothers her when she reaches behind her back area to assist with dressing. She also experiences discomfort when sleeping on her right side. Upon physical examination, you noticed she still has a pretty bad cough, and when asked if she has seen a physician for her respiratory problem, the patient indicates no. Upon further questioning, she said he is still coughing up phlegm that has a yellowish color.

The orthopedic exam reveals a positive Speed Test with point-specific tenderness over the long head of the biceps with tightness across her chest from the coughing. There are no other relevant findings.

After your evaluation, you determine that you need to do more research for about the upper respiratory tract infection to determine what your treatment approach should be. Please answer the following questions based on your research.

■ CASE STUDY QUESTIONS

1. Should you be concerned about a possible upper respiratory tract infection, and if so, what else should be examined?

2. What is the most common associated virus with an upper respiratory tract infection called?

3. Should all patients be prescribed an antibiotic for an upper respiratory tract infection?

4. How does influenza differ from an upper respiratory infection?

5. What functional tests would be beneficial to conduct on this patient at this time?

6. What laboratory tests would be ordered by a physician?

7. What appropriate diagnostic and imaging procedures should be performed at this time? What would a CT reveal for acute sinusitis?

8. What is the appropriate treatment for her pulmonary condition?

9. What is a Speed Test and how is it performed?

10. What other special tests are appropriate for diagnosing bicipital tendonitis?

11. How do you perform this additional test?

12. What are other associated problems with bicipital tendonitis?

29

VENTILATOR AND MOBILITY

Kyle Katz, PT, DPT

A 66-year-old Caucasian woman presented to a small community hospital with a 5-day history of shortness of breath, tachypnea, and cough. She had a history of recent exposure to an upper respiratory infection from a family member and was immediately transported to a university medical center and was admitted for respiratory failure. Her past medical history included pulmonary hypertension, hypothyroidism, scleroderma of the lungs, CREST syndrome or phenomenon, gastric esophageal reflux disease, and anxiety. She is married and lives with her two young sons in a one-story home with one step into the house. She is a former smoker of half a pack per day for numerous years but has recently quit. Her vital signs upon admission to the hospital were a blood pressure of 87/68 mm Hg, heart rate of 113 beats per minute, oxygen saturation of (SpO_2) 100% while on 2 L/min of oxygen via BIPAP (bilevel positive airway pressure), and a respiratory rate varying from 15 to 39 breaths per minute. Less than 6 hours upon admission she was intubated and sedated.

Lab testing revealed that she would not be a good candidate for a lung transplant due to excessively high levels of a panel reactive antibody (PRA). Over the next week, she was weaned from sedation meds with only one minor setback of a single seizure occurring 2 days postintubation. Eleven days postintubation she became interactive and began demonstrating active movement in all extremities for the first time since intubation. After an endotracheal intubation a tracheostomy was performed. A few days later she started to show improved range of motion including cervical range of motion as she was now lifting her head off the bed. On day 18 of her length of stay she was transferred from the intensive care unit to the progressive care unit.

A physical therapy evaluation was performed on day 20 of her length of stay. On examination, she presented with active range of motion within functional limitations and gross strength testing revealed at least a 4+/5 in all extremities but with minor weakness in hip flexion bilaterally. She also presented with decreased endurance, as she was only able to perform 5 minutes of active exercise with a heart rate increase of 40% before requiring a rest period. She required minimal assistance for bed mobility. Minimal assistance is defined as the patient's ability to perform at least 75% of the required work to perform the given task. She sat on the edge of the bed for approximately 10 minutes prior to ambulating 3 ft to a bed side chair with minimal assist. Her static sitting balance was rated as a "fair +" as she could hold herself independently without supervision or verbal cues without resistance for 10 minutes, measuring a 4 on the third item of the Berg Balance exam. She complained of mild generalized pain 3/10 in her upper and low back for which she was receiving medication. Her vital signs at rest in supine were a blood pressure of 116/66 mm Hg, heart rate of 106 beats per minute, respiratory rate of 26 breaths per minute, and a pulse oximetry of 93% while receiving 2 L of supplemental oxygen through a ventilator. With sitting, her blood pressure dropped to 108/56 mm Hg, heart rate 110 beats per minute, respiratory rate 22 breaths per minute, and a pulse oximetry of 92%. Her oxygen delivery was through a ventilator via a tracheostomy collar with a pressure regulated volume control (PRVC) of 70%, fraction of inspired oxygen (FiO_2) of 40%, and a positive end-expiratory pressure (PEEP) of 8.

■ CASE STUDY QUESTIONS

1. Describe the physiological changes associated with CREST syndrome.

2. What are panel reactive antibodies (PRAs) and how might they affect transplantation efforts?

3. How did this patient's medical history impact this hospitalization?

4. What is a ventilator? What do the settings FiO_2, PEEP, PRVC mean to the rehabilitation process?

5. What might be the plan of care for the next physical therapy session?

6. What would be appropriate short- and long-term goals at the time of evaluation?

7. How might her condition affect her ability to perform activities of daily living?

8. Are there any precautions that need to be taken during therapy?

9. How might her condition affect the rehabilitation process?

10. What medication was used to decrease her anxiety? What are the possible side effects for that medication?

11. Why is the monitoring of vital signs especially important with this patient?

12. What interventions would be useful for this patient?

13. How would this patient progress, without further medical complications during her length of stay, and what was her length of stay?

14. What assistance is performed during therapy to increase the patient's ventilator status?

15. What other test and measures would be useful?

16. What is the long-term medical care and prognosis?

17. What other advice would you give to this patient?

30

MYOCARDIAL INFARCTION

Eric Shamus, PT, DPT, PhD

Jennifer Shamus, PT, DPT, PhD

A 62-year-old male is performing rehabilitation on his left plantar fasciitis in the clinic. He had a negative history except for a hernia surgery years ago. He has been working on foot placement and lower extremity control with walking. You decide to place the patient on the treadmill to increase the speed to work on motor control. After 3 minutes he starts to sweat and look pale. You immediately slow down the treadmill and bring it to a stop and sit him in a chair. He has complaints of chest pain and a deep pressure behind the sternum, which is spreading to the left side of his neck. Immediately 911 emergency services are called. As the paramedics are arriving his chest pain has resolved and his color is coming back. The patient is brought to the emergency room for workup.

After your evaluation, you determine that you need to do more research for this disorder to determine what your treatment approach should be. Please answer the following questions based on your research.

■ CASE STUDY QUESTIONS

1. Did the therapist make the correct decision in calling emergency services?

2. What vitals should be taken?

3. What are the possible risk factors for myocardial infarction?

4. What are the common symptoms of myocardial infarction?

5. What are the common differential tests for myocardial infarction?

6. What types of medications may the patient be taking after diagnosis of myocardial infarction?

7. What are the common laboratory tests for myocardial infarction?

8. What are the common functional tests after myocardial infarction?

9. What are the common impairments from myocardial infarction?

10. What is the prognosis for a patient with myocardial infarction?

11. What medical procedures can be done following a myocardial infarction?

Jill Heitzman, PT, DPT, GCS, NCS, CWS, CEEAA, FACCWS

CHAPTER 5

Integumentary Cases

INTRODUCTION

THE AGING INTEGUMENTARY SYSTEM

The skin is the largest organ of the body and the outward appearance of an individual that identifies one cosmetically, allowing identification and body image of a person. Over the lifespan, the skin becomes drier, less elastic, less perfused, and vulnerable to damage from pressure, friction, shear, moisture, and malnutrition.[1,2] These changes can impact the overall function of the skin.[3]

The skin functions as a physical barrier to microorganisms to fight against infection, prevent excessive loss of fluids, provide sensation input, and is a storage for fat and water for metabolism and thermoregulation of the body.[1] Resident immune cells that participate in immune processes are present in the epidermis and dermis (Langerhans cells and dermal dendritic cells). The nerve endings present in the skin allow the ability to feel pain, pressure, heat, and cold. The skin functions as a thermoregulatory of body temperature through vasoconstriction, vasodilation, and sweating, allowing excretion of waste products, electrolytes, and water. Synthesis of vitamin D in skin exposed to sunlight activates metabolism of calcium and phosphates, which are important to bone formation and hormonal production and synthesis. A disruption in the skin, either directly or indirectly, as a result of underlying disease process, reaction to that process or medication, can alter the overall health of the individual. Underlying processes can also affect the healing phases of the integumentary system: inflammation, proliferation, and remodeling, including wound bed granulation, collagen formation, remodeling of the extracellular matrix, and reepithelialization.[4,5]

There are many factors that impact the skin and ultimately wound healing, both intrinsic (emerge from internal physiological abnormalities) and extrinsic (external to the body).[6] Intrinsic factors include genetics and the aging process. However, advanced age alone does not impact wound healing. The independent aging factors typically do not cross over threshold of wound healing, but can be the basis for the changes that can occur with stressors. The extrinsic factors along with the presence of risk factors are what impairs the integumentary repair system in the aging adult.[7] Extrinsic factors include ultraviolet exposure, environment, and lifestyle that includes smoking, nutrition choices, and alcohol. Risk factors that add to the aging skin issues include medications, obesity, comorbidities, decreased mobility, decreased mental status, and incontinence.[8] Once a wound occurs, the healing process is affected by all these factors plus added factors of external pressure and bacterial burden.[2]

Biological changes that occur with aging include a decrease in the vascularity, dermal tissue thickness, number and size of sweat glands and hair follicles, epidermal cell turnover rate, collagen density and elastin fibers, and number of Langerhans cells and melanocytes. These changes make the epidermis less effective in protecting the body from infection and dehydration. The changes in the basal cells lead to a flattening of the epidermal-dermal junctions. The risk for infection even from small wounds increases due to the mast cell decrease that alters the early inflammatory response. These changes also affect wound healing by altering skin permeability, decrease in the inflammatory and immunological response altering wound healing, and reduction in the skin strength and elasticity with less scar formation leading to durability reductions.[3,7]

The changes of the dermal tissue and basement membrane lead to a pallor color, decrease in skin temperature and regulation, thinning of the skin texture. Ultimately, this results in an increased risk for skin tears and moisture changes leading to dry flaky skin with a rough skin appearance. The added gravitational forces lead to facial creases, sagging folds, and wrinkles due to decreased turgor.[7]

Skin color changes occur as a result of the decrease in melanocytes. This reduces the efficiency of the skin barrier and increases photoaging damage, making the skin appear thin, pale, and translucent.[2] Vessel wall thinning also adds to the color changes. Loss of underlying hypodermal fat production in capillaries leads to purple patches occurring after injury due to blood leaking more easily into the skin tissues.

With less sebaceous glands, less sweat is produced, which can lead to overheating. The thinning of the subcutaneous fat reduces padding, which increases injury risk and reduces insulation thereby adding to the difficulty in maintaining body temperature as well as disrupting the absorption and distribution of fat soluble pharmaceuticals.[7]

Outward changes of the integumentary system that are noticed include hair and nail change. With the diminished melanin, color transitions to gray. Hair follicle reduction leads to thinning of hair. Rapid or diffuse hair loss may be accelerated with a patient who has cancer or taking pharmaceuticals such as heparin. Hair texture can become coarse and dry as a result of hypothyroidism or protein malnutrition.[5]

Nail changes can also be a good way to identify peripheral circulation and other issues that can affect wound healing. A bluish or purple nail bed can indicate cyanosis but any pale nail bed should be considered as a sign of reduced arterial blood. Slow growing with thick, brittle, or split nails can also indicate peripheral circulation reduction. Nutritional issues can manifest as bands across the nail (protein deficiency), white spots on the nail (zinc deficiency), and spoon-shaped nails (anemia). Unkempt appearance of nails could be a sign of mobility decline and/or visual changes.[9]

When assessing the external factors, the environment has a major impact, indoor and outdoor. Cold winds and low temperatures can cause vasoconstriction of the peripheral vascular system, contributing to dry skin.[10] Chronic ultraviolet or other light exposures can lead to a disorganization of elastin fibers and a reduction of collagen in the dermal extracellular matrix. This leads to a reduction in the skin's resilience and elasticity.[2] This chronic exposure is classified as photoaging and can lead to solar lentigo (liver spots or aging spots) appearing as dark brown flat clusters of macules on the face and hands. This can accumulate and is known as dermatoheliosis. The skin appears dry, leathery, wrinkling with irregular pigmentation. For those who spend a lot of time out in the sun (farmers, sailors), the leathery appearance of the skin is referred to as solar elastosis.[7] Understanding these aging changes can help in identifying other dermatological conditions that can develop as a result of allergies, disease, animal bites, and cancer.

Alcoholism affects the aging skin by dilating small blood vessels in the skin, increasing the blood flow to the skin's surface. These blood vessels can become permanently damaged, leading to flush appearance. This increases the risk to develop pressure ulcers.[8]

Smoking, even second-hand smoke, depletes the body of vitamin C, resulting in dry and wrinkle skin. Smoking also reduces blood flow to the area, increasing the risk of open wounds and delays healing. Since nicotine also binds to hemoglobin, there is reduced oxygen delivered to cells. Insulin resistance can occur in long-term smoking even if diabetes is not present. These effects of smoking increase risk of ulcerations and delayed healing.[8]

Nutrition is a major factor in not only wound healing but in the development of ulcers.[11] Inadequate nutrition can increase the risk of integumentary impairment.[12] Protein malnutrition is common in the aging population, especially those hospitalized, due to appetite decline due to sensory changes in taste and smell, ill-fitting dentures or inadequate dental management, depression due to loss of spouse and reduced socialization, GI changes, and inactivity, leading to a decline in metabolic rate. Lab values of albumin, prealbumin, and transferring need to be considered with wound management.[13] Protein is necessary for cellular repair. The low protein levels (protein malnutrition) have been associated with increased interstitial edema, which decreases the delivery of nutrients to damage tissue and an increase in risk for pressure ulcers and reduced tissue to protect the bony prominences from damaging the skin.[14,15] Comorbidities and pharmaceuticals can impact nutrition due to the many diet restrictions that accompany these.[12] Diet restrictions can then lead to inadequate nutritional needs leading to a diagnosis of Failure to thrive. This is defined as an imbalance of nutrient intake and body needs and leads to a loss of body weight, muscle wasting, poor wound healing, and loss of skin integrity. These body changes make a person at risk for spontaneous wound development and development of chronic wounds/infection. Patients with a 30% loss of lean body mass are at high risk for developing pressure ulcers due to the lack of soft tissue.[14]

Obesity is a risk factor that affects wound healing and has a greater risk for developing pressure ulcers. Many people with obesity are also malnourished, especially related to protein malnutrition. Those who are obese and bedridden for any length of time have greater risk for developing pressure ulcers due to the weight easily exceeding capillary closing especially if laying over bony prominences. Those who are obese and undergo surgery have longer surgery times due to the adipose tissue. This increases the risk for blood loss, decreases tissue perfusion and oxygenation, and increases intra-abdominal pressure from the immobility. Surgical incisions have a greater risk for dehiscence due to the stress on the incisions from the body weight.[16]

Medications can impact wound healing. Aging adults have a greater risk for medication effects on the skin due to the increased risk for multiple comorbidities requiring multiple pharmaceutical interventions. Many of these drugs have adverse effects (independently and as drug-to-drug interactions) that lead the skin to become more friable and susceptible to injury.[17] Some of the most commonly known medications that negatively affect the skin and wound healing are the corticosteroids (prednisone, cortisone, hydrocortisone). These drugs attenuate the inflammatory response, interfere with epidermal regeneration and collagen synthesis, decrease vascular permeability, and have a catabolic effect on bone, ligaments, tendon, and skin.[18] Immunosuppressive agents and antineoplastics both have side effects that include blood and skin disorders. Other drugs that impact wound healing include NSAIDs (aspirin, ibuprofen), COX-2 inhibitors, and disease-modifying antirheumatic drugs (methotrexate, D-penicillamine).[8,19] Many cardiac and psychotropic medications affect wound healing due to the effect on blood volume, cognitive issues, and insulin. Diabetic medications can affect glucose, which in turn affects wound healing.[20]

Systemic or local infection can impact the burden on the wound. While all wounds have some bacteria present, infection is classified as greater than 10^5 organisms/gram of tissue. Early identification of infection and proper classification of the type of bacteria present through culturing are important to avoid overuse of antibacterial agents that could lead to resistive strains.[21,22]

Some of the comorbidities commonly seen in aging adults impact the healing process (independent of the pharmaceuticals used). Any long-standing chronic disease can affect circulatory, nutrition, mobility, and sensation issues, which ultimately impacts the skin. Cardiac, vascular (arterial and venous), and pulmonary diseases can decrease the ability of oxygen to reach the injured area and reduce perfusion, resulting in an inadequate blood supply of nutrients to the wound area.[8,23] Diabetes damages white blood cells as well as damage to the macrovascular systems affects wound healing. The accompany neuropathy can lead to development of wounds. Diabetes can lead to dry skin, anhydrosis, which makes the skin more susceptible to fissures and breaks allowing bacteria to invade.[24] Disease or medication-induced immunosuppression affects collagen synthesis during the proliferation phase and the limited immune cells affect the inflammatory response phase.[8] Many neurological diseases affect the sensory system but also impact the mobility. This inactivity leads to obesity, diabetes, and risk of pressure ulcers. Unrelieved pressure against the skin by bony prominence or external devices contributes to local ischemia and tissue necrosis. Those at greatest risk for pressure ulcers include anyone with limited mobility, decreased sensation including spinal cord injury, stroke, cancer, brain injury, and diabetes.[25]

While incontinence (fecal and urine) is not a normal part of aging, many aging adults have incontinence as a result of comorbidities and medications. The chemical breakdown of the stratum corneum by the urine and feces macerates the skin and softens and separates the epidermal layers. A moist environment has been shown to increase the risk of pressure ulcer by altering the skin's integrity. This also increases the risk of candidiasis, a bacterium that burdens the wound further.[26,27]

Decreased mental status can also be a risk factor for poor wound healing. While cognitive impairments do not directly affect wound healing, an awareness of proper skin care, hygiene, and wound management factors of cleansing, dressing, and positioning is optimal to achieve wound healing. Those with cognitive issues need to be evaluated for identification of assistance necessary to achieve outcomes.

Although the basic wound healing process does not change in aging, the lower physiological reserve with the increased prevalence of risk factors (comorbidities, pharmaceuticals, etc) makes the aging adult more susceptible to delayed wound healing and increases the risk for infection.[6] Overall, wound healing will occur in aging adults but will be slowed/delayed. The aging process results in a delayed healing process up to four times slower than younger adults, but unless other comorbid factors are present, healing will occur. The effect on wound healing can affect all phases.[28] To understand wound healing, a look at the phases in normal healing and how aging and risk factors affect these phases are important.

Hemostasis occurs immediately following an injury to the skin. Platelets and platelet-derived growth factors along with inflammatory mediators come to the area. In aging, there is a marked reduction in cutaneous blood flow and dermal lymphatic drainage, which delays and then prolongs the inflammatory response. The inflammatory phase typically lasts 4 to 6 days and leukocytes (mainly neutrophils) and macrophages accumulate to destroy bacteria in the area. In the aging adult, this phase is delayed, which increases the risk for bacteria overload. The decrease in number and function of the antigen presenting cells also prolongs the inflammatory process. The prolonged inflammatory response can cause an increase in interstitial edema leading to reduction in blood flow through capillaries, which depletes the tissue of oxygen and essential nutrients necessary for the function of leukocytes and fibroblasts. This in turn stalls the wound. In the proliferations phase, granulation is generated to fill the wound. This consists of macrophages, fibroblasts (to stimulate collagen production), immature collagen, blood vessels, and ground substance. The wound begins to decrease in size by contraction of the margin. Because of the slowed cell turnover rate, in the aging adult the tissue regeneration is slowed. Delays in wound healing increase risk of injury and infection. The oxygen-carbon dioxide exchange is decreased due to the poor blood flow and this alters the perfusion rate to the local area. The epithelialization phase (also known as late proliferation phase) is the beginning of reestablishing the skin barrier. Keratinocytes migrate from the wound margins, divide, and become continuous. Matrix metalloproteinases (MMPs), such as collagenase, are important components of this phase. In aging adults, keratinocytes decrease in migration from the basal layer by 50%, which affects wound closure. Protein inhibitors may also be reduced, especially in protein malnutrition. The maturation phase (remodeling) can typically take 6 to 9 months. Collagen fibers are reorganized to improve the skin barrier strength. Fibroblasts, MMPs, and inhibitors of MMPs along with growth factors are needed for this process. Collagen provides tensile strength for the skin, and elastin provides for skin recoil. With aging, there is a reduction/delay in the production of collagen and the tensile strength of the closed wound is reduced, increasing the risk for reinjury. The elastin present with disordered morphology and reduces the integrity even further.[8,28-30]

The added intrinsic and extrinsic factors can add to the wound healing alteration. An understanding of the various lab values for blood tests, cultures, urinalysis, and other medical testing can assist in developing plans of care for effective wound healing.[13,31] The progressive loss of skin function can increase the skin's vulnerability to the environmental stressors and risks. There is an overall decrease in the homeostatic ability associated with aging, especially those with comorbidity issues. The subsequent issues result in a breakdown of normal tissue, impairment in acute wound healing, and predisposition to chronic wounds and infection. This results in poor wound healing, greater risk for infection, and altered inflammatory response.[32,33]

REFERENCES

1. Myer B. *Wound Management: Principles and Practice*. 3rd ed. Upper Saddle River, NJ: Pearson; 2012:411.
2. Irion G. *Comprehensive Wound Management*. 2nd ed. Thorofare, NJ: Slack; 2010: 290-291.
3. Irion G. *Comprehensive Wound Management*. 2nd ed. NJ: Slack; 2010:12-13.
4. Fore-Pflinger J. The epidermal skin barrier: implications for the wound care practitioner, Part II. *Adv Skin Wound Care*. November/December 2004;17(9)480-488.
5. Nigam Y, Knight J. Exploring the anatomy and physiology of ageing: the skin. *Nursing Times*. December 2008;104(49):24-25.
6. Rabbia J. Impaired integumentary repair. In: Guccione A, Wong R, Avers D, eds. *Geriatric Physical Therapy*. 3rd ed. St Louis, MO: Elsevier; 2012:359.
7. Rabbia J. Impaired integumentary repair. In: Guccione A, Wong R, Avers D, eds. *Geriatric Physical Therapy*. 3rd ed. St Louis, MO: Elsevier; 2012:355-356.
8. Myers B. *Wound Management: Principles and Practice*. 3rd ed. NJ: Pearson; 2012:31-33.
9. Irion G. *Comprehensive Wound Management*. 2nd ed. NJ: Slack; 2010:7-8.
10. Myers B. *Wound Management: Principles and Practice*. 3rd ed. NJ: Pearson; 2012:421-422.
11. Dorner B, Posthauer ME, Thomas D; National Pressure Ulcer Advisory Panel. The role of nutrition in pressure ulcer prevention and treatment: National Pressure Ulcer Advisory White Paper. http://www.npuap.org/wp-content/uploads/2012/03/Nutrition-White-Paper-Website-Version.pdf. Accessed June 30, 2015.
12. Rabbia J. Impaired integumentary repair. In: Guccione A, Wong R, Avers D, eds. *Geriatric Physical Therapy*. 3rd ed. St Louis, MO: Elsevier; 2012:360.
13. Hamm R. *Text and Atlas of Wound Diagnosis and Treatment*. New York: McGraw-Hill; 2015:298-299.
14. Hamm R. *Text and Atlas of Wound Diagnosis and Treatment*. New York: McGraw-Hill; 2015:307-308.
15. Myers B. *Wound Management: Principles and Practice*. 3rd ed. NJ: Pearson; 2012:178-181.
16. Hamm R. *Text and Atlas of Wound Diagnosis and Treatment*. New York: McGraw-Hill; 2015:306-307.
17. Wysocki AB. Anatomy and physiology of skin and soft tissue. In: Bryant RA, ed. *Acute and Chronic Wounds: Current Management Concepts*. 3rd ed. St Louis, MO: Mosby; 2007:39-55.
18. Hamm R. *Text and Atlas of Wound Diagnosis and Treatment*. New York: McGraw-Hill; 2015:301-302.
19. Hamm R. *Text and Atlas of Wound Diagnosis and Treatment*. New York: McGraw-Hill; 2015:303-304.
20. Hamm R. *Text and Atlas of Wound Diagnosis and Treatment*. New York: McGraw-Hill; 2015:305-306.
21. Hamm R. *Text and Atlas of Wound Diagnosis and Treatment*. New York: McGraw-Hill; 2015:300-301.
22. Myers B. *Wound Management: Principles and Practice*. 3rd ed. NJ: Pearson; 2012:28-29.
23. Irion G. *Comprehensive Wound Management*. 2nd ed. NJ: Slack; 2010:326.
24. Hamm R. *Text and Atlas of Wound Diagnosis and Treatment*. New York: McGraw-Hill; 2015:194-199.
25. Hamm R. *Text and Atlas of Wound Diagnosis and Treatment*. New York: McGraw-Hill; 2015:305-310.
26. Cakmak S, Gul U, Ozer S, Yigit A, Gonu M. Risk factors for pressure ulcers. *Adv Skin Wound Care*. September 2009;22(9):412-415.
27. Hamm R. *Text and Atlas of Wound Diagnosis and Treatment*. New York: McGraw-Hill; 2015:188.
28. Pittman J. Effects of aging on wound healing: current concepts. *J Wound Ostomy Continence Nurs*. July/August 2007;34(4):412-415.
29. Barr JE. Impaired skin integrity in the elderly. *Ostomy Wound Manage*. 2006;52(5):22-28.
30. Myers B. *Wound Management: Principles and Practice*. 3rd ed. NJ: Pearson; 2012:12-17.
31. Myers B. *Wound Management: Principles and Practice*. 3rd ed. NJ: Pearson; 2012:182-185.
32. Cheung C. Older adults and ulcers: chronic wounds in the geriatric population. *Adv Skin Wound Care*. January 2010;23(1):39-44.
33. Reddy M. Skin and wound care: Important considerations in the older adult. *Adv Skin Wound Care*. 2008;21(9):424-438.

1

SKIN TEAR AND DELAYED WOUND CLOSURE

Rose M. Pignataro, PT, PhD, DPT, CWS

Eric Shamus, PT, DPT, PhD

You have been asked to evaluate an 82-year-old female with a partial thickness wound of the left forearm. The patient reports that the wound occurred approximately 12 hours prior to consultation when she bumped into the armrest of her wheelchair while transferring back to bed. There is no longer any active bleeding at the wound site. Partial thickness damage is evident and the lower layer of the dermis is visible. There is moderate loss of the epidermal flap of approximately 50%.

Past medical history includes chronic obstructive pulmonary disease, inflammatory bowel syndrome, and hiatal hernia. Vital signs are unremarkable: temperature: 98.6°F, RR 16 breaths per minute, HR 76 beats per minute and regular, SpO_2 = 92%, and BP = 134/86 at rest in sitting. The patient's medications include fluticasone (Flovent Diskus) once a day, plus the use of a rescue inhaler (Ventolin) as needed for acute shortness of breath. The patient is independent in transfers and ambulation with use of a wheeled walker, distance limited by aerobic tolerance. The patient is able to walk 310 m (1017 ft) in a 6-Minute Walk Test.

During the course of your assessment, please consider the following questions and their impact on tissue vulnerability and healing based on this patient's medical history and clinical presentation.

■ CASE STUDY QUESTIONS

1. What are some of the physiologic changes involved in aging that make older adults more vulnerable to integumentary injury and delayed healing?

2. Describe the initial processes and cells involved in hemostasis and the acute phases of tissue repair.

3. How would you classify this type of tissue injury? What tool would you use?

4. Relate the classification of this tissue injury to the prognosis for healing.

5. Consider the patient's medical history and medications. Do steroids increase the likelihood of delayed healing?

6. Nutritional intake can have an impact on wound healing. What aspects of this patient's past medical history can affect the likelihood of delayed healing from a nutritional standpoint?

7. Are there any laboratory data that should be considered in identifying possible impediments to recovery?

8. What steps can be taken to assist in wound closure?

9. Explain how principles of moist wound healing may contribute to accelerated tissue repair.

10. Outline a comprehensive plan for preventing these types of tissue injuries from reoccurring.

11. Compared to other 82-year-old women, how is this patient's endurance?

12. Would you make recommendations for an exercise program?

2

DIABETIC FOOT

Rose M. Pignataro, PT, PhD, DPT, CWS

Eric Shamus, PT, DPT, PhD

A 68-year-old male was referred for physical therapy in the home care setting due to a non-healing ulcer on the plantar surface of the left foot. The patient is unable to identify the cause of the ulcer and denies trauma. The wound has been present for more than 6 weeks, is nonpainful, and was initially detected when the patient noticed some light pink drainage when removing his sock. The wound is located near the head of the third metatarsal. There is full-thickness damage revealing a pale wound base with no necrotic tissue or visible debris present within the wound. Wound margins are dry and callused. No drainage or odor is detected.

The patient is afebrile with unremarkable resting vital signs (HR = 80, RR = 16, SpO_2 = 96%, BP = 138/88). Past medical history is significant for DM2, hypertension, and seasonal environmental allergies. His BMI is 41.6. The patient is a retired accountant, does not exercise on a regular basis, and is "fairly" compliant with nutritional recommendations for glycemic control. He smokes approximately ½ ppd (packs per day), and has used tobacco since the age of 16.

Please use the above information as a basis for further research and clinical decision making as you consider the questions below.

■ CASE STUDY QUESTIONS

1. What types of additional medical data should be considered in completing a full patient assessment?

2. How would you evaluate this patient for signs and symptoms of diabetic peripheral neuropathy?

3. What objective tools or measures could be used to assess for diabetic peripheral neuropathy?

4. Does the appearance of this wound correspond with the expected clinical presentation of a diabetic foot ulcer? Relate the wound characteristics to pathophysiologic effects of prolonged hyperglycemia.

5. Given the patient's history, what are the imminent threats to healing?

6. How do lifestyle factors affect the prognosis for recovery? Explain how you would address these using patient education to promote changes in health-related behaviors.

7. What might you expect to find when assessing this person's gait? How might this relate to the location of the wound?

8. What types of dressings or topical agents could be used to facilitate wound closure?

9. How might adjunctive modalities be used to augment the plan of care?

10. Once the wound has been healed, what steps can be taken to prevent future recurrence?

3

PRESSURE ULCER (STAGE 3)

Jill Heitzman, PT, DPT, GCS, NCS, CWS, CEEAA, FACCWS

A 64-year-old African American female was recently hospitalized as a result of a fractured right patella for which she underwent surgical repair via a wire fixation and placed in a knee immobilizer. She was on bedrest for the first 24 hours postsurgery before being discharged to home. Prior to admission, she was using a walker to ambulate and living with her daughter in a two-bedroom first floor apartment. She has a history of type 2 diabetes, hypertension, and a BMI of 30. She presents 1 week later at the physician's office with a wound on the plantar surface of the right heel, which she reports as being warm to touch and painful. The wound is 4 cm × 3 cm and on the proximal edge of the calcaneus. The dermis and subcutaneous tissue are absent with a red wound bed, very minimal exudate, and minimal slough around the edges. The periwound is dry with edges and has even wound margins. Therapy has been requested to treat the wound and begin mobilization.

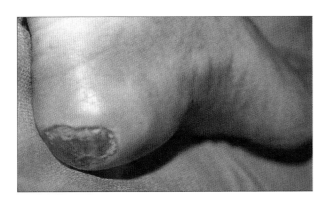

■ CASE STUDY QUESTIONS

1. Why did the ulcer develop on the heel?
2. What are the possible complications of diabetes that may cause additional problems?
3. What risk factors are present with this patient that lead to the development of the ulcer?
4. What tests and measures would have been beneficial to determine this patient's risk for developing pressure ulcers?
5. How is the wound staged as a pressure ulcer?
6. What tests and measures are most appropriate for this patient as a result of the wound and why?
7. From the picture or description, does this wound appear infected? Why or why not?
8. What would be an appropriate wound dressing for this patient?
9. What other interventions should be implemented for this patient?
10. What are the other high-risk areas for pressure ulcers?
11. If the patient is to be up ambulating, what precautions will be needed?

4

DEHISCED SURGICAL WOUND

Jill Heitzman, PT, DPT, GCS, NCS, CWS, CEEAA, FACCWS

A 75-year-old African American male with a history of type 2 diabetes mellitus was referred to outpatient physical therapy (PT) 10 days following a right total knee arthroplasty (TKA). The patient came to the PT wound clinic directly from the orthopedic surgeon's office where the surgical staples had been removed due to dehiscence. The wound was left open to allow healing by secondary intentions. The wound is currently packed with normal saline gauze. The periwound is discolored, painful, and edematous.

Upon examination, the surgical wound is on the anterior aspect of the right knee with discoloration (red, bruising) in the periwound region. The wound bed is red with slough present around the edges (about 25% of the wound) and moderate to heavy exudate is present. The wound is full thickness but bone is not exposed. The knee is edematous and the periwound is red and inflamed. The patient is having difficulty with ambulation using a standard walker demonstrating decreased weight bearing by 25% due to antalgia on the right. The gait pattern also lacks heel strike on the right leg. He was recently prescribed ciprofloxacin (Proquin XR) and is also taking glyburide (DiaBeta), metformin (Glucophage), and naproxen (Naprosyn). His vital signs are HR 74, RR 16, BP 138/88, SpO$_2$ 96%.

■ CASE STUDY QUESTIONS

1. Based on his medication profile, what is the concern with this patient?
2. What does the therapist need to be observing in this patient to prevent a more serious risk from the infection occurring?
3. What is wound dehiscence?
4. What would be the intervention most appropriate for this wound?
5. Why would silver be used as a form of the foam dressing?
6. How is negative pressure wound therapy (NPWT) applied?
7. As the wound is closing, what is he at high risk for developing based on his ethnicity?
8. What are the warning signs of abnormal scarring?
9. How are scars assessed?
10. How can abnormal scarring be treated?
11. What does healing by second intention mean?

5

OPEN WOUND POSTERIOR KNEE

Jill Heitzman, PT, DPT, GCS, NCS, CWS, CEEAA, FACCWS

A 72-year-old female had a right CVA 5 years ago, resulting in left upper and lower extremity weakness. She lives at home with her husband and has been able to walk with a large-based quad cane, a plastic hinged ankle-foot orthosis (AFO), and ADLs were slow but independent. Her history also includes a myocardial infarction (MI) 3 years prior to the stroke, which required a CABG ×2. Her medications since the stroke include propranolol hydrochloride (Inderal) 100 mg bid, verapamil hydrochloride (Calan-SR) 200 mg bid, chlorothiazide (Diuril) 250 mg daily, atorvastatin (Lipitor) 10 mg daily, and alprazolam (Xanax) 0.5 mg tid.

She is coming to physical therapy to improve her walking to get to use a "fancy cane" for their 50th wedding anniversary cruise. She also states that she has been on a diet for this trip too as she wants to lose 50 lb. She has already lost 15 lb. Her current BMI is 34. She reports that approximately 5 days ago she developed dizziness and that any rapid change in position would bring on the dizziness. She contacted her family physician who prescribed meclizine hydrochloride (Antivert) 25 mg daily. Her vital signs are HR 74, RR 18, BP 148/84, SpO$_2$ 97%. She is noted to have the wound on the back of her left knee as noted in the picture.

had complaints of paresthesia and pain distal to the injury and diminished dorsal pedis and posterior tibialis pulses. The physician performed an emergency fasciotomy and packed the wound with saline moistened gauze to be changed three times per day (tid). He was put on IV antibiotics, anti-inflammatories, and hydrocodone.

The patient's medical history includes type 2 diabetes mellitus with medications of sliding scale insulin and oral hypoglycemic medication. He is referred to physical therapy (PT) on day 3 of the hospitalization in preparation for him to go home on oral antibiotics and Bactrim DS. This patient has only been transferring to bedside chair and commode prior to PT being ordered. His pain is poorly controlled and he is unable to put weight on the RLE without excruciating pain. The patient is anxious as he reports this is planting season and he needs to get back to work. Upon dressing removal, the wound is beefy red, granulating, and has a moderate amount of drainage.

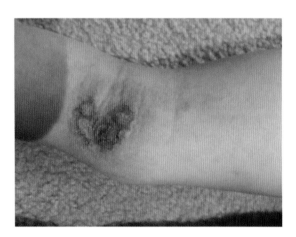

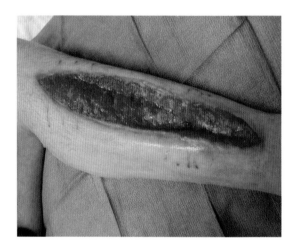

 CASE STUDY QUESTIONS

1. What are the medical issues related to this case?
2. What are the medication issues related to this case?
3. How could her losing weight on the diet have played an issue in the current status of dizziness?
4. What else could be a factor in the dizziness complaints?
5. What could be the causes of the wound noted in the picture?
6. What tests and measures need to be performed prior to intervention?
7. How would this wound be classified?
8. What wound dressings would be most appropriate?
9. What are the education issues needed in relation to the AFO?
10. Are there other referrals needed for this patient?

 CASE STUDY QUESTIONS

1. What are the concerns for activity that are needed to be addressed?
2. What factors are going to affect the healing of this wound?
3. What major risk concerns are present?
4. What interventions are needed besides wound care?
5. What weight bearing status would the PT plan of care if the physician has ordered WBAT?
6. What services would be appropriate for this patient after discharge?
7. Is the saline moistened dressing tid a realistic dressing for this patient once discharged?
8. What patient education is needed for this patient at home?
9. Is he at risk for a deep venous thrombosis (DVT)? How would this be determined?
10. Discuss the relationship between using Bactrim DS and insulin.

6

FASCIOTOMY

Jill Heitzman, PT, DPT, GCS, NCS, CWS, CEEAA, FACCWS

A 62-year-old farmer was admitted to the hospital as a result of a farm machine accident to the right lower extremity (RLE), below the knee. The right calf had an area of 12 cm × 6 cm, which was red, warm, and hard to touch. Edema was noted as 4+. The patient

7

SKIN TEAR

Jill Heitzman, PT, DPT, GCS, NCS, CWS, CEEAA, FACCWS

An 83-year-old female is referred to you in home health following a surgical procedure for an open reduction, internal fixation (ORIF) as a result of a fractured right femur from a fall at home. She is noted to have an open wound on her hand (see below). She says she hit her hand on her dresser that morning when getting dressed. She self-applied a self-adhesive bandage to the area. Her medications include atenolol, Celebrex, Femiron, Levoxyl, fluoxetine, Lipitor, Lotensin, and omeprazole. She is also reporting increased pain in her hip with walking toe-touch weight bearing on the right using a standard walker. The incisional line of the hip is fiery red with induration, no drainage, and fever in the periwound region. The incision is held in place with staples.

The patient is alert, oriented but only able to one-step commands. Her strength is grossly 4+/5 except for the right hip, which is painful with active movement. She has a slight kyphosis, which limits shoulder flexion to 155° bilaterally. Otherwise ROM is within normal limits except for left hip extension, which is 0°, and bilateral dorsiflexion, which is 5°. Right hip ROM was not measured secondary to pain and recent surgery. Vital signs are HR 72, RR 17, BP 136/82, SpO$_2$ 96%, temp 98.9°F. Sensation to light touch is intact. She is only able to ambulate 20 ft before stopping due to the pain in her hip, which is rated as 8/10 on a verbal analog scale.

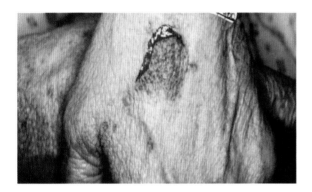

■ CASE STUDY QUESTIONS

1. What are the aging issues that make her at a greater risk for the skin tear?

2. How does aging issues affect healing?

3. What is the risk of using an adhesive Band-Aid on this wound?

4. How would this hand wound be classified according to the Payne-Martin Classification for Skin Tears?

5. What is the most appropriate dressing for this skin tear?

6. Based on the presentation of this patient, what else is present?

7. How do you determine if there is a systemic or local infection?

8. What could have been the cause of her hitting the dresser?

9. How do the pharmaceuticals in this case affect the physical therapy plan of care?

10. What other interventions are indicated for this patient based on her original diagnosis?

8

BURN: ARM

Jill Heitzman, PT, DPT, GCS, NCS, CWS, CEEAA, FACCWS

A 71-year-old male was working in his yard burning leaves 3 days ago. The fire got out of control and his shirt caught fire with him sustaining a partial thickness burn to his right arm. He had gone to

the ER where he was given 1% silver sulfadiazine and the arm was wrapped in gauze. He was given a prescription of hydrocodone at that time and was referred to physical therapy.

He lives and functions independently in the community and lives in a single-story home with his wife who is dependent on her husband for IADL and most ADL care following a stroke last year. The patient has no chronic diseases and only takes one 81 mg aspirin per day. His vital signs at rest are HR 72, BP 124/78, RR 15, SpO$_2$ 99%. Sensation to light touch is intact distal to the wound.

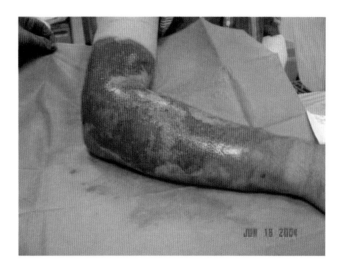

JUN 18 2004

■ CASE STUDY QUESTIONS

1. How is this burn classified?

2. What is the risk of using silver sulfadiazine?

3. What is the risk of taking hydrocodone?

4. How will this injury affect function?

5. What are the issues that need to be considered regarding home health or skilled placement?

6. What treatment intervention is most appropriate for this wound?

7. What dressings are most appropriate?

8. What are the risks involved with this patient?

9. What education needs does he have at this time and postdischarge?

10. Will this patient require extra fluids? If so, how much?

11. What specific diet recommendations should be made?

12. What other interventions besides wound management are needed?

9

PLANTAR WOUND

Jill Heitzman, PT, DPT, GCS, NCS, CWS, CEEAA, FACCWS

A 71-year-old white male has had a history of digital amputation of his right fourth and fifth digits as a result of type 2 diabetes mellitus and hypertension. He had a 52-year history of 1 pack per day smoking, but quit after his amputations 2 years ago. He has been taking insulin regular (Novolin R), metformin (Glucophage), lisinopril (Zestril), and mannitol (Osmitrol). His blood sugar levels have been averaging 180 mg/dL for the last few months. He states he has had a callous on his foot for about 2½ months but got concerned when he noticed blood on his socks one evening. He went to the emergency room where it was determined he had a *Staphylococcus aureus* infection, was prescribed cefuroxime (Ceftin) via IV, and admitted. He is now being seen in acute care for wound management.

His lab values are: Hgb = 11.0 g/dL, Hct = 31%, WBC = 13000/μL, platelets = 13000/μL, random blood glucose = 300 mg/dL, urine glucose = negative, x-ray = old fracture but negative for current fracture or osteomyelitis. His BMI is 31. Vital signs are HR 80, RR 18, BP 144/92, SpO$_2$ 98%, temp 99.7°F.

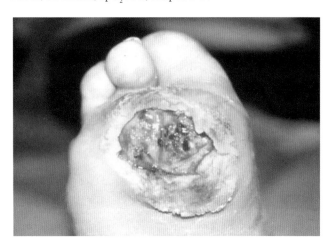

■ CASE STUDY QUESTIONS

1. What do his lab values indicate?

2. What tests and measures are needed to be performed?

3. How do you test for sensation?

4. How would you test for circulation?

5. What gait pattern would you expect to see him utilize and what would be recommended for gait?

6. What are his risk factors for developing this wound and future wounds?

7. What is uncontrolled diabetes?

8. What will affect wound healing for this patient?

9. What wound classification scales would be appropriate to utilize with this patient?

10. What would the wound bed preparation (wound care) consist of?

11. What is the progression of the wound interventions?

12. What preventative risk tool can be used on this patient to determine future interventions?

13. What would be implemented once the wound closes?

10

PSEUDOMONAS

Jill Heitzman, PT, DPT, GCS, NCS, CWS, CEEAA, FACCWS

An 82-year-old patient has been coming to the wound clinic for open wounds on his both medial and lateral malleoli of the left lower extremity (LLE). He has swelling that is off and on

in the LE and significant moisture in the surrounding area. He has reported he has not walked as much as he used to due to the heavy sensation and aching with walking especially at the end of the day. The patient has been receiving multilayer gauze dressings two times a week. Today upon removal of the dressings he presents with greenish-colored drainage and a fruity odor is noticed. His toenails are bluish-green in color. The therapist suspects *Pseudomonas* and calls the physician. The physician orders a swab culture. During the conversation, orders are also received to use electrical stimulation.

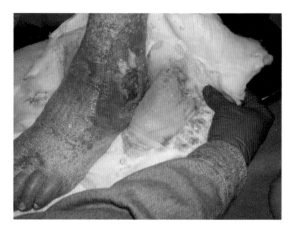

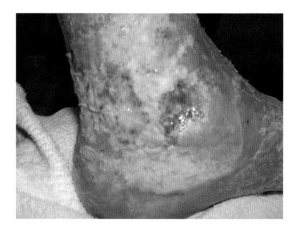

■ CASE STUDY QUESTIONS

1. What do you know about *Pseudomonas* presentation?

2. What is a possibility that the *Pseudomonas* developed?

3. How is a culture performed on this wound?

4. What is the *most* likely primary underlying condition for this patient?

5. How would you classify this wound?

6. What type of dressings will need to be applied at this time?

7. How would you utilize a multilayer dressing system if the ABI was found to be 0.8 and he had strong pulses?

8. Due to the chronic nature of this wound, the therapist discussed with the physician the use of electrical stimulation. What considerations are needed to apply electrical stimulation?

9. The physician decides to order a silver-impregnated gauze for the dressing. How will this affect the electrical stimulation usage?

10. What other education is needed for this patient?

11

END OF LIFE SKIN FAILURE

Jill Heitzman, PT, DPT, GCS, NCS, CWS, CEEAA, FACCWS

A 72-year-old male with pulmonary fibrosis developed pneumonia and was admitted to the hospital. He subsequently was determined to be at end-stage pulmonary fibrosis and was admitted to hospice care. Despite regular repositioning by the nurses, the patient developed the skin condition in the sacral area as shown in the picture and this developed quickly over a 24-hour period.

Vital signs are HR 88, RR 30 on 5 L O_2 nasal, BP 144/68, SpO_2 90%, temp 99.5°F. The patient has limitations in ROM throughout, gross muscle strength of 3/5, in nonambulatory, and requires maximal assistance for transfers and bed mobility.

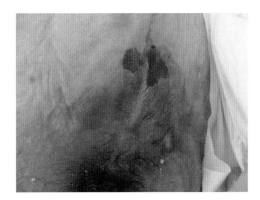

■ CASE STUDY QUESTIONS

1. What is this condition called?
2. Why did this ulcer develop?
3. What are the criteria for hospice according to Medicare rules?
4. What services are allowed under hospice?
5. How does the diagnosis of pulmonary fibrosis affect healing of this condition?
6. What is palliative care?
7. How does palliative care relate to this wound?
8. What are the most important considerations for wound management in this case?
9. What can increase the risk of further deterioration in this case based on the location and medical condition?
10. What other issues are at risk for developing in this patient and how can they be addressed?

12

SKIN RASH

Jill Heitzman, PT, DPT, GCS, NCS, CWS, CEEAA, FACCWS

A 61-year-old female comes to physical therapy with an open wound on the leg, as shown in the picture. She states she was playing at the park with her grandson and the next day the rash developed. She complains of itching and burning sensation that started about 2 days later. She reports no other medical history and only takes vitamins, calcium supplements, but is allergic to sulfa.

Vital signs are HR 78, RR 18, BP 136/82, SpO_2 98%, temp 98.7°F.

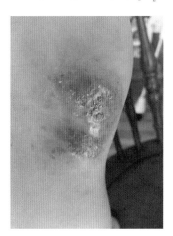

■ CASE STUDY QUESTIONS

1. What is the most likely cause of this wound?
2. How do you differentiate between the various potential diagnostic conditions including eczema, dermatitis, psoriasis, and vasculitis?
3. Does the itching onset give you more information to differentiate the diagnosis?
4. Does her allergy have any impact on the wound management plan of care?
5. What phase of healing is this patient presenting?
6. What is the risk as the wound heals, especially if she has darker pigmented skin?
7. What is the best management for this wound?
8. How would you rule out an underlying venous issue being present?
9. How do you distinguish an acute episode from a chronic episode?
10. Are there any pharmaceuticals that would benefit this patient?

13

TRAUMATIC WOUND

Jill Heitzman, PT, DPT, GCS, NCS, CWS, CEEAA, FACCWS

A 69-year-old male was injured at work when a cable fell on his arm. The x-ray is negative for fracture. However, upon return to the physician 4 days later, he had a large open hematoma with necrotic tissue covering the hematoma. The physician ordered blood tests and his PT was 15 seconds and INR was 1.5. Coumadin-induced necrosis was suspected so Coumadin was discontinued until after the wound is healed and this patient was prescribed a 6-day course of prednisone. He is referred to your outpatient wound clinic for debridement and pulsatile lavage.

During the initial evaluation, you discover he had been on warfarin (Coumadin) due to having had a mild myocardial infarction 2 years ago, which he describes "being no big deal." During conversation with him, you discover he eats highly garlic seasoned foods on a daily basis and does not take his medication regularly. However, he did report he had taken some Advil after the injury due to the pain and swelling. He now reports some paresthesia in his hand and fingers and has had increased pain in his arm with a feeling of pressure in his wound area but is very hypersensitive to touch. He reports that he has to continue to work due to personal and family issues. His BP is 135/84, HR: 82 beats per minute, RR: 26, SpO₂ 99%.

His left arm was not tested for strength and ROM due to the acuteness of the wound, but other extremities have normal strength and ROM.

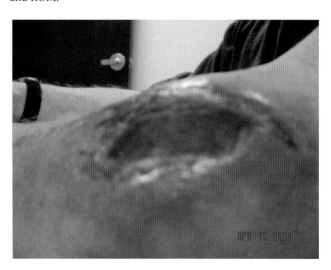

■ CASE STUDY QUESTIONS

1. Why is Coumadin prescribed?

2. What do his PT and INR indicate?

3. What impact does his history profile have on the effects of Coumadin?

4. What is Coumadin-induced necrosis (CIN)?

5. What were the most likely causes of CIN developing?

6. What were some of the symptoms that lead to the diagnosis?

7. How is a 6-day course of Prednisone administered?

8. Why was Prednisone prescribed?

9. What impact does this diagnosis have on the chosen intervention?

10. What type of intervention is appropriate for this patient?

11. What type of dressing is appropriate?

12. What education needs are appropriate for this patient once the wound is healed?

13. Are there any other foods that could affect the use of Coumadin?

14

DIFFERENTIATION OF TWO WOUNDS

Jill Heitzman, PT, DPT, GCS, NCS, CWS, CEEAA, FACCWS

An 80-year-old male of Hispanic decent is a resident of the long-term care facility as a result of left cerebral vascular accident (CVA middle cerebral artery) with resultant right hemiparesis

occurring 8 weeks ago. Past medical history includes a fractured left hip 2 years ago with resultant total hip arthroplasty (THA), chronic cough, hypertension, and gastroesophageal reflux disease (GERD). His medications include calcium, multivitamins, warfarin (Coumadin), omeprazole (Prilosec), atenolol (Tenormin), and using a Alka-Seltzer Heartburn relief regularly. He has a 40-year history of 1 to 2 packs of cigarettes/day. His BMI is 32. His Braden Scale is 12/23 and has open areas on his buttocks as shown in the picture. He also is noted to have the open areas on his right lower leg and lateral malleoli. His vital signs include BP: 172/92, HR: 110 beats per minute, RR: 15 breaths per minute, SpO₂: 91%.

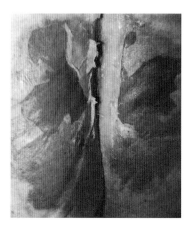

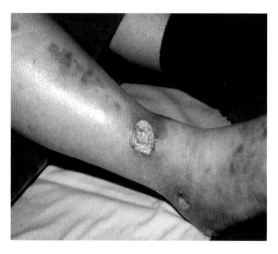

■ CASE STUDY QUESTIONS

1. What does the Braden Scale indicate?

2. What is the difference between the Braden, Norton, and Gosnell Scales for assessing pressure ulcer risk?

3. How would the buttock wound be classified?

4. What was the risk of this wound developing?

5. What condition could be present to have led to the leg ulcer indicate?

6. What test and measure would you utilize to determine if the leg ulcer is due to this other condition?

7. How would you document the leg wounds?

8. What risk factors does he have present that would affect healing?

9. How do the medications he is taking affect healing?

10. Due to his history, what other conditions will affect his PT interventions?

15

BACK PAIN AND LESIONS

Jill Heitzman, PT, DPT, GCS, NCS, CWS, CEEAA, FACCWS

A 67-year-old African American male comes to physical therapy with complaints of low back pain (LBP) of 1 week duration with increased tingling and pain on the right side of his trunk over the last 3 days. His past medical history included type 2 diabetes mellitus and hypertension. He reports taking oxycodone (Percodan) for pain relief and propranolol (Inderal LA) for his hypertension. He states the diabetes is controlled through his diet and oral glyburide (DiaBeta). His glucose levels have been at 124 mg/dL and the HbA1c at 6%. However, he reports this morning his glucose level was at 210 mg/dL, which has him concerned. During the interview, you notice pruritic lesions of various stages of vesicles, ulcerations, and dryness along the T11-T12 dermatomes on the right side. His vital signs are: BP 146/84, HR 88 beats per minute, RR 20 breaths per minute.

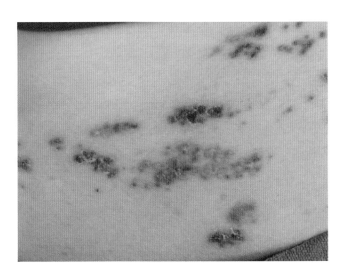

■ CASE STUDY QUESTIONS

1. What is most likely new problem present with this patient?
2. What other medical conditions could have a similar clinical presentation?
3. What question would be most indicative to differentiate this condition from other dermatological conditions?
4. Discuss the etiology progression of this new condition.
5. What is of the utmost importance regarding this patient and the wider community?
6. What do you need to consider if you plan to continue treating him for his LBP?
7. How are these wounds managed?
8. What does his medical history tell you that he is most at risk for developing as the lesions resolve?
9. What is a potential treatment to assist this patient with postlesion (long-term) issues?
10. One of the medications to treat the condition is prednisone. What long-term effects can this drug have on this patient?

16

PRESSURE ULCER

Jill Heitzman, PT, DPT, GCS, NCS, CWS, CEEAA, FACCWS

A 78-year-old female who lives alone in her home of 52 years fractured her right lower leg (tibia and fibula) falling down stairs at home. She was found the next day by her son and brought to the emergency department. An external fixation device was applied to the lower leg by the orthopedic surgeon and she was placed on bedrest for 5 days due to developing bacterial pneumonia. She was treated with azithromycin (Zithromax) and put on 2 L of nasal oxygen. She is in acute care hospital setting and is referred to physical therapy to begin mobility training. Her medications include benazepril (Lotensin), Humulin 70/30, meperidine (Demerol) via a patient-controlled analgesic (PCA) infusion pump. She is unable to move independently in bed due to the appliance on her lower leg. She has pain complaints of 8/10 in the lower leg with movement. Upon turning the patient, the patient is noted to have intact nonblanchable reddened areas as shown in the picture. Her BP is 106/90, HR is 92 beats per minute, RR is 20 breaths per minute, SpO_2 is 94% at rest off the oxygen, and temp is 99.7°F.

Prior to the fall she lived independently in the community and ambulated independently without an assistive device. Strength and ROM of the noninjured extremities are within normal limits. Sensation to light touch is diminished in the soles of both feet. She is alert and oriented to self, place, and time.

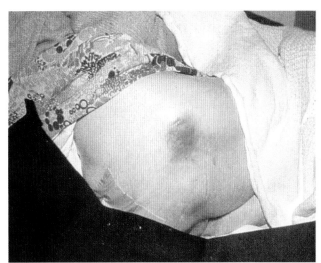

■ CASE STUDY QUESTIONS

1. How would this wound be classified?
2. What risk factors were present for the wound to occur?
3. What do her medications tell you about her underlying conditions?
4. What are some of the signs and symptoms of bacterial pneumonia?
5. What risks did she have to develop bacterial pneumonia?
6. Once Physical therapy begins, what is she at risk for developing and how would you determine this?
7. What is a PCA pump?
8. What is the therapist's role in the PCA pump?

9. How would this wound be addressed?

10. How do you determine post-acute care placement?

11. If this patient's goal is ultimately to go home, what environmental issues need to be addressed based on the causative factor of the fall?

10. What interventions would be indicated for the wound?

11. Based on the presentation of back pain and leg symptoms, what also could be present?

12. What other tests and measures would be indicated?

13. What other interventions are needed by PT?

14. Are there any referrals indicated for this patient?

17

FOOT DEFORMITY

Jill Heitzman, PT, DPT, GCS, NCS, CWS, CEEAA, FACCWS

An 80-year-old female is in a nursing home with a diagnosis of Alzheimer disease and has comorbidities of gout, hypertension, osteoarthritis, and atrial fibrillation. Her medications are: furosemide (Lasix) 80 mg daily, haloperidol (Haldol) 5 mg at bedtime, allopurinol (Aloprim) 300 mg daily, warfarin (Coumadin) 5 mg daily, Tylenol 325 mg every 6 hours as needed for pain. She has developed a urinary incontinence with resultant urinary tract infection three times in the last 6 months for which she was prescribed darifenacin (Enablex). She recently started using a rolling walker and requires assistance for mobility. The nursing home staff has reported the patient has fallen three times in the past week. She has complaints of back pain that increases with breathing, weakness in her legs, and cramping at night. Upon removal of her shoes, the therapist notes a wound on the top of the second digit on the left foot. She is noted to 3+ pitting edema in the left foot. Her resting vital signs are: BP 162/92, HR 100 beats per minute, RR 34 breaths per minute and shallow, SpO_2 94%.

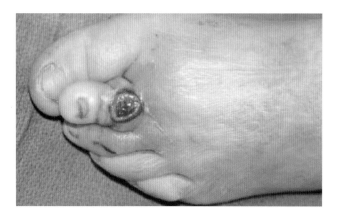

■ CASE STUDY QUESTIONS

1. What is the risk of Lasix on this patient?

2. What is the risk for this patient of each of the medications?

3. What is the risk of Aloprim on this patient?

4. What is the risk of Coumadin on this patient?

5. What is the risk of Enablex on this patient?

6. What else could be the cause of the urinary incontinence in this patient?

7. How would you describe her foot?

8. What most likely caused the wound?

9. What would be the tests and measures needed for this patient regarding her wound?

18

TISSUE INJURY

Jill Heitzman, PT, DPT, GCS, NCS, CWS, CEEAA, FACCWS

A 70-year-old female who lives in her daughter's home is referred to physical therapy for strengthening and mobility. She has the wound as shown in the picture on the left malleoli. Her history includes rheumatoid arthritis, type 2 DM, neuropathy, nephropathy, hypertension, and arteriosclerosis. She had a cardiac stent placement 2 years ago and a transient ischemic attack (TIA) 3 years ago. Her medications include insulin aspart (NovoLog), metformin (Glucophage), chlorothiazide (Diuril), propranolol (Inderal LA), warfarin (Coumadin), gabapentin (Neurontin), and prednisone. She has fallen two times in the last 3 months, requiring her daughter's assistance to get up off the floor. She has been recently wearing a plastic solid insert ankle-foot orthosis (AFO) for the month. Her vital signs are: BP 152/88, HR 92/min, respiration 28/min, SpO_2 96%.

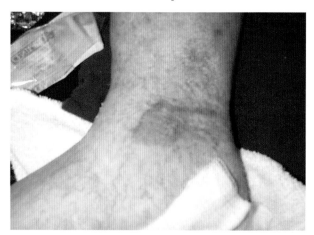

■ CASE STUDY QUESTIONS

1. What type of wound is present in this patient?

2. What could be the cause of this wound?

3. What medications would most affect wound healing?

4. What would be the reason for the AFO usage based on her medical history?

5. What is the intervention for this wound?

6. What other tests and measures are needed for this patient?

7. How would you determine if she needs an assistive device to ambulate?

8. What home issues need to be evaluated?

9. What do her comorbidities indicate with regard to future risks?

10. What is proper diabetic foot care?

11. What other education is needed for this patient?

19

BURN: LOWER LEG

Jill Heitzman, PT, DPT, GCS, NCS, CWS, CEEAA, FACCWS

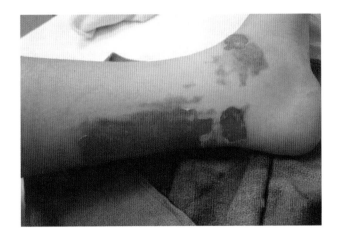

A 75-year-old female, who has been taking warfarin (Coumadin) and chlorothizide (Diuril) for her cardiac condition, lost her spouse to cancer 1 year ago. The patient's daughter reported to the physician that she had noted frequent episodes of crying by her mother and a continued withdrawal from all of her social activities. The doctor prescribed lorazepam (Ativan) for this problem. Within 6 months, the woman was no longer able to care for herself, often forgetting her meals, medications, and even who the family members were. She moved in with her daughter and the physician prescribed donepezil (Aricept).

She is now admitted to the hospital 3 months later with burns on the plantar surface of her left foot (not pictured), ankle, and over the Achilles tendon. She has been referred by her physician to physical therapy to increase her mobility. The daughter has reported that her mother had made her own bath water and gotten into the tub even though the water was too hot. The patient was prescribed hydrocodone + acetaminophen (Lortab) on admission. Her vital signs are: BP 162/80, HR 90 beats per minute, RR 16 breaths per minute, SpO$_2$ 96%, temp 98.6°F.

Her strength and ROM are grossly within normal limits except for the left ankle, which is painful with active or passive movement in any direction. Sensation to light touch is intact.

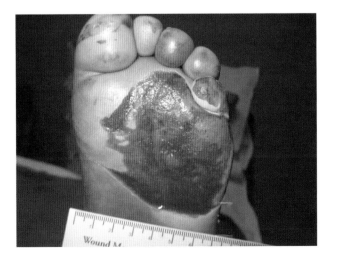

Wound M

■ CASE STUDY QUESTIONS

1. How is this wound classified?
2. How is this wound size determined?
3. What cardiac issues are present in this case based on the medications?
4. What is Ativan prescribed for?
5. What is Aricept prescribed for?
6. What is Lortab?
7. What social issues are present in this case?
8. What impact does the medications have on this case?
9. What referrals are needed for this patient and caregivers?
10. Was donepezil an appropriate medication for this patient's condition?
11. What risks are present in this patient?
12. What treatment is most appropriate for this patient's wounds?
13. How can physical therapy proceed with the physician orders?
14. What other physical therapy interventions should be provided?
15. What other medical interventions are needed?
16. What considerations are needed regarding her discharge placement?

20

BUTTOCKS ULCERS

Jill Heitzman, PT, DPT, GCS, NCS, CWS, CEEAA, FACCWS

You are providing home health care in a rural area. You arrive at the new patient's home 30 minutes earlier than scheduled. You notice the door is wide open so you knock while announcing who you are. You hear a soft "come in" and enter the home. The patient is home alone sitting slouched in a wheelchair leaning over the left arm rest and looking out the window.

The patient is an 82-year-old female and has comorbidities of right cerebral vascular accident (CVA) secondary to a brain tumor which was surgically excised. She has left hemiplegia as a result of the CVA. She was discharged against medical advice from a rehabilitation care setting 3 weeks ago upon her husband's insistence. The husband had refused home health care for therapy until recently when the patient's daughter from out of town called in to request services. According to the medical records at the time of discharge, the patient required 24-hour care. During the therapist's visit, this patient appears anxious and keeps looking over to the window. She transfers to the bed from the wheelchair with maximal assistance of 1. You notice an odor of feces and upon rolling the patient to her side, there is new and old fecal material present and the buttocks are as shown in the picture. Vital signs are: BP 110/70, HR 64 beats per minute, RR 32 breaths per minute, SpO$_2$ 97%, temp 99.2°F.

The patient is alert and oriented to person, time, and place. She has a flaccid left upper extremity and proximal left lower extremity strength of 2/5 grossly in the hip and knee. Sitting balance is poor as she is unable to remain upright without trunk support. Sensation to light touch is absent on the left, present on the right. DTRs are 2+ on the right 0 on the left.

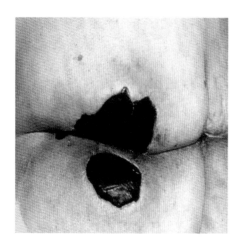

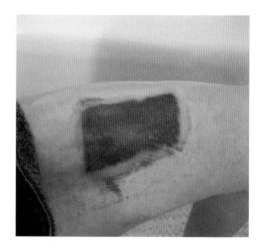

■ CASE STUDY QUESTIONS

1. How would you classify this wound?
2. What are the risk factors leading to this wound?
3. What are the pressure ulcer risk assessment scales that should be utilized?
4. What is the most appropriate treatment for this wound?
5. What are the key factors for preventing pressure ulcers?
6. What is the Pressure Ulcer Scale for Healing?
7. What is the Bates-Jensen Wound Assessment Tool and how does this compare to the PUSH?
8. What other issues are present in this case?
9. What is the therapist's responsibility in this case?
10. What referrals are needed for this patient?

■ CASE STUDY QUESTIONS

1. What is a CD4+ count?
2. What does the CD4+ count level of this patient indicate?
3. What does his pharmaceutical profile indicate?
4. What type of lesion was most likely present to require the surgery?
5. What does the health care provider need to know regarding spread of this disease?
6. Why is a skin graft utilized?
7. What are the steps of healing for a skin graft?
8. What are the various forms of skin grafts? How are they classified?
9. What type of graft is presented in this wound?
10. What are the risks for graft failure?
11. What type of dressing intervention could be done in this case?
12. How could a negative pressure wound therapy system be used on the graft site?
13. What treatment is appropriate for the donor site?
14. What other interventions are needed for this patient?
15. What educational needs are appropriate for this patient?

21

WOUND WITH HIV

Jill Heitzman, PT, DPT, GCS, NCS, CWS, CEEAA, FACCWS

The 70-year-old patient developed a cutaneous purple nodular lesion on the posterior aspect of his calf that kept getting larger. This was surgically removed. A skin graft was applied with the skin taken from the patient's thigh used as a donor site. His goal is to return to bicycle riding. Six months ago his CD4+ count was 525 cells/mm³, and his last CD4+ was 300 cells/mm³. His vital signs are as follows: BP: 138/80, HR: 76 beats per minute, RR: 24 breaths per minute. His medication profile following surgery includes Atripla, lithium (Lithobid), and hydrocortisone (Cortef).

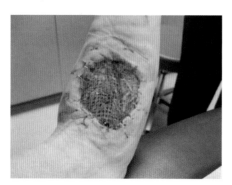

22

LYMPHEDEMA: PART 1

Jill Heitzman, PT, DPT, GCS, NCS, CWS, CEEAA, FACCWS

A 70-year-old male is working part-time as a janitor in an elementary school. He is referred for treatment of his open wounds on the left lower extremity. Upon the initial visit, he is noted to have open draining wounds with slough present on the medial aspect of his left lower calf. He reports he has had wounds on his legs off and on for years. He is noted to have edema with lipodermatosclerosis present bilaterally and reports some swelling in his groin. His medication profile includes furosemide (Lasix), amlodipine (Norvasc), and baby aspirin. His doctor recently prescribed amoxicillin (Amoxil). His medical history includes hypertension and he had surgery for prostate cancer 5 years ago.

His BP is 168/90, HR 100 beats per minute, RR 32 breaths per minute and shallow. ROM of the ankle is limited from 3° dorsiflexion to 18° plantar flexion, otherwise within normal limits. Strength is 4/5 in the ankle and 5/5 throughout the rest of the extremities. Sensation is diminished to light touch in the left lower extremity. He ambulates without any assistive device but states as the day wears on his leg gets tired and he has to do a lot of leaning on the cleaning equipment.

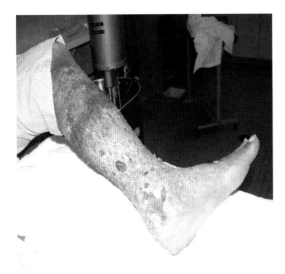

CASE STUDY QUESTIONS

1. What is lipodermatosclerosis?
2. What causes the lipodermatosclerosis?
3. How is his job affecting this chronic condition?
4. How is his pharmaceutical profile affecting the condition?
5. What conditions are present to lead to the presentation seen in this lower extremity?
6. What tests and measures will you utilize for the chronic condition?
7. What is the Stemmer sign?
8. How is this lymphedema classified?
9. What is the treatment needed for this patient?
10. Discuss the pros and cons of using a whirlpool with this patient?
11. Discuss the use of a pneumatic compression pump on this patient?
12. What will need to be provided prior to discharging this patient?

23

LYMPHEDEMA: PART 2

Jill Heitzman, PT, DPT, GCS, NCS, CWS, CEEAA, FACCWS

A 65-year-old female is 12 months postoperative for a left modified radical mastectomy. She underwent both chemotherapy and radiation therapy, which were completed 4 months ago. She is referred to your clinic due to severe edematous left upper extremity. Brawny tissue is palpated in the upper arm. She reports having some blistering and skin peeling right after completion of the radiation therapy but that resolved. She is currently taking Tamoxifen. Her vital signs include: BP 140/84, HR 82 beats per minute, RR 24 breaths per minute, temp 98.6°F.

Her left upper extremity is 4 cm greater in circumferential measurements than the right. Her shoulder range of motion is decreased in flexion and abduction by 30°. Strength is normal except for shoulder motions, which is 4/5, and elbow movements, which is 4/5. She reports some transient numbness and tingling in her left hand and fingers. She also complains that she is easily fatigued trying to complete her household chores.

CASE STUDY QUESTIONS

1. What happens during a modified radical mastectomy?
2. What are the risks of developing breast cancer?
3. How is breast cancer staged?
4. What is chemotherapy?
5. What effects does radiation have on the skin?
6. What is brawny tissue?
7. Why does edema form in the affected UE?
8. How do the pharmaceuticals used for the chemotherapy (as well as her current medication) impact this patient?
9. What is complete decongestive therapy (CDT)?
10. What phase of CDT would this patient be in at this time?
11. What exercises are appropriate to assist lymphatic flow?
12. What type of bandaging is needed during phase 1?
13. How is a customized garment fitted?
14. What other interventions are needed?
15. What is she at risk for developing?
16. What education is needed for this patient before discharge?

24

SKIN CANCER

Jill Heitzman, PT, DPT, GCS, NCS, CWS, CEEAA, FACCWS

A 66-year-old male, with no other medical issues, had noticed an unusual change in the appearance of a lesion around an abnormal mole following a bug bite on the posterior calf. He went to his physician who subsequently performed an excisional biopsy. The pathology report indicated he had squamous cell carcinoma and the physician injected interferon alfa-2b (Intron A) into the open area a week later. The area is presenting with slough and swelling as shown in the picture. He reported that he had burned his legs about 20 years ago while burning leaves, which resulted in a skin graft.

His BP is 140/80, HR 82 beats per minute, RR 25 breaths per minute, SpO₂ 98%, temp 98.5°F. Strength and ROM are normal. Sensation to light touch is intact, all DTRs are 2+. What does a physical therapist need to know about skin lesions?

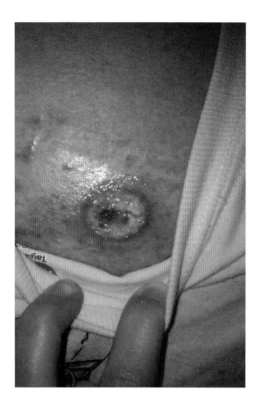

CASE STUDY QUESTIONS

1. What changes in appearance would have indicated the need to see the doctor?

2. What is the acronym to assist educating the public to assist in self-assessment of skin lesions?

3. What other conditions could be present from abnormal skin color?

4. What are the different forms of skin cancer?

5. What are the risks for developing skin cancer?

6. What is an excisional biopsy?

7. How are skin cancers staged?

8. What should the patient look for on the rest of his skin?

9. What is the risk of this patient developing a Marjolin ulcer?

10. Why was Intron A injected into the lesion?

11. What are the various forms of treatment for squamous cell carcinoma?

12. How would you describe this wound?

13. What interventions are appropriate for this wound?

25

PERIPHERAL ARTERY DISEASE (PAD)

Jill Heitzman, PT, DPT, GCS, NCS, CWS, CEEAA, FACCWS

A 71-year-old retired male lives alone in his own trilevel home and drives himself daily to the community center for senior activities that include lunches, billiards, cards, and gardening. He is referred to physical therapy following a percutaneous transluminal angioplasty and stent placement. The incisional wound has dehisced along the lateral aspect of the calf and the physician has ordered a negative pressure wound therapy system (wound VAC) for this patient.

Foot wounds that would not heal. He had smoked a pack of cigarettes each day prior to surgery and reports he is now down to a pack lasting him 3 days. He is taking albuterol (AccuNeb), tiotropium (Spiriva), digoxin (Lanoxin), benazepril (Lotensin), simvastatin (Zocor), furosemide (Lasix), and spironolactone (Aldactone). He recently was put on clopidogrel (Plavix), acetaminophen + oxycodone (Percocet), and levofloxacin (Levaquin). His BMI is 32. His right leg is swollen compared to the left and 2+ pitting edema. His vital signs are: BP 168/90, HR 92 beats per minute, RR 28 breaths per minute and shallow, SaO$_2$ 96% via pulse oximetry, temp 98.8°F. His right ABI is 0.6. The patient states that if the wound does not heal, he has been told he will have to have an amputation. During the treatment, small staple-like material was found loose in the wound.

Right ankle ROM is limited to 2° dorsiflexion and 14° plantar flexion, otherwise ROM is within functional limits. Muscle strength of the right ankle is 3/5 within the limited range and painful with any resistance. Grossly strength is 4+/5 in the other extremities. The patient is able to ambulate with an antalgic gait pattern using a straight cane. He is able to ambulate only short distances of 100 to 120 ft before requiring a rest due to calf pain. Sensation to light touch is absent in a stocking-type distribution to the midcalf in the right lower extremity.

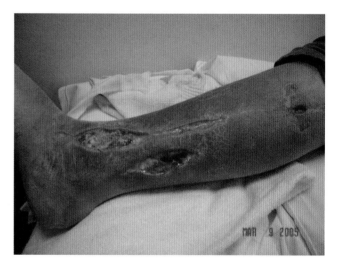

CASE STUDY QUESTIONS

1. What is a percutaneous transluminal angioplasty?

2. What risks are associated with this procedure?

3. What is peripheral arterial disease (PAD)?

4. What risk factors does he have for PAD?

5. What does his pharmaceutical profile indicate regarding other comorbidities?

6. What are some potential causes for the dehisced incision?

7. How is the Wells criteria used to determine his deep vein thrombosis (DVT) risk?

8. How is an Ankle Brachial Index (ABI) determined?

9. Explain the values for the oxygen saturation in relation to his history.

10. What was the staple material found in the wound?

11. What technique is needed to apply a negative pressure wound therapy system to these wounds?

12. What referrals are needed if this wound is expected to heal?

13. What type of amputation is most likely to be performed on this patient and why?

14. What is the risk following amputation?

15. What are the advantages and disadvantages of post-surgical dressings following an amputation?

16. What considerations are needed in determining the proper prosthesis?

17. What is physical therapy's role in postamputation and prosthesis care?

26

TRANSTIBIAL AMPUTATION

Jill Heitzman, PT, DPT, GCS, NCS, CWS, CEEAA, FACCWS

A 68-year-old male continues to live and work on his family farm with his 40-year-old son and 19-year-old granddaughter. During harvesting of the wheat, the combine became jammed. While the patient was clearing the blades, he slipped, resulting in a traumatic crush injury to the left lower leg. He was rushed to the hospital and a transtibial amputation was performed. A morphine PCA was started in recovery where a bolus was given along with ondansetron (Zofran). Ciprofloxacin (Cipro) and clindamycin (Cleocin) were started intravenously at that time as well.

His current status includes a BMI of 18.7 (he is 6 ft 3 in weight 150 lb). Vital signs: BP 132/84, HR 82 beats per minute, RR 22 breaths per minute, SaO$_2$ 97%, temp 98.6°F. After 24 to 48 hours the goal was to put him on oral oxycodone + aspirin (Percocet) and move the IV antibiotic to oral medications. Upon arriving on the floor, the nurse requested an order for a CBC with differential to be ordered. On postoperative day 1, this patient is confused, disoriented, and very agitated, so the nurse gave lorazepam (Ativan) IM. Zofran was available for the patient to have PRN.

■ CASE STUDY QUESTIONS

1. How is an amputation classified as a traumatic crush amputation?

2. What are important factors following a traumatic crush injury?

3. What would a CBC differential lab test indicate?

4. What is the difference between SaO$_2$ and SpO$_2$?

5. What does his medication profile indicate?

6. What risk factors does he have that will impact wound healing?

7. Does this patient have delirium, depression, or dementia?

8. How will the emotional/mental status of this patient affect physical therapy?

9. What are the physical therapy needs post-surgical for this patient?

10. What are important considerations when using an elastic bandage with a patient who has a transtibial amputation?

11. How will pain impact physical therapy?

12. What are the positioning needs for this patient?

13. What are the pros and cons of using a walker or crutches?

14. What would his Medicare Functional Classification K level be in deciding the proper prosthesis?

15. What is the Amputee Mobility Predictor (AMP)? How is it used?

16. What is the basic skin care education needed for this patient?

17. What are some common problems, potential causes, and care needs associated with residual limbs once prosthetic is obtained?

18. What are the pressure areas to be mindful of regarding a transtibial prosthesis?

19. What considerations does he need to take into account as a farmer?

27

TUBERCULOSIS

Jill Heitzman, PT, DPT, GCS, NCS, CWS, CEEAA, FACCWS

A 72-year-old male is referred to PT for wound therapy. The wound is located on the lateral right calf and presents as a large kidney–shaped wound with slough in the center and yellow cottage cheese–like substance surrounding the wound edges. The pathology report indicates that he has tuberculosis (TB) of the bone and vancomycin-resistant *Enterococcus faecium* (VRE). The patient is receiving IV infusion therapy with linezolid (Zyvox). He is also taking celecoxib (Celebrex), isoniazid (INH), pyrazinamide (PZA), rifampin (Rifadin), and ethambutol (Myambutol). His past history includes TB of the lung 15 years ago while still in his home country of Vietnam. He moved to the United States when he retired 7 years ago to join his children.

He reports drinking four to six bottles of beer daily and was diagnosed with type 2 diabetes mellitus 3 years ago and prescribed glipizide (Glucotrol). His BMI is 17. His BP is 148/88, HR 84 beats per minute, RR 26 breaths per minute, SpO$_2$ 96%, temp 98.9°F. He has signs of arthritic deformities in his hands and has decreased range of motion in both knees and ankles. He uses a straight cane for ambulation and has decreased weight bearing on the right with circumduction of the RLE through swing.

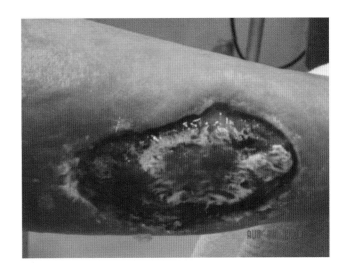

■ CASE STUDY QUESTIONS

1. What is TB of the bone?

2. Who is most at risk for developing TB of the bone?

3. What are the signs and symptoms of TB of the bone?

4. What are the risks involved with TB of the bone?

5. What is vancomycin-resistant *Enterococcus faecium* (VRE)?

6. How is VRE spread prevented?

7. How does the pharmaceutical profile affect his plan of care?

8. What does the yellow cottage cheese appearance on the edges of the wound indicate?

9. How does his medical history (outside of the TB and VRE) affect his plan of care?

10. Discuss the use of negative pressure wound therapy on this wound.

11. Discuss hyperbaric oxygen therapy use for this patient.

12. What other therapy needs and education are needed?

CHAPTER

6

Medically Complex Cases

INTRODUCTION

COMPLEX MEDICAL PROBLEMS IN THE OLDER ADULT

William H. Staples, PT, DHSc, DPT, GCS, CEEAA

This chapter will investigate the geriatric client that may present with multiple comorbidities that can complicate the rehabilitation process. As life expectancy grows, chronic illness has become more common and is a hallmark of modern health care. A physical therapist has a great deal to consider when assessing the geriatric client. Conditions of normal aging such as difficulty with heat regulation, loss of eyesight and hearing can make assessment and intervention more difficult. Decline in physical reserve (homeostasis) may transform mild problems such as a cold into those that are life threatening. According to the Centers for Disease Control and Prevention, early 80% of older adults (over 65) have been diagnosed with one chronic condition and more than 50% of older adults have three or more comorbidities including chronic diseases.[1,2] Older adults with multiple health problems have higher rates of death, disability, adverse effects, institutionalization, use of resources, and a poorer quality of life.[3] A comprehensive review of all systems and a biopsychosocial or patient-centered approach must be utilized when assessing and planning intervention for these clients. Health is best understood in terms of a combination of biological, psychological, and social factors rather than purely in biological terms. This concept was first put forth by Dr Gorge Engel.[4] Older adults may have multiple medical problems and will benefit from this comprehensive approach that is multidisciplinary in scope. Physical therapists must not only understand internal factors such as physical abilities, cognition, and pharmacological interaction, but also how external factors such as environment, financial resources, and social support will affect the therapeutic relationship and eventual outcome.

Not all older adults' problems can be classified into specific disease categories. A term "geriatric syndrome"[5] has been utilized to categorize many of the most common health interrelated problems in older adults. Geriatric symptoms do not fit neatly into distinct categories; that is why they are classified as a syndrome. Geriatric syndromes are a group of chronic symptoms or problems that are logically connected, associated with old age, have a multifactorial etiology. There can be progressive decline, increased vulnerability to outside stressors, and an increased risk for adverse health outcomes. Often, the syndrome becomes a vicious circle and it leads to a decline in the human abilities and independence. So when treating geriatric patients, health care providers need to consider four domains inclusive of medical, psychological, functional, and social domains. Supportive services, such as assistance with food preparation, shopping, maintaining a checkbook, or transportation, may need to be provided by an outside agency or family member and are vital to success.

Geriatric syndromes include falls, incontinence, delirium, and functional decline and represent a state of impaired health.[5] These complex syndromes are multifactorial and associated with poor outcomes, loss of mobility (hypomobility), frailty, dependence, and significant morbidity. A change in health status may be precipitated by one of the interrelated conditions. For instance, an episode of pneumonia might lead to hospitalization and the development of orthostatic hypotension, which may then cause a fall that results in a fractured hip and then develop a deep vein thrombosis, which could be fatal. Or this patient might develop a fear of falling which self-limits mobility and leads to a cycle of decline when returning home. Poor nutrition affects the overall condition of every person. Malnutrition leads to muscle atrophy. Malnutrition can lead to worsening of a disease, impair wound healing, and slow overall recovery (prolongation of hospitalization), which could only increase the number of complications and mortality and morbidity rates. Dehydration is common in older adults because they do not feel as thirsty as a younger person does physiologically. Some people may limit their fluid intake for fear of an incontinence. Hypodipsia is a condition in which homeostasis is threatened by an abnormally low fluid intake.[6] Hypodipsia is often related to dysfunction of the thirst osmoreceptor in the anterior hypothalamus.[6] Dehydration may also be caused by psychological factors such as depression or dementia. Dehydration is a frequent cause of decompensation of chronic disease and subsequent hospitalization.

Some cognitive declines, such as confusion and memory loss, may be attributable to acute illnesses or conditions that are reversible if caught early enough. They include urinary tract infections, vitamin B_{12} deficiency, pneumonia, or hypothyroidism, all of which are common in the elderly. Confusion and cognitive symptoms can also be caused by heart attacks, stroke, and some infectious diseases.

The geriatric population is a unique group to work with because of the aging and disease processes that interact to produce a wide variation in each individual. The increasing number of older adults combined with the increasing rates of diabetes, obesity, and other chronic diseases may overwhelm our already stretched health care system. Physical therapists, as health care providers, are also health educators and health promoters and will continue to play an ever more important role in the provision of health care services. Time should be spent to teach, counsel, and modify the behaviors of individuals that if left unattended, would lead to dysfunction. Some of the concerns that can affect the older adult, such as nutritional concerns, psychosocial problems, and limited finances, may fall outside the immediate practice of physical therapists, but must be addressed in order to maximize therapeutic outcomes. The geriatric practitioner must also understand reimbursement issues to better serve their clientele. Rather than working in a vacuum, communication and team work must be utilized for the best overall care of the patient or client. Geriatric rehabilitation offers a huge challenge to the talent and creativity of each therapist. As the geriatric population continues to grow, so will the challenges.

REFERENCES

1. Centers for Disease Control and Prevention. *The State of Aging and Health in America 2007*. Whitehall Station, NJ: The Merck Company Foundation; 2007.
2. Anderson G. Chronic care: making the case for ongoing care. Robert Wood Johnson Foundation 2010. http://www.rwjf.org/files/research/50968chronic.carechartbook.pdf. Accessed October 2, 2014.
3. Boyd CM, Fortin M. Future of multimorbidity research: how should understanding of multimorbidity inform health system design? *Public Health Rev*. 2011;32:451-474.
4. Engel GL. The need for a new medical model: a challenge for biomedicine. *Science*. 1977;196:129-136.
5. Inouye SK, Studenski S, Tinetti ME, Kuchel GA. Geriatric syndromes: clinical, research, and policy implications of a core geriatric concept. *J Am Geriatr Soc*. 2007;55:780-791.
6. Miller PD, Krebs RA, Neal BJ, McIntyre DO. Hypodipsia in geriatric patients. *Am J Med*. September 1982;73(3):354-356.

1

ACUTE DELIRIUM

William H. Staples, PT, DHSc, DPT, GCS, CEEAA

You are a therapist assigned to the intensive care unit (ICU) and are asked to see a 75-year-old woman who was admitted 1 week ago in acute respiratory distress. She has been medically stable for the last 3 days and mechanically ventilated until yesterday. The physician has requested physical therapy to mobilize the patient. When you begin your assessment, you find that the patient has difficulty staying attentive to your questions and when she does answer them the answers were rambling and make no sense. The nurse performs a Confusion Assessment Method short form to assess delirium and the patient scores a 5/7.

Although confused, the patient is able to sit over the side of the bed with maximal assistance and her strength is grossly 4/5 in all four limbs. She requires only minimal support to remain sitting and her vital signs as monitored by the ICU remain stable.

■ CASE STUDY QUESTIONS

1. What is delirium?
2. What is the pathophysiology of developing delirium in the intensive care unit (ICU)?
3. What are the risk factors for someone developing acute delirium in the ICU?
4. What is the incidence of someone having acute delirium in a hospital?
5. Are the immediate outcomes for someone with delirium worse than those who do not have delirium?
6. What are the long-term outcomes of someone having acute respiratory distress syndrome?
7. Is there a way to determine who might have delirium during a hospital admission?
8. How is the CAM-S screening device scored?
9. Can delirium be prevented outside of the ICU?
10. Is there an effective medical treatment for treating people with delirium in the ICU?
11. What are the clinical practice guidelines for the management of delirium, established by the Society of Critical Care Medicine that physical therapy should be aware of?
12. Was this the appropriate time to start physical therapy?
13. What should the therapist do now?

2

ALZHEIMER DISEASE: BIOPSYCHOSOCIAL ISSUES

William H. Staples, PT, DHSc, DPT, GCS, CEEAA

The therapist has a referral to see a 76-year-old African American male (Mr B) due to recent physical decline including several falls at home. During a physician visit last week, he was diagnosed with Alzheimer disease after a thorough medical workup and a Mini Mental Status Examination (MMSE) score of 21/30. In addition to his newly diagnosed Alzheimer disease, the patient has a history of a mild right cerebrovascular accident, high blood sugar, and hypertension. Mr B currently controls his blood sugar through diet, which his wife regulates. The patient is a poor historian and his wife, Mrs B, intercedes to assist the therapist during the evaluation. Mr B had been a truck driver for a large merchandise chain and retired 10 years ago. Mrs B is a 74-year-old African American woman who reports that she stayed home to raise the three children she had with Mr B. After the children got to high school, Mrs B began work as a certified nursing assistant in a long-term care facility near their home. She retired a few years ago, around the time her husband started to show the first signs of confusion. They live in the house they have owned since getting married and share it with one of their daughters and her two teenage sons. Mrs B was actively involved with her faith community as a volunteer but has been unable to find any extra time in the past 6 months. Mrs B has no history of chronic illness, but was recently diagnosed with elevated blood pressure (150/96). She reports recent lack of sleep due to her husband pacing in the home at night and rummaging through the cabinets and refrigerator, which affects his blood sugar readings. Yesterday he ate a half box of cookies at 3:00 AM. Mrs B complains of being "tired" much of the day. She also shares that she has recently lost several pounds of weight.

On evaluation Mr B has no deficits in strength (manual muscle test) or range of motion but shows deficits in standing balance, with a Berg Balance Score (BBS) of 44/56 and Timed Up and Go (TUG) test of 14 seconds. He is able to complete four repetitions sit-to-stand in 30 seconds. A 2-Minute Step Test to test for endurance is

46, with the patient having to be reminded to continue to step as he stops frequently. His heart rate increases from 78 at rest to 130 during this test. He is able to complete his ADLs independently, but his wife reports that some days it takes Mr B an hour to get dressed in the morning. After dressing, he generally sits in a chair watching television for the majority of the day.

CASE STUDY QUESTIONS

1. Is the Mini Mental Status Examination (MMSE) a good predictor of Alzheimer disease?
2. What would some areas that a physician would screen in a medical workup to rule out a diagnosis of Alzheimer disease?
3. What should the interventions be focused on?
4. Describe the Berg Balance Scale and what it measures. What does a score of 44/56 mean?
5. Describe the Timed Up and Go Test and what it measures. What does a score of 14 seconds mean?
6. Describe the 30-Second Sit-to-Stand Test and what it measures. What does a score of four repetitions mean?
7. Describe the 2-minute Step test and what it measures. What does a score of 46 steps in 2 minutes mean?
8. What does the change in heart rate indicate?
9. What are the common signs of caregiver stress? Does Mrs B have any of them?
10. Should Mrs B be referred for any assistance?
11. Is there anything that can be done to prevent Mr B from eating outside of his recommended diet?

3

MILD COGNITIVE IMPAIRMENT/ ALZHEIMER DISEASE

William H. Staples, PT, DHSc, DPT, GCS, CEEAA

PART 1

A 76-year-old woman walks into the clinic about 30 minutes late for a scheduled appointment with a complaint of right shoulder pain, stating that she almost forgot about the appointment, and that she was lucky she wrote it down in her calendar. Her vital signs are heart rate 70, blood pressure 122/74, respiratory rate 14, and pulse oximetry (SpO_2) is 96. She has a 3/10 pain in her right shoulder using a verbal analog scale. She has slight limitations in right active shoulder range of motion (ROM) in external rotation and abduction as compared to the left. The anterior shoulder is slightly warm to the touch and tender to palpation. She is taking 325 mg of acetaminophen (Tylenol) three times per day for pain relief. As you begin your physical examination, you also make a mental status assessment: She is carefully dressed, well groomed, poised, with good eye contact. She is cooperative throughout interview, somewhat guarded when discussing feelings. She smiles appropriately, but carefully choosing her words when answering questions. Mood is stable and affect is appropriate; she is somewhat hesitant when asked how she "feels." No evidence of delusions/hallucinations or incoherent thought process. She is alert, oriented to time, place, and person, with good long-memory recall, but has difficulty with more recent information as to how and when she hurt her shoulder.

You determine that she has a mildly strained right rotator cuff (supraspinatus) muscle. You decide to give her a mental status screening tool, the Montreal Cognitive Assessment (MoCA) to determine how you would proceed with giving her a home exercise program. She scores a 22/30 on the MoCA. She has three treatments consisting of ice, range of motion exercises, and manual therapy and reports no pain and returns to normal activities and she is discharged with a maintenance exercise program.

PART 2

About 1 year later the same woman comes into your office again with a complaint of right shoulder pain. Upon examination you determine that this time she has developed adhesive capsulitis. In reviewing her history, you find that the patient is now taking 10 mg of donepezil (Aricept) in addition to 500 mg acetaminophen (Tylenol) four times a day. Her vital signs are heart rate 102, blood pressure 124/76, respiratory rate 14, and pulse oximetry (SpO_2) is 96. Her right shoulder pain is 6/10 with passive ROM on a verbal analog scale. Range of motion is limited in a capsular pattern and she has great difficulty with her activities of daily living. After your evaluation is complete, you decide to do some further study into this patient's condition and medication.

Namzaric
↓
Donepezil + Memantine

... ng her

... n?

... n you

1\. ... eimer

2. What are pathological manifestations of AD?
3. What are the medications that are FDA approved to treat AD?
4. What is donepezil (Aricept)?
5. What are the side effects of this medication?
6. For patients undergoing physical therapy, what is the most significant side effect?
7. Are there any foods or supplements that people may choose to use for treatment?
8. What should the physician tell the patient about the medications?
9. What percentage of people with MCI go on to develop AD?

4

BPH, ORTHOSTATIC HYPOTENSION

Bill Anderson, PT, DPT, GCS, CEEAA, COS-C

Amy M. Lilley, PT, GCS, CEEAA

EXAMINATION

You are seeing a patient in the home health setting. He is an 84 y/o retired widow who lives with his son. He has a past medical history of benign prostatic hyperplasia (BPH), hypertension, cerebrovascular accident (CVA) 3 years ago with residual right lower extremity weakness, smoking history of ½ pack per day (ppd) × 60 years, bilateral carotid artery stenosis, and hyperlipidemia. His past surgical history includes a left total hip replacement 8 years ago. The patient's son reported that his father has been having some difficulties managing his checkbook lately. The son reported that the patient has had a progressive worsening of his balance since having his total hip replacement and CVA. He has experienced an increased frequency of falls recently. He had recently seen his urologist and had some adjustments to his medications. The patient reports his chief complaint to be light-headedness when he stands and unsteadiness and fatigue when walking. His goals are to return to walking to the local diner every morning.

CURRENT MEDICATIONS

1) Metoprolol succinate (Toprol-XL) 25 mg: one tablet in the morning with breakfast

2) Simvastatin (Zocor) 10 mg: one tablet in the evening

3) Aspirin/dipyridamole (Aggrenox) 25/200 mg: one capsule every 12 hours

4) Terazosin (Hytrin) 10 mg: one capsule at bedtime _BPH - relax smooth muscles of bladder &_

5) Acetaminophen (Tylenol) 325 mg: One to two tablets every _bladder neck to improve urine flow_ 4 hours as needed, not to exceed 4 g/day

ENVIRONMENT

The patient lives in a single family home with stairs to enter with a bedroom and a half bathroom on the first floor but his shower is on the second floor with 12 steps to access. The son lives with the patient but works during the day and does all of the shopping and yard work. Currently the patient has been getting his own meals during the day and his son provides stand-by assist for bathing and performance of stairs.

SYSTEMS REVIEW

Cardiopulmonary: BP (rest, sitting) 110/68, HR 60. Edema: trace pedal bilaterally.
Neuromuscular: Gait: Patient ambulates with a 2-point step-through pattern without assistive device with a wide base of support and using upper extremities for proprioceptive feedback.
Musculoskeletal: Pain in his right hip with ambulation and stairs 4/10. Bilateral upper extremities AROM: symmetrical and the

patient able to don and doff his shirt. Bilateral lower extremity AROM: able to tie shoes with some difficulty and pain with right hip while performing. He rises from a chair with armrests in two attempts.
Integumentary: Clubbing of digits, pale color throughout, absence of hair bilateral upper extremities and lower extremities. Bilateral feet skin intact but dry.
Gastrointestinal/genitourinary: Reports of increased urinary frequency and nocturia. No changes in bowel function from his norm of once a day.
Communication: Alert and oriented × 4. Affect: pleasant and follows multistep directions, is not aware of the names of his medications or their purpose. The patient is a high school graduate.
Vision/hearing: He wears glasses for reading, able to hear whispers.

TESTS AND MEASURES

Berg Balance Scale (BBS): The patient was unable to complete all components of the test due to light-headedness. Not scored.
Timed Up and Go Test (TUG): 36.7 seconds without device and 42.6 seconds using a straight cane.
Five Times Sit-to-Stand Test (FTSST): unable to complete due to light-headedness and balance loss.
St Louis University Mental Status Examination (SLUMS): 27/30 points
Orthostatic hypotension: BP (rest, sitting) 110/68 HR 60, BP (initial standing) 70/38 HR 62, BP (3 minutes standing) 74/44 HR 66 with complaints of light-headedness throughout standing.

EVALUATION

The patient presents with impairments in balance, altered cardiovascular response to position change, resulting in an increased fall risk and decreased ability to perform locomotion safely.

■ CASE STUDY QUESTIONS

1. What is benign prostatic hyperplasia (BPH)?

2. What patient population tends to have a higher incidence of BPH? _60+_

3. What are the symptoms associated with BPH?

4. What are the typical medication classes used to treat BPH, and how do they work?

5. What is the Beers List?

6. In addition to medications, what herbal therapies or procedures are reported to be used to help treat BPH?

7. Define symptomatic orthostatic hypotension.

8. Which medication's side effects is most likely interfering with the patient's functional status? Why? _→ Metoprolol_

9. Regarding the medication from the previous question (if this medication could not be discontinued), what other medical management can be utilized to decrease the side effects of orthostatic hypotension?

10. What did each of the functional tests tell you?

11. What would your physical therapy intervention include for this patient?

5

BREAST CANCER: PART 1

William H. Staples, PT, DHSc, DPT, GCS, CEEAA

Linda R. Staples, RN, BS, MA

A 60-year-old woman has been treated for ER/PR (estrogen receptor and progesterone receptor) positive invasive ductal carcinoma.

She underwent a partial left mastectomy, or lumpectomy, and a sentinel lymph node biopsy 8 months ago. Then she had a course of chemotherapy and radiation. For the last 6 months, she has been on hormonal therapy with exemestane, generic for Aromasin.

She fatigues quite easily and has had some physical therapy to improve her functional mobility and endurance. She also reports multiple areas of joint pain for which she is taking diclofenac sodium (Voltaren) 75 mg twice a day. She rates the pain in her hips and knees 5/10 and both hands 4/10 on a verbal analog scale. Range of motion is not limited and muscle strength is grossly 4+/5 in the extremities. Trunk musculature is 4−/5. She has no abnormal neurological signs. Her vital signs are pulse 74, blood pressure 134/72, respiratory rate 16, and SpO₂ is 96. She has a body mass index (BMI) of 29. She has expressed fear that exercising will increase her joint pain.

■ CASE STUDY QUESTIONS

1. What is invasive ductal carcinoma?
2. What does it mean for a tumor to be ER/PR positive?
3. What is removed when a person has a partial mastectomy or lumpectomy?
4. What is a sentinel node biopsy and why is it done during surgery?
5. What are some negative after effects of having a partial mastectomy or lumpectomy?
6. Why is lymphedema present following mastectomy or lumpectomy?
7. What are some negative side effects of chemotherapy?
8. What are some negative side effects of radiation?
9. What are aromatase inhibitors and what do they do?
10. What are some negative side effects of aromatase inhibitors?
11. Are there other medications for breast cancer?
12. What are some negative long-term side effects of surgery and radiation?
13. Can physical therapy help following breast cancer surgery and use of aromatase inhibitors?
14. Should patients exercise during chemotherapy?
15. Should people postcancer exercise?

6

BREAST CANCER: PART 2

William H. Staples, PT, DHSc, DPT, GCS, CEEAA

Linda R. Staples, RN, BS, MA

A 60-year-old woman has been treated for ER/PR (estrogen receptor and progesterone receptor) positive invasive ductal carcinoma.

You originally saw her 10 months ago for 1 month to set her up with a home exercise program. To review she underwent a partial left mastectomy, or lumpectomy, and a sentinel lymph node biopsy 18 months ago. Then she had a course of chemotherapy and radiation. For the last 16 months, she has been on hormonal therapy with exemestane, generic for Aromasin. The cancer returned and now has had a total left mastectomy 8 weeks ago. Her physician has recommended physical therapy.

She originally sought out physical therapy because she fatigued quite easily and wanted to improve her functional mobility and endurance. She also reported multiple areas of joint pain for which she is taking diclofenac sodium (Voltaren) 75 mg twice a day. She rated the pain in her hips and knees 5/10 and both hands 4/10 on a verbal analog scale. Today her pain is in the 2-3/10 range in her proximal left arm and 2/10 distally. She also complains of pain in the lateral chest and back. Range of motion was limited in the left shoulder to 120° of flexion and abduction, and slight losses of flexion in the elbow wrist and hand due to swelling. Muscle strength is grossly 5/5 in the extremities except the left arm which is 4/5. Trunk musculature is 4−/5. She has no abnormal neurological signs. Her vital signs are: pulse 74, blood pressure 134/72, respiratory rate 16, and SpO₂ is 96. She has a body mass index (BMI) of 29. She has expressed fear that exercising will increase her joint pain.

■ CASE STUDY QUESTIONS

1. What is now going on with the patient's symptoms?
2. After mastectomy, are there any restrictions?
3. Why would the arm be swollen?
4. Is the arm the only location that can be affected by the edema?
5. What can physical therapy do to help the lymphatic system?
6. What is complete decongestive therapy?
7. Describe where and how the massage for the lymph system should be performed.
8. Describe the deep breathing exercises you would utilize.
9. Describe the postural exercises you would instruct.
10. Describe some of the arm mobility exercises you would instruct.
11. How is edema measured?
12. What can be done long term to reduce the reoccurrence of the lymphedema?
13. Can patients utilize resistive exercise training?

7

CHRONIC PAIN: PART 1

William H. Staples, PT, DHSc, DPT, GCS, CEEAA

A new referral for home health is a 61-year-old female who was hospitalized for 3 days from home after bending over to pick up her dog (12 lb) and feeling a "popping" sensation in her back. She had severe pain and inability to ambulate since that event. Prior to this injury she was functioning independently. An MRI at the hospital revealed herniated disks at L4 and L5. After hospitalization, she was discharged to a skilled nursing facility to undergo rehabilitation but was not able to participate in therapy due to a complaint of

9-10/10 pain and inability to get out of bed, and therapy was discontinued. She is now at her home with her husband in a hospital bed in her first floor dining room. Two adult daughters have temporarily come home to help care for their mother during the day when the husband is at work. The home has 1 step into the front door and 14 steps to the second floor where her bedroom and bathroom with a tub/shower are. There is a first floor half-bath and a bedside commode.

Her previous medical history includes adhesive capsulitis both shoulders, coronary artery disease, chest pain (angina), fibromyalgia, migraines, shoulder, hip, and knee pain. Previous surgical history includes appendectomy, C-section times two, tonsillectomy, breast reduction surgery. Family history includes mother and two aunts with breast cancer, and another aunt with uterine cancer. She does not smoke or drink alcohol.

CURRENT MEDICATIONS

Tenormin (atenolol) 25 mg oral, bid
Lipitor (atorvastatin) 80 mg oral, daily
Cymbalta (duloxetine) 30 mg delayed release oral, daily
Nitropaste 2% ointment dermal application for chest pain
Ranexa (ranolazine) 500 mg extended release oral, daily
Topamax (topiramate) 200 mg oral, daily
Dilaudid (hydromorphone) 4 mg oral, every 6 hours
Tylenol (acetaminophen) 650 mg oral, every 4 hours

EXAMINATION

The patient examination began with the patient supine in a hospital bed. Vital signs are heart rate 66, blood pressure 116/72, respiratory rate 14, and pulse oximetry 98%. The patient is alert and oriented with a current subjective complaint of pain at rest in both hips (8/10), bilateral low back (9/10), left lateral leg from the buttock to the calf (7/10), right shoulder (5/10) and states this is the best that the pain gets. The patient describes the pain as "aching" but changes to "sharp" with any movement. Asked what makes the pain better she responds "nothing" and to what makes the pain worse she states "everything." Palpation of the painful areas did not alter pain. The right shoulder has limitations in range of motion to 85° of flexion and abduction, and 40° of external rotation and 75° of internal rotation with end feels capsular. The patient states that these shoulder limitations have been present for almost 2 years. Lasègue test is positive at 45° on the right and 50° on the left. The patient states that she has had pain for more than 5 years mostly in her hips and back "from the fibromyalgia."

Strength is 4−/5 in limited range of right shoulder otherwise 4/5 throughout. Sensation is intact to light touch and sharp/dull all lower extremity dermatomes and reflex testing was 2+ bilateral knees and ankles. Coordination is normal. No edema noted in the lower extremities.

The patient was moved to sitting with moderate assist to assess trunk mobility and sitting balance with the patient letting out a loud yell. The patient had slumped sitting posture with forward head posture but was able to correct with physical and verbal cueing. The patient did complain of increased pain in the back and hips with postural changes. She states she has not been sleeping well because the pain wakes her up and she is "tired all the time."

The patient is very anxious about attempting to stand but did so with maximum assistance of one and the patient was able to support her weight on the lower extremities while clutching the therapist's arms very firmly. As the patient stood longer, she was able to decrease her grip on the therapist and stood for 2 minutes before starting to visibly shake her lower extremities.

The patient's goals are to decrease the pain to 1/10, walk in the home including upstairs to take a shower. Currently, her daughters help her with all ADLs.

■ CASE STUDY QUESTIONS

1. What is Lasègue sign?
2. Are there any other tests that could be performed today to determine the cause of the back pain?
3. Are there any other tests that could/should be performed today?
4. Would you describe this patient as being a chronic or acute pain patient?
5. How is a patient with chronic pain best described?
6. How many people in the United States have some form of chronic pain?
7. What is the neuromatrix theory of pain?
8. What interventions would you start with?
9. When would be the best time to take her pain medication?
10. What is Ranexa?
11. Would you consider spinal manipulation?
12. Will her lack of sleep affect physical therapy? Why or why not?
13. Are there any other services that should be added to the home care team?

CHRONIC PAIN: PART 2

William H. Staples, PT, DHSc, DPT, GCS, CEEAA

One month ago you received new referral for home health is a 61-year-old female who was hospitalized for 3 days from home after bending over to pick up her dog (12 lb) and feeling a "popping" sensation in her back. She had severe pain and inability to ambulate since that event. Prior to this injury, she was functioning independently. An MRI at the hospital revealed herniated disks at L4 and L5. After hospitalization, she was discharged to a skilled nursing facility to undergo rehabilitation but was not able to participate in therapy due to a complaint of 9-10/10 pain and inability to get out of bed, and therapy was discontinued. She is now at her home with her husband in a hospital bed in her first floor dining room. Two adult daughters have temporarily come home to help care for their mother during the day when the husband is at work. The home has 1 step into the front door and 14 steps to the second floor where her bedroom and bathroom with a tub/shower are. There is a first floor half-bath and a bedside commode.

Her previous medical history includes adhesive capsulitis, both shoulders, coronary artery disease, chest pain (angina), fibromyalgia, migraines, shoulder, hip, and knee pain. Previous surgical history includes appendectomy, C-section times 2, tonsillectomy, breast reduction surgery. Family history includes mother and two aunts with breast cancer, and another aunt with uterine cancer. She does not smoke or drink alcohol.

MEDICATIONS

Tenormin (atenolol) 25 mg oral, bid
Lipitor (atorvastatin) 80 mg oral, daily

Cymbalta (duloxetine) 30 mg delayed release oral, daily
Nitropaste 2% ointment dermal application for chest pain
Ranexa (ranolazine) 500 mg extended release oral, daily
Topamax (topiramate) 200 mg oral, daily
Dilaudid (hydromorphone) 4 mg oral, every 6 hours (discontinued)
Tylenol (acetaminophen) 650 mg oral, every 4 hours

The original patient examination found the following information. The patient was alert and oriented with a subjective complaint of pain at rest in both hips (8/10), bilateral low back (9/10), left lateral leg from the buttock to the calf (7/10), right shoulder (5/10) and stated this is the best that the pain gets. The patient described the pain as "aching" but changes to "sharp" with any movement. When asked what makes the pain better, she responded "nothing" and to what makes the pain worse she states "everything." Palpation of the painful areas did not alter pain. The right shoulder had limitations in range of motion to 85° of flexion and abduction, and 40° of external rotation and 75° of internal rotation with end feels capsular. The patient states that these shoulder limitations have been present for almost 2 years. Lasègue test was positive at 45° on the right and 50° on the left. The patient stated that she has had pain for more than 5 years mostly in her hips and back "from the fibromyalgia."

Strength was 4−/5 in limited range of right shoulder otherwise 4/5 throughout. Sensation was intact to light touch and sharp/dull all lower extremity dermatomes and reflex testing was 2+ bilateral knees and ankles. Coordination was normal. No edema was noted in the lower extremities. The patient complained of fatigue and lack of sleep.

The patient's goals on admission were to decrease the pain to 1/10, walk in the home including upstairs to take a shower. Currently, her daughters help her with all ADLs.

The patient made very slow, limited progress with therapy the first 2 weeks. Use of moist heat, exercise, and a TNS for the lumbar spine were able to decrease pain by 2 to 3 points but was still considered to be the primary barrier to improved mobility. In consultation with the patient's primary care physician, a corticosteroid injection was performed in the lumbar spine 2 weeks ago and Dilaudid was discontinued. Over the last 2 weeks the patient has made much progress. The patient is now able to ambulate with a rolling walker independently in the home and exhibits good posture during gait. All transfers and bed mobility are also independent. The exercise program has been designed to increase lower extremity strength in order to enable the patient to climb stairs. Pain in the low back and hips is now 3/10 with no pain extending below the buttock. Occupational therapy has completed her treatments and the patient is independent in ADLs including the use of the first floor bathroom. The right shoulder only has pain at the end range of abduction, flexion, and external rotation, which have only increased by 5° to 10° with moist heat and joint mobilizations.

You believe that the patient is ready to progress to stair climbing. There are handrails on both sides of the stairwell. After first giving verbal instructions on stair climbing, you begin with having the patient step up and down (backward) from one step five times. The patient is successful with this and is praised for her efforts. After a few minutes of rest, you attempt to have the patient go up and down three steps but now the patient at first balks at this suggestion and appears to become quite anxious. After calming the patient down, you chose to attempt more stairs. On the attempt to step up a second step, the patient begins to breathe rapidly and shake her whole body saying "I can't, I can't, I have to sit down." When you try to give her confidence, she begins to complain of chest pain and increased pain in other areas and she wants to return to the bed.

CASE STUDY QUESTIONS

1. What can be done for the chest pain?
2. What do you think is going on with the patient psychologically?
3. How would you try to calm this patient down and have this patient progress with the program?
4. Would screening for anxiety be helpful?
5. What are the rates of anxiety in adults?
6. What are the symptoms of anxiety?
7. What causes anxiety?
8. If the pain is due to the anxiety, should you ignore it?
9. Are there medications that should be given for anxiety?
10. What are some guidelines and goals for people with chronic pain receiving physical therapy?
11. What is a biopsychosocial approach to patient care?
12. Have you encountered any techniques that might assist this patient?

9

COMPLEX MEDICAL DIAGNOSIS WITH COMPLICATIONS

Lucy H. Jones, PT, DPT, MHA, GCS, CEEAA

Richard is 62 years old and discharged from the hospital following a myocardial infarction. While hospitalized, he developed a pulmonary embolism. With diagnostic workup, a small mass was found in the right lower lobe and surgically removed. During the surgery, his large intestine was "nicked" and was followed by a right colectomy and end ileostomy. Within 1 day, a wound vacuum (vac) was inserted due to fluid collection in the abdomen as a result from these surgeries.

His previous medical history includes end-stage liver disease (ESLD) with a liver transplant in 2012, hepatitis C, type 2 diabetes mellitus, coronary artery disease, previous myocardial infarction, left upper extremity arterial-venous fistula, and end-stage renal disease (ESRD) requiring 3× a week dialysis.

Vital signs at rest are BP 128/78, RR 18/ min, HR 64/min, SpO$_2$ 96%, RPE 4/10.

His medications include aspirin 81 mg, carvedilol (Coreg), apixaban (Eliquis), tacrolimus, (Prograf), alprazolam (Xanax), Lisinopril (Zestril), and omeprazole (Prilosec OTC).

The patient's ROM is grossly within normal limits. Strength is grossly 4/5. The patient has history of low activity level and states he never exercises. Therapy has been ordered to mobilize the patient and progress to discharge to the appropriate venue.

CASE STUDY QUESTIONS

1. What is the indication, side effects, of the medication Prograf?
2. What is rate of perceived and exertion (RPE), and how can it be helpful with providing an exercise prescription for Richard?
3. How does a wound vacuum work, and what precautions would be indicated with movement and exercise?
4. What are the characteristics of end-stage liver disease, and what are precautions indicated for exercise?

5. What is an exercise prescription that could affect the endurance and exercise capacity of those with ESLD?

6. What is an arteriovenous (AV) fistula? What would be the indications for its use, and is it reversible?

7. Richard's cardiac ejection fraction was 40%. What does this mean to his cardiac health and to feasibility of exercise training?

8. How feasible is it for someone with an ejection fraction below 50% to exercise and regain strength?

9. What is a colectomy? Can it be reconnected?

10. What is an ileostomy? Can it be reversed?

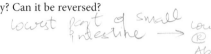

10

CONCUSSION

William H. Staples, PT, DHSc, DPT, GCS, CEEAA

During a follow-up visit with a 73-year-old male home health patient, his wife states that she had to help get him up after a fall last night. His referral diagnosis was for a right total knee replacement. The patient denies any new knee pain. His medications include Xarelto (rivaroxaban) and Vicodin (hydrocodone and acetaminophen). You first check his knee for damage to the suture line, additional bruising and find no new injury.

Evaluation 1 week ago: On his evaluation last week you noted no cognitive deficits. Pulse 72 beats per minute, respiratory rate 14 breaths per minute, blood pressure 130/80 mm Hg, and pulse oximetry 98%. The patient was alert and oriented, and anxious to return to his previous level of function. The knee surgical incision was clean, without any drainage and staples in place. Gait was weight bearing as tolerated and independent with a rolling walker in the home. Neurological system was intact with no deficits noted. Single leg stance on the left was 30 seconds eyes open and 22 seconds eyes closed.

Today's visit: Vital signs are similar to the measures taken last week with pulse 72 beats per minute, respiratory rate 14 breaths per minute, blood pressure 132/82 mm Hg, and pulse oximetry 97%. He is able to follow instructions but slow to perform. He cannot remember anything about the fall. He denies any vomiting but does complain of nausea. He has a reddened, bruised, and swollen area over the right orbit and laterally, which is painful to palpation. He denies dizziness but complains of a headache. His single leg stance is 24 seconds eyes open and unable to perform with eyes closed. Cranial nerve testing reveals difficulty with eye movements but otherwise intact.

■ CASE STUDY QUESTIONS

1. What is a concussion?

2. What is the mechanism of injury for a concussion?

3. Do older adults get concussions?

4. How dangerous are concussions in older adults?

5. What are the signs of a concussion?

6. Are all the signs of a concussion immediately recognizable?

7. What should you do if you suspect a concussion in this patient?

8. What should you not do, if you suspect a concussion?

9. What signs and symptoms would be considered an absolute medical emergency?

10. How is a concussion diagnosed?

11. How is a concussion treated?

12. Are multiple concussions a problem?

13. Are there any long-term complications of a concussion?

14. Are there physical therapy interventions that can assist with recovery?

15. What functional outcome tools might be utilized to measure progress in the rehabilitation of a patient following a concussion?

11

DEPRESSION: PART 1

William H. Staples, PT, DHSc, DPT, GCS, CEEAA

You are working in a skilled nursing facility and are seeing a 73-year-old man who fell and fractured his left hip (intertrochanteric) and status post open reduction open fixation (ORIF) with a screw, plate, and nails 1 week ago. He is alert, oriented, and cooperative with the rehabilitation program and eager to return home. He was widowed last year and prior to the fracture he was living independently in a senior community. He is hard of hearing but otherwise appears to be doing well except for the weakness and pain (5/10) in his left hip well. He has begun gait training non-weight bearing with a standard walker 25 ft times 4 with only minimal assistance and verbal cueing for correct weight bearing. He is taking furosemide (Lasix) 40 mg twice a day and acetaminophen and hydrocodone (Lortab) (2) 300/5 mg every 6 hours.

Week 2 begins with continued improvement and gait has increased to 50 ft, but by the end of the week he needs more and more encouragement to attend therapy, he complains of fatigue, and is irritable. You speak with nurse who states that the patient has not been eating well. You think that this patient may be becoming depressed.

■ CASE STUDY QUESTIONS

1. What are the signs and symptoms of depression?

2. How common is depression in the elderly?

3. What are some risk factors for developing depression?

4. Did the hip fracture contribute to the depression?

5. How do patients with late-onset depression compare to those with an initial diagnosis earlier in life?

6. Would you want to screen this person for depression? How?

7. What is another screen for depression?

8. Is depression usually diagnosed by the primary care physician?

9. What is the recommended for the initial evaluation in elderly patients suspected of having depression?

10. What types of antidepressants are used and what is considered the first-line pharmacologic treatment for late-life depression?

11. Is there a role for brain stimulation in treating late-life depression?

12

DEPRESSION: PART 2

William H. Staples, PT, DHSc, DPT, GCS, CEEAA

You have received a referral for a home health patient who has been diagnosed with Parkinson disease 4 years ago, but the symptoms are now worsening and impacting his mobility. He is 77 years old and has no other actively treated medical condition. He is now taking a controlled-release (CR) Sinemet (carbidopa and levodopa 25-100 mg) three times a day, in addition to Requip (ropinirole HCl) 0.75 mg three times daily, which he has been taking since his initial diagnosis.

During your initial visit, the patient appears lethargic, but oriented and cooperative. He is upset about the worsening of his disease and his wife is not pleased that he will not be able to help around the house as much as he used to. They both understand that this is a chronic progressive disease. He has a forward flexed head posture and rounded shoulders, but ambulates without an assistive device, slight left upper extremity resting tremor, and slight rigidity in both upper extremities. He is lacking 30° of bilateral shoulder flexion and abduction and 0° of hip extension. Muscle strength is grossly 4+/5 throughout. He is able to perform 9 sit-to-stand repetitions in 30 seconds. His favorite hobby was fishing which he has been unable to do for the last year. He states "I'm pretty much useless now."

To maximize the patient's ability to exercise you schedule your next visit in the morning to take advantage of the prime effect of his Sinemet. During the second visit, you find that the patient and his wife have been involved in a loud arguing over where to keep the breakfast cereal boxes. The wife does not want to keep the cereal boxes on the kitchen counter where the patient has easy access, but on the shelf in the cabinet "where they belong." The patient replies to his wife, "You would be better off if I just died." After calming the couple, a discussion ensued over the course of the visit, and together we (patient, wife, and therapist) made a goal of the patient independently using a three-step ladder with an arm handle, to climb up and retrieve his cereal from the cabinet and the wife would put them back. During the next two visits, the patient did not perform the ladder task as well as had been expected, but at the start of the third week, the patient became quite motivated and showed rapid improvement and became independent in the task after 3 weeks. You are quite pleased with you work and the patient's progress in all areas and plan discharge from physical therapy after one more week to upgrade the home exercise program of postural, mobility, and strengthening exercises. The patient is also very pleased and asks if he can give you the mounted bass that you admired on his wall as a thank you gift.

You get a call from the home health agency the next day that unfortunately the patient took the ladder out the garage, which enabled him to hang himself.

■ CASE STUDY QUESTIONS

1. What is depression?
2. What causes depression?
3. Is it important that you know the signs and symptoms of depression?
4. Are there screening devices that can be utilized by a therapist for depression?
5. If the screen is positive, what do you say to your patient?
6. When would the best time to see the patient in relation to his dosing of Sinemet?
7. What do patients think about when they consider depression?

8. Can suicidal tendencies be a side effect of taking Sinemet?
9. What are the epidemiology/demographics of suicide?
10. Is it important that you know the signs and symptoms of people contemplating suicide?
11. What do you do if a patient tells you that they are considering suicide?
12. What are the legal ramifications for someone who attempts suicide?

13

DIFFERENTIAL DIAGNOSIS (FIBROMYALGIA)

William H. Staples, PT, DHSc, DPT, GCS, CEEAA

A 55-year-old female postal worker presents with joint pain and fatigue of about 14 months duration. Her diffuse pain and stiffness lasts all day long in both upper and lower extremities, but is worse in the arms and hands. The pain, stiffness, and swelling in her hands never diminish. The patient reports that her overall pain makes it difficult for her to keep up and keep track of her work tasks in the post office. She states that she wakes up two to three times at night to urinate, which adds to her fatigue. She does not currently exercise.

The patient does not report any recent illnesses such as the flu or a cold. Because the patient has a family history of colon cancer from her mother, she recently underwent colonoscopy that was reported as normal. She has had intermittent constipation and abdominal discomfort but says that her stools have been more regular since taking a fiber supplement containing methylcellulose recommended by the physician who performed the colonoscopy. She also reports a history of arthritis, hypothyroidism, hyperlipidemia, and depression. She has not had recent mammography screening although it has been recommended by her primary care physician (PCP).

She recently revisited her psychologist who does not think her depression has worsened and has not recommended any medication, but thought that an exercise program may help with some of the pain and sleeplessness. She has taken a nonsteroidal anti-inflammatory drug (Tylenol) since the onset of pain, but it does not seem to help. At her last physical 6 months ago, her PCP told her that her thyroid and hypercholesterolemia were well controlled with the current medications and that weight loss would help with her arthritis. The patient brings results of a previously obtained (6 months ago) complete blood count, basic metabolic panel, liver function tests, thyroid testing, and erythrocyte sedimentation rate (ESR), all of which are within normal limits. She denies tobacco/alcohol/recreational drug use. She also went to an orthopedic surgeon for radiographs of her knees; the report states that the films did not show any abnormalities.

MEDICATIONS

levothyroxine (Synthroid) 250 μg daily, simvastatin 20 mg daily, ibuprofen (Tylenol) as needed for pain, and a multivitamin.

PHYSICAL EXAMINATION

The patient vital signs are pulse 74 beats per minute, respiration 15 breaths per minute, blood pressure 138/86 mm Hg, pulse oximetry 98%, and temperature 98.5°F. She is overweight, with a body mass

Dsss of fibromyalgia: 11 out of 18 tender points, widespread pain

index of 28 kg/m². Cardiac and pulmonary sounds are normal. Bowel sounds are normal.

Range of motion and strength are grossly within normal limits for the extremities. Abdominal strength is 3/5. The patient has multiple soft-tissue tender points on palpation that include the bilateral mid-upper trapezius muscles, cervical paravertebral muscles, lateral epicondyles, upper lateral thighs, and medial portions of both knees just proximal to the joint line. Large joint examination is remarkable for diffuse tenderness (3/10 verbal analog scale) without warmth, swelling, or joint effusions. She does complain of mild tingling in her hands. No deformities are present in the hands. Reflexes are normal (2+) and symmetric in the upper and lower extremities. Cranial nerves are intact. No rash/bruises/open areas are noted on integumentary examination.

■ CASE STUDY QUESTIONS

Fever, headache, fatigue, chills eye 14

1. On the basis of the history and examination and using your skills at differential diagnosis, why or why wouldn't you suspect Lyme disease? → *Flu like symptoms, morning*
2. Why would or why wouldn't you suspect rheumatoid arthritis? → *morning swelling warmth → ANA*
3. Why would or why wouldn't you suspect myositis? → *ANA*
4. Why would or why wouldn't you suspect polymyalgia rheumatica disease? *Wide spread aching & stiffness*
5. Why would or why wouldn't you suspect osteoarthritis?
6. Why would or why wouldn't you suspect systemic lupus erythematosus? *Fever, fatigue, weight loss, butterfly rash, ANA*
7. Why would or why wouldn't you suspect depression?
8. Why would or why wouldn't you suspect fibromyalgia? *Pain, fatigue*
9. Should you send this patient to a specialist to get a specific medical diagnosis?
10. Why is it important to recognize and diagnose this disease?
11. The patient would like to avoid taking additional medications for treatment and asks whether she should look into acupuncture as a treatment for her chronic pain syndrome. What would you tell her?
12. Should you discuss the increased use of pain relievers with her primary care physician?
13. What medications are typically used to treat this disease?
14. What program would be the best for this patient?
15. Can and should people with this diagnosis exercise?

CRP ESR
↑ myorg → higher stiffer

Aquatic
Anti epileptics - typical, gabapentin (Neurontin) Anti depressants, analgesics

14

DIFFERENTIAL DIAGNOSIS (COMPLEX PAIN ASSESSMENT AND MANAGEMENT)

Lise McCarthy, PT, DPT, GCS

REFERRAL HISTORY

This patient's primary care physician has referred her for massage therapy for chronic neck pain. Her care manager has requested the expertise of a physical therapist as she thinks her 87-year-old client's needs are particularly complex and beyond the scope of a massage therapist so she makes a direct referral to a geriatric physical therapist in private practice who provides primary physical therapy care in the home under Medicare Part B.

PSYCHOSOCIAL

The patient, Lucille, identifies herself as an 87-year-old African American and a retired professor. She has no children but she has an older sister who lives on the East Coast. She was widowed 6 months ago having married her life partner 5 years before. Four months ago she fell into her glass shower door in an alcoholic stupor, and other than multiple superficial cuts and bruises, no further injuries were found during her 2 day hospital stay. She was discharged home with 24/7 home care services, which are still in place since she stopped walking right after the fall. She is currently bed bound with her caregivers providing assistance for personal hygiene care and meal prep. She has continued to drink alcohol, which is judiciously controlled by her caregiver under specific physician orders. She enjoys spending time watching television and talking with friends on the phone. She is not currently receiving services from a home health agency and she has not seen a medical health care professional since her hospitalization. Her primary caregiver reports Lucille has not changed in her presentation in the past 4 months.

MEDICAL CONDITIONS

TIA (diagnosed 2 years ago), cataracts (diagnosed 2 years ago), mild cognitive impairment (diagnosed 3 years ago), osteoporosis (diagnosed 4 years ago), left hip replacement (surgery 4 years ago), neuropathy (diagnosed 5 years ago), bilateral rotator cuff tears (diagnosed 8 years ago), osteoarthritis (diagnosed 10 years ago), atrial fibrillation (10 years ago), pacemaker (implanted 10 years ago), and cholecystectomy (removed 16 years ago).

MEDICATIONS (COMMON SIDE EFFECTS)

81 mg aspirin daily (bruising), 300 mg Neurontin 3×/day (dizziness, depression), 2 TUMS daily, calcium and vitamin D 600 to 400 tab daily.

CHIEF COMPLAINTS

She reports having "sore" neck pain that encompasses her posterior neck from the base of her head to her shoulders, as well as an "achy" headache on the top of her head. She also reports having "maybe tingling" in her right leg, and nausea and dizziness when lying on her right side so she tries to avoid this position and sleeps on her left side or on her back with a big pillow under her head.

FUNCTIONAL DEFICITS/LIMITATIONS

She is able to lift her head off the bed and hold her head up unsupported in a semi-reclined position. She is able to assist with rolling to either side. Her right leg feels "funny" and she acknowledges it feels "like it's tingling" but that she is not sure since she has not had much feeling in her legs for the past couple of years. She is able to laterally swing her legs and perform heel slides, but she is otherwise unable to lift them off the bed against gravity. She is only able to lift her arms to touch her forehead. Her hand grips are weak (right side worse).

ALLEVIATING/AGGRAVATING FACTORS

She is unable to turn her head to the right past midline or laterally bend her head in either direction without feeling something "strange" in her right leg. Cervical right rotation, right lateral side

15

Dizziness

bending and extension, and SLUMP test all increase her neck and right lower extremity symptoms. She expresses feeling dizzy when her upper cervical spine is palpated. She denies any increase or decrease in her symptoms when rest of her spine is palpated. She is not able to spend more than a couple of minutes lying on her right side due to nausea and dizziness. Her headache increases with attempts to cough.

OBSERVATIONS

She is a thin woman lying semi-reclined in bed who holds her head stiffly and slightly cocked to the left. She looks sad, her facial expressions overall are flat, and she speaks in a soft voice. She grimaces and verbally acknowledges feeling pointed tenderness with gentle palpation of her upper cervical spine, levator scapulae, and upper trapezius muscles, and along her nuchal ridge. Visual inspection and palpation of her back and lower extremities confirm there are no apparent signs of pressure wounds, joint inflammation, or signs of injury or infection. She describes the sensation of being touched on her legs as "I think I can feel something." She has a slight resting tremor in her left hand.

VITAL SIGNS (RESTING, SEMIRECLINED)

BP (left arm) 94/62, PR 70, O_2 sat 97%, RR 12, neck pain "mild," temperature is 97.9° Fahrenheit.

VITAL SIGNS (SITTING, TRUNK UNSUPPORTED)

BP (left arm) 82/50, PR 70, O_2 sat 93%, RR 24, neck pain "moderate."

FUNCTIONAL OUTCOME TESTS

Mini-Cog score = normal clock, unable to remember three words (ie, boat, apple, justice).
Function in Sitting Test (FIST) score = 12/56.
Pain Assessment in Advanced Dementia (PAINAD) score = 4/10.

INITIAL CARE PLAN AND OUTCOME

Diagnosing the presence of cervical dystonia, cervicalgia, and headache, but not knowing the cause, the physical therapist recommends use of a soft cervical collar as a protective measure and contacts the primary care physician to discuss the need for further diagnostic testing. Because Lucille is bed bound, arrangements are made for her to be transported by ambulance to the hospital for radiographic imaging of her spine and MRI of her brain. The results of these tests reveal an unstable C2 cervical fracture and associated soft tissue swelling with extensive white matter disease, ventricular swelling, and two small strokes in the area of the left basal ganglia and cerebellum. Review of her prior hospital records shows her neck and brain were not imaged. She is not a candidate for surgery, and so she is sent home with a cervical collar and a referral for physical therapy.

■ CASE STUDY QUESTIONS

1. On the basis of the history and examination and using your skills at differential diagnosis, why or why wouldn't you suspect cervical dystonia (CD)?

2. Why would or why wouldn't you suspect degenerative joint disease?

3. Why would or why wouldn't you suspect new onset of transient ischemic attack (TIA) or stroke?

4. Is there any evidence that supports the possibility that her cognitive impairment has advanced or that she may have delirium and/or depression?

5. Why was the Mini-Cog performed?

6. Why was the FIST performed?

7. Why was the PAINAD performed?

8. Can you use the International Classification of Function (ICF) model to outline elements supporting the need for physical therapy care management?

9. Given the findings on the physical therapy examination, what diagnostic imaging tests should be considered and why?

10. Given her new onset of unstable C2 fracture, what are four physical therapy care management services appropriate to provide during this first month, and what are the associated billing codes?

15

DIZZINESS

William H. Staples, PT, DHSc, DPT, GCS, CEEAA

A 70-year-old woman comes to your outpatient clinic complaining of having some unsteadiness, including a couple of near-falls and wanted to be proactive by going to physical therapy. During her evaluation, she states that "sometimes I get the feeling that things around me are spinning, especially in the morning when I get out of bed." She also reports that these "dizzy spells" only last about 30 seconds. She is taking furosemide (Lasix) for hypertension and a potassium supplement, otherwise she is in excellent health. She does not drink alcohol or smoke. She has no complaint of pain.

Her strength, range of motion, and endurance are all normal. She scores a 53/56 on the Berg Balance Score with difficulty when turning 360° in either direction. She is able to single leg stance with eyes open for 30 seconds and eyes closed for only 2 seconds. Her vital signs are as follows:

	Sitting	Standing
Heart rate	70 beats per minute	72 beats per minute
Blood pressure	128/82	124/80
Respiratory rate	16 breaths per minute	16 breaths per minute
SpO$_2$ (room air)	98%	98%

■ CASE STUDY QUESTIONS

1. What differential diagnoses would need to be made to assist this patient?

2. What is most likely the cause of the feeling that the room spinning for this patient?

3. What procedure/test can be done to help develop a physical therapy diagnosis for this patient?

4. How is the maneuver for benign paroxysmal positional vertigo performed?

5. What specific interventions can be given for this problem?

6. What is the prevalence of dizziness and falls in the population?

7. Most falls are multifactorial, so there is not one thing that necessarily is contributing to them. What are some other factors that can contribute to a fall?

8. What other types of treatment can be given to reduce the risk of falls?

9. What other tests or measures could you utilize in your examination of this patient?

10. Would you consider any referrals or discussions with the patient's physician?

11. Is there a scale to measure dizziness?

16

EMERGENCY DEPARTMENT REFERRAL

William H. Staples, PT, DHSc, DPT, GCS, CEEAA

You are a physical therapist working in the emergency department (ED) of a large hospital. A 63-year-old man walked into the ED with a fever of 100.9°F (38.3°C) and a chief complaint of left lower extremity pain and discoloration (erythema). He reported associated knee pain for the previous 3 days. He has been taking 650 mg of Tylenol (acetaminophen) for his pain and fever four times per day and just before coming to the ED. The intake nurse gives an initial diagnosis of "possible cellulitis with knee joint injury." Blood work was begun with a complete blood cell (CBC). The nurse referred the patient to the ED physical therapist to rule out knee injury as the source of the pain and erythema and to recommend further care of the injury.

On examination, the patient stated that he had 3 days of unilateral lower extremity pain with slight edema to the calf since playing softball this past weekend. His stated pain was 8 on a 0 to 10 pain intensity rating scale, and the pain was not relieved by the acetaminophen. He has been unable to go to work for the last 2 days and has been lying on a couch for most of the time. As for an inciting event for this injury, he was hurt sliding into second base on a close play. He states that he did not feel any significant pain until the next day. He reported minor cold symptoms but denied history of recent travel, trauma, surgery, hospitalization, chest pain, shortness of breath, or hemoptysis. He did report recent unintentional weight loss of about 10 lb in the last 3 months. His family history was positive for breast cancer. He had a one-pack-per-day smoking history for 20 years but quit 3 months ago when started his new exercise program, which included playing softball along with jogging 2 to 3 miles per day. His gait is slightly antalgic and he has not been able to jog since the injury. He reported a strong history of alcohol (2-3 drinks per day) use. He had no allergies and is taking no medications.

Vital signs in the ED were BP 128/74 mm Hg; heart rate 118; respiratory rate 20; and SpO$_2$ 94% on room air. He was alert and oriented and was in no apparent distress. The examination was unremarkable except for the left lower extremity evaluation. An area of ecchymosis measuring 4 cm in diameter was noted on the inner to posterior aspect of the left calf. This mark had no scabbing but visible surrounding erythema. His left inner calf and popliteal fossa had palpable warmth and moderate tenderness. Active range of motion (ROM) is normal; passive ROM is painful at end of flexion. The knee ligaments and menisci appear intact with testing. No masses were noted in the posterior popliteal area, and he had a negative Homans sign. His left knee was tender but without warmth, erythema, or loss of motion. His pedal pulse was intact.

■ CASE STUDY QUESTIONS

1. What else would you want to evaluate with this patient? Radiographs?

2. Is his self-dosing of Tylenol correct?

3. Are there side effects of Tylenol that you should be aware of?

4. What tests would you utilize to rule out ligamentous or meniscal injury to the knee?

5. What else is significant about the mechanism of injury?

6. Why would you ask about history of recent travel, trauma, surgery, hospitalization, chest pain, shortness of breath, or hemoptysis?

7. Are you concerned about his vital signs?

8. What mass are you screening for in the posterior popliteal area?

9. What is a Homans sign? Is this the best test to use?

10. Why is checking the pedal pulse important?

11. What would you say to the patient about the alcohol use?

12. How might the patient be treated?

17

STUCK IN THE EMERGENCY DEPARTMENT

William H. Staples, PT, DHSc, DPT, GCS, CEEAA

An 81-year-old woman and resident of an assisted living facility (ALF) with a history of right cerebrovascular accident 2 years ago was seen in the emergency department (ED) on a Friday afternoon with neck pain after falling forward out of her standard wheelchair at the ALF while trying to pick up a dropped deck of cards. She was diagnosed with fractures of the lamina of the right C3 and C4 vertebrae and contusions to her right shoulder and head. A neurosurgeon saw her and recommended only a soft cervical collar as there were no neurological deficits, and follow-up as an outpatient in 3 weeks. As the physical therapist on duty in the ED, the physician asks you for a consult to determine if it would be safe to send the patient home that evening. Her residual deficits, from the stroke, include a nonfunctional left upper extremity, which is held in a flexed position (synergistic pattern) due to increased tone. Ambulation before the fall required minimal assist of one person using a hemiwalker, but transfers in and out of the chair, toilet, and bed were all independent. She was also independent in wheelchair propulsion in the ALF. During your evaluation, the patient is found to have neck and right shoulder pain that limits her ability to propel her wheelchair or utilize her right arm to assist with any ADLs or transfers. The patient also complained of pain with swallowing. The ALF in which she resides requires that its residents must be independent in mobility either ambulating or in a wheelchair/powerchair to live there. Her pain on the right side is 7/10 using a verbal analog scale. Her daughter lives 60 miles away, but will be there in the morning. The patient lives on Social Security and modest savings. She has Medicare Parts A and B. You determine that she would be unable to be successful at the ALF in her current condition.

That evening, a hospitalist (MD) was contacted for patient admission based on the patient's status, the emergency physician's and therapist's concerns about pain control, and the need for assistance with mobility, feeding, bathing, and toileting. The hospitalist evaluated her but recommended discharge back to the ALF because she did not meet criteria for Medicare inpatient admission. The hospitalist suggested that speech therapy and additional physical therapy evaluations in the morning might be useful to guide the daughter on how to care for her after release from the hospital. On day 2, the speech evaluation is completed and it was determined that she could swallow liquids and food safely, but would require a soft diet for the next 2 weeks. A second physical therapist began to instruct the patient's daughter in proper care including transfers and mobility. The hospital discharged the patient to the care of her daughter the third day after another session of physical therapy without ever being admitted to the hospital as an inpatient.

■ CASE STUDY QUESTIONS

1. How does Medicare pay for admitted patients?
2. If the hospital does not admit the patient, how is the care provided by the hospital paid for?
3. Why didn't the hospital admit this patient?
4. Why isn't a skilled nursing home admission a possibility?
5. How many older adults visit the emergency department?
6. Would people not admitted to the hospital stay in the ED until discharge?
7. What happens to these patients who are not admitted?
8. What about home health care back in her ALF as an immediate option?
9. Will Medicare pay for home health care without a hospital admission?
10. On day 2 after the speech evaluation and physical therapy treatment, a meeting was conducted with a social worker, the speech and physical therapist, and the daughter. The hospital plans to release the patient tomorrow (day 3) without admission. What appears to be the best option at this time?
11. Why is a social worker involved in the discharge meeting?

18

END-STAGE RENAL DISEASE

William H. Staples, PT, DHSc, DPT, GCS, CEEAA

Your patient is a 64-year-old African American woman with diagnoses of type 2 diabetes, end-stage renal disease (ESRD), hypertension (HTN), peripheral vascular disease (PVD), and aortic stenosis (AS). She is currently living independently in the community and receiving hemodialysis as an outpatient at your hospital. Over the past several months, the patient has a self-reported lack of energy to perform IADLs, a loss of 10 lb, weakness in all four extremities. Her physician wants her to start an exercise program to regain strength and endurance.

The evaluation findings are as follows. Vital signs are HR 76, BP 154/90, RR 18, SpO$_2$ 96%. She has a shunt in her left arm (nondominant). Strength is grossly 4/5 with the left arm not tested against resistance except grip strength. Grip strength of the left hand is 12 lb, the right 16 lb of force measured with a dynamometer. Range of motion is within normal limits, except the left shoulder, which

is limited to 126° in flexion and 121° in abduction. She is able to complete five sit to stands in 30 seconds. A Timed Up and Go is 18.3 seconds. She ambulates independently without an assistive device, but requires a handrail to negotiate stairs.

■ CASE STUDY QUESTIONS

1. What are some of the consequences of kidney disease?
2. What is chronic kidney disease bone mineral disorder?
3. What is uremic arterial calcification (calciphylaxis)?
4. According to Fried et al (2001), what are the five signs of frailty?
5. Does this patient have frailty?
6. Are people with end-stage renal disease typically frail?
7. What do the functional tests performed tell the therapist?
8. What is dialysis?
9. What is the typical frequency and duration of dialysis?
10. What is the role of exercise in end-stage renal disease?
11. What precaution must be taken when performing exercise with a patient receiving dialysis?
12. What can exercise improve in a patient with end-stage renal disease?
13. When is the best time to exercise a patient end-stage renal disease?
14. Can someone exercise while simultaneously having dialysis? Are there any precautions for this?
15. What type of exercises can be performed while undergoing dialysis?
16. Can people undergoing hemodialysis actually build muscle mass?
17. What are the ACSM guidelines for exercise prescription for people with renal disease?

19

MEDICALLY COMPLEX WITH COMORBIDITIES

William H. Staples, PT, DHSc, DPT, GCS, CEEAA

You are referred a 78-year-old female patient for home health care with a primary complaint of lower mid back pain—right side. Her daughter, with whom she lives, took her to an immediate care clinic 5 days and again 3 days ago due to complaints of nausea and dizziness. She was put on two antibiotics Cipro (ciprofloxacin) and Levaquin (levofloxacin) but cultures came back negative so she was informed today to discontinue the antibiotic medication and start physical therapy to begin to mobilize the patient. The patient does not smoke or drink alcohol.

Her previous medical history includes hypertension, previous episodes of lower back pain, obesity, diffuse osteoarthritis, osteoporosis, and systemic lupus erythematosus. She has received vaccines for influenza and pneumonia. Surgical history includes an appendectomy 40 years ago, cholecystectomy 35 years ago, history of right hip hemiarthroplasty 5 years ago, and two (T-10, T-12) spinal percutaneous vertebroplasty injections 3 years ago. Mammogram screening performed 6 months ago was negative. Family history includes lung cancer in a sister that smoked, and cardiac-vascular disease in both her parents. Her husband is deceased from a cerebral vascular accident suffered 12 years ago.

She has not been out of bed, except to visit the immediate care clinic in the last 10 days.

The following are listed as current medical active problems under treatment:

1. Arthralgias in multiple sites
2. Benign essential hypertension
3. Chest pain
4. Congestive heart failure
5. Constipation
6. Costochondritis (Tietze syndrome)
7. Diarrhea two to three times per week
8. Dyspnea
9. Fibromyalgia
10. Hypertension
11. Inflammatory myopathy secondary to disseminated lupus erythematosus
12. Insomnia
13. Joint pain, localized in both hips
14. Osteoarthritis of the right knee
15. Obesity
16. Osteoporosis
17. Dysuria
18. Pancreatic disorders
19. Sebaceous cyst
20. Systemic lupus erythematosus
21. Recurrent urinary tract infections

She is currently taking the following medications for the previous active medical problems:

1. Calcium + D 400 mg tabs twice daily
2. Carvedilol (Coreg) 12.5 mg oral tablet; one tablet twice daily
3. Docusate (Colace) 50 mg oral: one tablet four times daily
4. Folic acid 1 mg oral tablet; one tablet twice daily
5. Furosemide (Lasix) 20 mg oral tablet; take one tablet daily
6. Hydroxychloroquine sulfate (Plaquenil) 200 mg oral tablet; one tablet by mouth twice a day
7. Ibandronate (Boniva) 150 mg oral tablet; one tablet per month
8. Klor-Con M20 (potassium chloride) 20 mEq oral tablet extended release; three tablets twice daily
9. Multivitamin tab; one tablet daily
10. Oxycodone-acetaminophen 7.5-325 mg oral tablet; one to two tablets twice daily every 4-6 hours as needed for pain.
11. Prednisone (Sterapred) 5 mg oral tablet; one tablet daily
12. Phenazopyridine (Pyridium) 200 mg oral tablet; three times daily as needed for burning sensation
13. Sulfamethoxazole-trimethoprim (Bactrim) 400-80 mg oral tablet; one tablet daily
14. Vitamin D (Ergocalciferol) 1.25 mg (50,000 units) oral capsule; one tablet weekly
15. Zolpidem tartrate (Ambien) 10 mg oral tablet; one tablet at bedtime daily as needed for insomnia

Her vital signs are: heart rate 81 regular; respiratory rate 20; blood pressure 126/82, temperature 97.8°F; oxygen saturation 93% on room air. Her height is 5 ft 4 in; weight 218 lb; calculated BMI 37.42.

On examination, she is alert, oriented ×3, in no acute distress (except for pain complaint), and does not appear to be acutely ill. Trunk: abdominal tenderness, but abdomen soft, normal bowel sounds, no guarding/rebound, no costovertebral angle tenderness, and no apparent distention. She is tender to palpation right of midline level of T10-12, no muscle spasm, nontender with spinal movements. The patient does complain of 5/10 pain (verbal analog scale) in the left hip and lumbar spine, and she states that the pain medications have had no dampening effect on the pain in her low back. Palpation of the low back pain in sideling does not illicit an increase in pain, but moving to sitting in bed increases pain to 7/10 in the low back and hip. The patient states that she has only been out of bed to use a bedside commode in the last 2 weeks because of the pain. She requires assistance for all activities of daily living. The patient expresses that she is tired all the time and wants to improve her ability to move around her apartment.

Musculoskeletal assessment reveals slight limitations in shoulder flexion and abduction with generalized weakness 4−/5 in the trunk and all four extremities and 3/5 in the axial (core) muscles.

Integument: No rash or open areas. There is slight reddening in the sacral area.

Neuromuscular: Intact to light touch, denies any numbness or tingling in the extremities. Reflexes are 2+ biceps, triceps, quadriceps, and gastrocnemius. Hearing and corrected eyesight (glasses) are normal.

Cardiovascular and pulmonary: Cardiac auscultation reveals normal heart rhythm with no murmur; lung auscultation reveals clear breath sounds in all lung fields. Deep breathing does increase spinal pain.

Mobility: Bed mobility from her standard bed is independent and is able to transfer independently in a squat pivot from bed to commode and wheelchair. Sit-to-stand transfer requires moderate assistance of one. She is able to sit on the edge of the bed using upper extremities for support. Unable to accurately assess standing balance due to assistance required to stand. She gets into her wheelchair only two times per day for meal preparation and stays up for less than an hour each time.

Assessment: The patient is generally lethargic, but cooperative with the evaluation process. Your primary goal is to mobilize the patient to prevent further complications.

■ CASE STUDY QUESTIONS

1. Can you make any preliminary judgment of this patient (what would you expect to see or not see) considering her previous medical history and needed rehabilitation?
2. What do you know about the variety of diagnoses that this patient has?
3. Are there any medical tests you would like to see the results for?
4. What can you determine from the multiple medications: possible side effects or interference with the rehabilitation process?
5. What additional physical therapy tests would you wish to perform?
6. What "red flags" would want to be aware of during the course of treatment?
7. What interventions would you start with?
8. What can be done to decrease the pain?
9. What are the complications of immobility?
10. What could be the cause of constipation and how can it be treated?

11. Why should a physical therapist worry about constipation?

12. Can you have both constipation and diarrhea at the same time?

13. What are the two medications she is taking for bladder problems?

14. What are the signs and symptoms of a urinary tract infection?

20

GAIT ABNORMALITY

Timothy L. Kauffman, PT, PhD, FAPTA, FGSA

As a physical therapist in an outpatient physical therapy clinic, you are about to evaluate a married 78-year-old female with the primary diagnosis of gait abnormality. You walk with her to your examination room. You notice a slight unsteadiness of gait, slight hesitation of forward progression of her gait, and she is using a single point cane in her right hand.

As you take her medical history, you learn that she has secondary diagnoses of (1) bilateral lower extremity peripheral neuropathies due to diabetes; (2) wet, age-related macular degeneration in both eyes; (3) left total knee arthroplasty 18 months ago; (4) osteoporosis with a vertebral compression fracture (L1) 9 months ago, which was repaired with a kyphoplasty. Additionally, your patient complains of symptoms including weakness, fatigue, unsteadiness, and she has had one fall without injury 8 weeks ago. She denies pain, dizziness, light-headedness, and cardiovascular diagnoses. Medications include insulin isophane and insulin regular (HumuLIN 70/30), alendronate (Fosamax), acetaminophen (Tylenol), and aflibercept (Eylea) injection every 8 weeks.

PHYSICAL THERAPY EVALUATION

Vital signs at rest: HR 74 beats per minute regular, BP 132/82 mm Hg, RR 18 breaths per minute, SpO_2 95%, temp 98.6°F.

The patient's static stance without the use of her cane appears safe. There is a moderate dorsal kyphosis and the distance from the wall to the occiput is 6½ in. The functional reach is 3 in left, right, and forward.

She becomes less steady with the Romberg test, but it is negative. The unsteadiness also increases with a tandem stance. She is able to maintain the sharpened Romberg position (one foot in front of the other) for only 1 second. She is unable to attain the sharpened Romberg position with her eyes closed without assistance.

A 128-Hz (cycles per second) tuning fork is applied to her right ulnar stylus and she feels it for 11 seconds. The tuning fork is applied to her left lateral malleolus and she does not feel it. The same response is found at the right lateral malleolus. She does feel it for 1 second at the right tibial tuberosity and for 2 seconds at the left.

She performs a 360° turn in 14 steps without the use of her cane. She maintains a one leg stance for 2 seconds on the right lower extremity and 1 second on the left.

With the use of her cane her score on the Modified Gait Abnormality Rating Scale is 9/21 with 0 being the best possible score. Without her cane, her score is 10 and persons who score over an 8 are a greater risk of falling.

Her self-selected gait velocity is 0.77 m/s with the use of her cane and 0.69 m/s without the use of her cane. Her Timed Up and Go (TUG) score is 14.1 seconds when using a cane. She performs a sit to stand five times in 18.8 seconds. Her score on the Modified Gait Abnormality Rating Scale is 10/21 without her Cane.

Her lower extremity strength on the manual muscle test (MMT) is essentially 4/5 when measured in the seated position. You do detect weakness in the end range of knee extension more on the left than on the right. The patient does reach full knee extension with force without extensor lag in both knees. She is unable to perform a one leg heel rise for plantar flexion strength testing. In the seated position manually, you score her ankle dorsiflexion and plantar flexion at 4/5 and you note the variation from the standard MMT. Ankle inversion and eversion are scored 3+/5.

■ CASE STUDY QUESTIONS

1. How is gait abnormality defined?

2. Why did the neurologist diagnose your patient with a gait abnormality?

3. What findings of your physical examination corroborate the patient's symptoms of weakness, fatigue, and unsteadiness?

4. Why is the patient at risk for falls?

5. What is the importance of the gait velocity?

6. What other testing might you perform?

7. What strength interventions will you employ to improve your patient's mobility?

8. Is the macular degeneration a possible factor in the diagnosis of gait abnormality?

9. How common is gait abnormality in persons age 65 years and older?

10. What is the potential for improvement in persons with a gait abnormality?

21

CLAW/HAMMER TOES

Meri Goehring, PT, PhD, GCS, CWS

William H. Staples, PT, DHSc, DPT, GCS, CEEAA

Ray is a 65-year-old man who lives alone in his two-story home. Ray is a retired carpenter, and has one daughter in the area whom he has dinner with once a week. In his retirement, Ray enjoys building birdhouses and cooking gourmet meals. Ray has a BMI of 29. He knows that he should exercise more, but has a hard time getting started. He found it difficult to maintain a regular walking program, and has a history of falls over the last 2 years. At his last physical examination, his physician discovered open wounds on his toes and feet. His physician told Ray that some of his toes have claw and hammer deformities. Even though he has not had much pain from the toes, he has open wounds on the superior aspects of four toes. Ray's physician gave him dressings and bandages and referred him to physical therapy. Ray is willing to try conservative treatment before considering surgical treatment to realign his toe joints. Ray has a history of cardiovascular disease (CVD), type 2 diabetes mellitus with peripheral neuropathy, and hypertension. He had a mild myocardial infarction (MI) 3 years ago which led him to retire. His current medications include Tenormin (atenolol), Capoten (captopril) 25 mg tid, Farxiga (dapagliflozin) 10 mg daily (which was increased from 5 mg at the last physician visit), and daily 81 mg aspirin.

When you see Ray in your outpatient orthopedic clinic and do a systems review, his ratings are: HR 84, RR 14, BP 124/72, and SpO$_2$ 96%. Light touch is impaired on both lower extremities to his knees with no dermatomal or peripheral pattern, and inability to localize a 6.10 monofilament pressure. He has diminished strength distally, and is unable to walk on his heels or toes when asked. There is some mild edema at bilateral ankles, leading to dorsiflexion limited to neutral position. On Ray's left foot, his second digit has a nonfixed hammer toe malformation, and his third and fourth digits have the claw toe deformities. On his right foot, he has another hammer toe on the second digit, and claw toe only on the third. On each of these toes with the deformities, there are wounds where the superior parts of the toes touch Ray's shoes, all with dry and cracking periwound. All deformed toes but the second digit on the left foot are moveable through passive range, whereas the left hammer toe is more rigid. Ray's proprioception is impaired in all of his toes and left ankle.

■ CASE STUDY QUESTIONS

1. In which toes are hammer or claw deformities most common?
2. What does a hammer toe look like?
3. What does a claw toe look like?
4. What other foot deformities may be associated with a hammer toe?
5. What are the most common reasons for these toe deformities?
6. In what types of individuals is this deformity most common?
7. What types of symptoms are present in individuals with these types of toe deformities?
8. Are balance problems associated with these deformities?
9. What is Tenormin (atenolol), and what does it do?
10. What is Farxiga (dapagliflozin), and what does it do?
11. What is Capoten (captopril), and what does it do?
12. Are there any medications for a diagnosis that this patient has that should not be taken with Captopril?
13. What balance tests might you perform?
14. What does the inability to localize a 6.10 monofilament pressure mean?
15. What type of shoes would you recommend?
16. What else can be done for these toe deformities?

22

LEFT CEREBROVASCULAR ACCIDENT (CVA) AND SLEEP APNEA

William H. Staples, PT, DHSc, DPT, GCS, CEEAA

A 72-year-old male with a history of hypertension and left cerebrovascular accident (CVA) with right hemiplegia, 15 years ago, comes to outpatient physical therapy at the urging of his wife due to recent difficulties with basic ADLs and community ambulation. She complains of hurting her back to get him into and out of the car last week. He is currently not performing any exercises or activities.

The patient also has expressive aphasia, sleep apnea, and hypercholesterolemia. He arrives in a standard wheelchair, which he

propels using his left arm and leg, but brings a large-based quad cane and is wearing a right ankle-foot-orthosis (AFO) with a hinged ankle joint with a plantar flexion stop. After the CVA, he received extensive physical and occupational therapy for 8 months and became an independent community ambulatory. During the last 3 years, he has decreased his activity level and gained 50 lb and has a BMI of 35. He is on the following medications:

Carbamazepine (Tegretol)	200 mg bid
Cozaar (losartan)	100 mg daily
Coumadin (Heparin)	(2) 5 mg + (2) 2 mg M&F and (2) 5 mg + (1) 2 mg Su, T, W Th, Sa
Indapamide (Lozol)	1.25 mg daily
Diltiazem (Cardizem)	360 mg daily
Lipitor (Atorvastatin)	40 mg daily
Travatan (Travoprost)	0.004% One drop each eye, daily

Examination reveals a flaccid right upper extremity with a one-finger glenoid-humeral subluxation. Range of motion (ROM) is limited in shoulder flexion and abduction to 100° with no other passive limitations. The right hand is edematous. The right lower extremity strength is as follows: hip flexion 4−/5, abduction 2/5, extension 2/5, adduction 4/5; knee flexion 2/5, extension 2/5; ankle plantar-flexion 1/5, dorsiflexion 0/5. The left upper and lower extremities are within normal limits for strength and ROM. There is no swelling in the left hand.

Gait: He is able to independently ambulate on level surfaces using a wide-based quad cane on which he leans heavily during the swing phase of the right leg. The right knee is in extension during swing phase and the leg circumducts. He is able to ambulate 40 ft with standby assistance and occasional verbal cues to increase hip flexion as he tires in order to clear the right foot before tiring and requests to sit down.

Vital signs at rest are HR76, RR 20, BP 146/92, SpO$_2$ 96%, rate of perceived exertion (RPE) 1/10. With activity (gait), vital signs are HR 80, BP 150/96, SpO$_2$ 92%, RPE 7/10.

He is able to follow all commands but has great difficulty in responding due to his aphasia. He is able to respond correctly to yes/no questioning.

■ CASE STUDY QUESTIONS

1. How common are strokes in the United States?
2. How would you objectively measure the swelling in the right hand?
3. What is the most probable cause of the swelling in the right hand?
4. What do the vital signs tell you?
5. Can this person be put on an exercise program?
6. What limitations need to be followed with this patient?
7. Can this person be put on a weight loss program?
8. What is sleep apnea?
9. How common is sleep apnea?
10. Is there a relationship between sleep apnea and stroke risk?
11. Can an untreated sleep disorder affect the rehabilitation process?
12. How is sleep apnea treated?
13. Why is sleep important?
14. What some tools to screen for sleep disorders?

23

MEDICATION RECONCILIATION—A THERAPIST'S JOB?

William H. Staples, PT, DHSc, DPT, GCS, CEEAA

Your new patient is a 78-year-old woman who has undergone bilateral total knee replacements 5 days ago and you are seeing her for the first home health session. She has a previous medical history including osteoarthritis, hypothyroidism, gastroesophageal reflux disease (GERD), depression, migraines, type 2 diabetes mellitus, peripheral neuropathy, insomnia, a BMI of 34, and hypertension. She has recently tried to improve her diet with increased raw fruits and vegetables, and began drinking diet sodas in an effort to counteract the obesity and diabetes prior to her knee replacements. Along with the traditional evaluation of range of motion, strength, vital signs, and function, you should perform a medication reconciliation by reviewing all the medications she is taking, both prescription and over the counter (OTC). The medications that you found include all of the following:

Prescribed:

Xarelto (rivaroxaban) 10 mg, daily
Vicodin (hydrocodone and acetaminophen) 300 mg-7.5 mg: one
    tablet orally every 4 to 6 hours as needed for pain
Nexium (esomeprazole) 20 mg, daily
Synthroid (levothyroxine), 100 μg, daily
Belsomra (suvorexant) 10 mg, daily before bedtime
Lasix (furosemide) 100 mg bid
Lyrica (pregabalin) (prescribed 2 months ago), 100 mg tid
Neurontin (gabapentin) (prescribed 6 months ago) 300 mg tid
Glucophage (metformin) 500 mg tid with meals
Elavil (amitriptyline) 50 mg, daily at bedtime

Over the counter (OTC):

Omega-3 fish oil 1000 mg daily
Motrin 800 mg, bid
Calcium citrate with vitamin D 630 mg/500 IU, daily
dl-α tocopherol (synthetic vitamin E) 1000 mg (1500 IU), daily
Pharmacy brand "Non-Drowsy Cold & Sinus Relief" PRN for
    nasal congestion

■ CASE STUDY QUESTIONS

1. Why do therapists need to review the medications that the patient is taking?

2. Why are therapists in a good position to see all the medications a patient is taking?

3. What are over-the-counter (OTC) medications?

4. Are there any possible problems with the pain medications she is taking?

5. What is rivaroxaban (Xarelto), and what is risks involved with it?

6. What are the side effects of the antihypertensive medications that she is taking?

7. What are Lyrica and Neurontin used for? Can they be taken together?

8. What medications may cause problems when taken with Lyrica?

9. What is Nexium for?

10. What is Belsomra (suvorexant), and what are the side effects?

11. Do therapists need to know what vitamins and minerals patients are taking?

12. Are there any concerns about the patient's new diet?

13. What are the ingredients of a pharmacy brand "Non-Drowsy Cold & Sinus Relief" that she is taking PRN for nasal congestion? Can these affect the rehabilitation process?

14. What is a tricyclic antidepressant?

15. Are there any problems associated with tricyclic antidepressants?

16. Why is the patient taking Glucophage, and are there any possible drug interactions?

24

MULTIPLE MYELOMA

James R. Creps, PT, DScPT, OCS, CMPT

Walt is a 68-year-old man referred to physical therapy for evaluation and treatment of unremitting back pain. He reports that his pain began approximately 4 months ago without any traumatic incident. In addition to his complaints of back pain, Walt reports that his symptoms are worse at night, and that they often occur in conjunction with a low-grade fever. He also reports that his weight has been decreasing even though he has not been watching his diet.

Upon examination by his physical therapist, Walt experiences point tenderness to palpation at T9-T12, although normal lower extremity reflex and strength testing is noted. Investigation of a biomechanical cause to his symptoms is unremarkable, although vital sign testing reveals an elevated temperature indicative of a fever of undetermined etiology. Because of these findings, the physical therapist refers Walt back to his primary care physician for further evaluation. After diagnostic imaging and lab tests, it is determined that Walt has diffuse osteoporosis of the thoracic spine, anemia, hypercalcemia, and abnormal monoclonal paraprotein. A diagnosis of multiple myeloma is made.

Walt is referred on to an oncologist and started on lenalidomide, bortezomib, and dexamethasone. After several months of treatment, his monoclonal protein peak is rapidly declining, although he has become agitated, has developed a serious skin rash, and is sleeping poorly. Walt is seen by his oncologist for follow-up, and the decision is made for Walt to undergo autologous stem-cell transplantation (ASCT). Two weeks post-ASCT, Walt feels profoundly fatigued and reports that his quality of life is very poor. As a result of this, he is referred back to his therapist for physical conditioning to include both aerobic and strength training. Walt and his wife receive instruction in a basic home exercise program, which she assures the therapist that she and her husband will complete together.

■ CASE STUDY QUESTIONS

1. Is multiple myeloma more common in the elderly?

2. Are Walt's signs and symptoms consistent with the usual presentation of multiple myeloma?

3. What is the underlying cause of Walt's skin reactions?

4. What is contributing to Walt's agitation and insomnia?

5. Is autologous stem cell transplantation (ASCT) a therapeutic option for the treatment of multiple myeloma?

6. Does ASCT give Walt a significant chance for long-term survival?

7. Is it common for Walt to feel poorly so soon after receiving his ASCT?

8. Is it better for home exercise programs in this patient population to be simple or more complex?

9. Does aerobic training reduce cancer-related fatigue?

10. Will physical exercise improve quality of life and reduce depression in patients with multiple myeloma?

3. What is a urinary tract infection (UTI)?

4. Are UTIs more common in men or women?

5. What is the most common form of a UTI?

6. What are the common signs and symptoms of a UTI?

7. What are some of the risk factors for a UTI?

8. How is the diagnosis of a UTI made?

9. What is a typical treatment for UTIs?

10. Do people with diabetes have a higher risk for UTIs? Why or why not?

11. Are symptoms in older adults the same as a younger person?

12. Are there ways to reduce the incidence of UTIs?

25

MYOCARDIAL INFARCTION OR URINARY TRACT INFECTION

William H. Staples, PT, DHSc, DPT, GCS, CEEAA

An 84-year-old woman residing in a skilled nursing facility has been referred for physical therapy evaluation due to worsening of her "Alzheimer symptoms" with "increased confusion, and loss of independent gait status" in the last 2 days with a fall yesterday. She had no complaints of chest or urinary pain. No injuries are reported from the fall. She also has diagnoses of type 2 diabetes mellitus and hyperthyroidism. On admission 4 months ago, an MMSE was 24/30. Vital signs are HR 92 beats per minute, RR 18 breaths per minute, BP 118/74, SpO$_2$ 94%, temp 99.8°F, and is not short of breath when transferring with moderate assist from the bed to a bedside chair.

At the time of the therapy evaluation, she had difficulty following simple commands or responding verbally to questioning. The therapist decided to curtail the evaluation and request that the physician order blood and urine labs before continuing the evaluation. The labs returned were as follows:

Blood Labs (Cardiac Biomarkers)		Urinalysis	
AST (Aspartate transaminase)	63 U/L	Specific gravity	1.040
Troponin I	8 µg/L	Glucose (mg/dL)	50
Glucose	110 mg/dL	pH	7.0
LDH (lactic dehydrogenase)	125 U/L	Leukocytes	++
Creatine kinase	1.3 mg/dL	Nitrite	Positive
WBC	6.3K/mm³	Protein (mg/dL)	Trace
RBC	4.2 M/mm³	Ketones	+Small
Myoglobin	50 (ng/mL)	Bilirubin	Negative
		Blood (ery/µ)	Positive
		Color	Amber
		Appearance	Cloudy

■ CASE STUDY QUESTIONS

1. What do each of the categories under urinalysis measure?

2. Does it appear that this patient has a UTI or MI? Why or why not?

26

GAIT ABNORMALITY WITH FALLS: CASE 1

William H. Staples, PT, DHSc, DPT, GCS, CEEAA

A referral is made to your home health agency for an 88-year-old woman who is living with her daughter and has a recent history of falls. The reports state that the patient did not strike her head during the falls and they occurred when the patient was trying to get to the bathroom. She lives with her daughter in a two-story home, and is independent in all ADLs. She began having episodes of urinary urgency, incontinence, and falls starting about 4 months ago and obtained a rolling walker. The daughter reports episodes of confusion and some paranoia. She still drives, but her daughter has concerns about this. She had walked around the block daily up until a few months ago when she got "too tired" to complete the walks. She received a new diagnosis of Alzheimer disease and now takes Aricept (donepezil). Other current medications are furosemide and acetaminophen.

Her previous medical history includes a 70-year 1 pack/day smoking and peripheral vascular disease, bilateral total knees 15 years ago, and hypertension. She is not diabetic and has not been involved in any exercise program.

She was referred for home health physical therapy for strengthening, endurance, coordination, balance, and gait training.

On examination, you encounter an alert, pleasant woman who is not oriented to time and has difficulty remembering recent events. She is also somewhat slow in responding to verbal commands. Her vital signs were a heart rate 74 beats per minute sitting and 80 when standing, respiratory rate 15 breaths per minute, blood pressure (sitting) 128/80 mm Hg, (standing) 116/70 mm Hg, and an O$_2$ saturation 97%. The patient has 1/10 pain in both knees. Her current medications are furosemide and acetaminophen. Strength and range of motion are all within functional ranges, with the knees limited to 106° to 108° bilaterally.

The patient is able to stand and transfer independently from a bed, chair, and toilet. The patient uses a rolling walker but has difficulty initiating gait. The gait pattern presents with three primary deficits including reduced stride length bilaterally, reduced foot to floor clearance, and a prominent loss of dorsiflexion at the terminal swing phase of the gait pattern. There tends to be a shuffling pattern using a wide base and short, slow steps with markedly diminished angular joint movements. At points during ambulation she appears to "freeze" and verbal cueing does not appear to help "unfreeze" her or stop the "freezing." She was unable to ambulate without the rolling walker. She is unable to stair climb, even with railings. Her functional reach is 6 in. Sensation is diminished in a stocking-type pattern in the lower extremities, and no resting or intention tremors are present. There is no spasticity or rigidity. Deep tendon reflexes are 2+/4 throughout.

■ CASE STUDY QUESTIONS

1. Does this patient have orthostatic hypotension?
2. What does the functional reach distance tell you?
3. What other balance test would you consider? Why?
4. How is the test you chose performed?
5. She has peripheral vascular disease, how would you check the severity of the disease?
6. What other medical problems might a person have who has peripheral vascular disease?
7. Does this patient have classic signs of Alzheimer disease?
8. Would you screen for dementia? How and why or why not?
9. What classic signs and symptoms of Parkinson disease might you use to differentiate this diagnosis?
10. What are the classic signs and symptoms of dementia with Lewy bodies?
11. What are the classic signs and symptoms of frontotemporal lobar degeneration?
12. What are the classic signs and symptoms of normal pressure hydrocephalus?
13. What is urinary urgency?
14. Why do you think that this person is incontinent?
15. How many fall risks can you determine?

27

GAIT ABNORMALITY WITH FALLS (NORMAL PRESSURE HYDROCEPHALUS): CASE 2

William H. Staples, PT, DHSc, DPT, GCS, CEEAA

A 76-year-old woman who began having mobility problems in her home recently moved into a continuing care community. Over the course of the last 3 months, she had been having difficulty with gait and had fallen several times while trying to get to the bathroom. One month later she had become essentially wheelchair bound, incontinent of urine, and more confused. Other than hypertension and mild osteoarthritis in both knees she had been in excellent health. Her daughter, who is active in her care, took her mother to the patient's physician and she was diagnosed with dementia and orthostatic hypotension. The patient's daughter was talking to the nurse in the facility about moving her mother to assisted care because of her increasing disability. The nurse told the daughter that it seemed to be a pretty fast advancement of dementia and suggested a more thorough medical workup from a neurologist. After seeing a neurologist and subsequent testing,

a diagnosis of normal pressure hydrocephalus was made. The neurologist wanted the patient to have 4 to 6 weeks of physical therapy to gather baseline data and to determine if improvements could be made conservatively prior to any possible surgery. The patient was referred for home health care under Medicare provisions.

On examination, you encounter an alert, pleasant woman who is not oriented to time and has difficulty remembering recent events. Her vital signs were a heart rate 74 beats per minute sitting and standing, respiratory rate 15 breaths per minute, blood pressure (sitting) 128/80 mm Hg, (standing) 116/76 mm Hg, and an O$_2$ saturation 97%. The patient has 1/10 pain in both knees. Her current medications are furosemide and acetaminophen. Strength and range of motion are all within normal ranges. The patient is able to stand and transfer independently from bed to the wheelchair and to the toilet from the wheelchair. The patient has a quad cane but has difficulty initiating gait and is unable to ambulate without moderate assistance and verbal cueing with the cane to ambulate 15 ft. Her functional reach is 4 in. Sensation is intact.

You order her a rolling walker from a local durable medical equipment (DME) supplier and commence therapy the next day. Over the course of the next 4 weeks, she makes steady progress. Gait progressed to 25 ft (I) with the rolling walker, able to get the bathroom, but not far enough to get to meals in the facility's dining room. Her functional reach improved to 6 in. She remained confused and episodes of incontinence increased, requiring the patient to wear adult diapers. The physician decides that surgery is the best option.

■ CASE STUDY QUESTIONS

1. Does this patient have orthostatic hypotension?
2. How would the rolling walker be paid for?
3. What does the functional reach distance tell you?
4. What is normal pressure hydrocephalus?
5. What are the classic signs and symptoms of normal pressure hydrocephalus?
6. Is there more than one type of normal pressure hydrocephalus?
7. How is normal pressure hydrocephalus diagnosed?
8. What makes the diagnosis of normal pressure hydrocephalus difficult?
9. What other diseases might share some of the symptoms causing a misdiagnosis?
10. What signs and symptoms differ between normal pressure hydrocephalus and Parkinson disease?
11. How common is normal pressure hydrocephalus?
12. Are there any risk factors for developing normal pressure hydrocephalus?
13. What is the primary reason for referral for undiagnosed patients?
14. How does this cause problems with ambulation?
15. What does the "typical" gait pattern look like for someone with normal pressure hydrocephalus?
16. What disease shares similar gait deviations? Which deviations?
17. What is the medical treatment for normal pressure hydrocephalus?
18. What is the desired post-surgical outcome?
19. What are signs that a shunt may be causing overdrainage?

28

OBESITY: PART 1

William H. Staples, PT, DHSc, DPT, GCS, CEEAA

A 62-year-old obese African American woman comes to your clinic to get advice about starting an exercise program. She has been to a surgeon because she is considering gastric bypass surgery. She has been told by the surgeon that she needs to start an exercise program first because the surgeon wants her to continue the exercises after surgery. Her vital signs are heart rate 88 beats per minute, respiration 20 breaths per minute, blood pressure 150/92 mm Hg, pulse oximetry 98%, and temperature 98.7°F. Her height is 5 ft 5 in, and weight is 312 lb. She is a type 2 diabetic and her medications include Levemir two units daily, Lasix (furosemide), and Cozaar (losartan). She is hesitant to start an exercise program and has several questions for the therapist. What is your knowledge pertaining to obesity?

■ CASE STUDY QUESTIONS

1. What is her body mass index?
2. Does this patient have hypertension?
3. What is Levemir?
4. What is Cozaar?
5. Is obesity a disease?
6. Is obesity a factor in cause of death?
7. Is diabetes related to obesity?
8. What other comorbidities associated with obesity?
9. Is cancer associated with obesity? If yes, what types?
10. Are some ethnic groups associated with higher rates of obesity than others?
11. Which country has the highest obesity rate?
12. Are all states equal in their rates of obesity?
13. What is the annual medical cost of obesity in the United States?
14. Your patient says her obesity is due to genetics, how would you respond?
15. Should your patient start an exercise program prior to surgery?

29

OBESITY: PART 2

William H. Staples, PT, DHSc, DPT, GCS, CEEAA

In Part 1, a 62-year-old obese African American woman comes to your clinic to get advice about starting an exercise program. She has been to a surgeon because she is considering gastric bypass surgery. She has been told by the surgeon that she needs to start an exercise program first because the surgeon wants her to continue the exercises after surgery. Her vital signs are heart rate (rest) 86 beats per minute, respiration 20 breaths per minute, blood pressure 150/92

mm Hg, pulse oximetry 98%, and temperature 98.7°F. Her height is 5 ft 5 in and weight is 312 lb. She is diabetic and her medications include Levemir two units daily, Lasix (furosemide), and Cozaar (losartan). She comes back for a second visit with several questions because she is still worried about the safety of starting an exercise program.

■ CASE STUDY QUESTIONS

1. Is it safe for people with obesity to exercise?
2. How do you determine someone's exercise intensity using the Karvonen method?
3. What are the guidelines put forth by ACSM about exercise for obesity?
4. Is there a link to increased risk for orthopedic conditions and surgical complications with obesity?
5. What are the effects of exercise for someone with obesity and diabetes?
6. Would diet alone enable weight loss?
7. What kind of exercise would work the best for weight loss?
8. How far would you have to walk/jog to burn 1 lb of fat?
9. Does exercise need to be continued to maintain weight loss in obese individuals?
10. How many blood vessels (length) are in 1 lb of body fat?
11. Why would bariatric surgery be good for a patient like this?
12. What do you know about bariatric surgery?

30

OBESITY: PART 3

William H. Staples, PT, DHSc, DPT, GCS, CEEAA

In Parts 1 and 2, a 62-year-old obese African American woman came to your clinic to get advice about starting an exercise program. She has now had the Roux-en-Y gastric bypass surgery 5 weeks ago and has been cleared medically to upgrade her exercises. She has been told by the surgeon that she needs to continue an exercise program to help with weight loss and overall health. Her vital signs are heart rate (rest) 86 beats per minute, respiration 20 breaths per minute, blood pressure 150/92 mm Hg, pulse oximetry 98%, and temperature 98.7°F. Her height is 5 ft 5 in and weight is 297 lb having lost 15 lb since surgery. She is diabetic and her medications include Levemir two units daily, Lasix (furosemide), and Cozaar (losartan). The patient believes that the surgery is a cure for her diabetes and weight problem and maybe she does not need to do anything else. Currently she walks 5 minutes in the morning and afternoon.

■ CASE STUDY QUESTIONS

1. How would you address her concern that her surgery is a cure?
2. Are they any specific precautions for exercise following gastric bypass?

3. How might the patient start an exercise program and be compliant?

4. What activity recommendations might you make to decrease a sedentary lifestyle?

5. What functional outcome tool would you choose to measure her endurance?

6. Are there any specific considerations during exercise that you would make to someone post-bariatric surgery?

7. What kind of diet do people need to follow after gastric bypass?

8. Are there any specific medications that will need to be added or adjusted?

9. What is "dumping syndrome," and how can it be avoided?

10. Is hypoglycemia a problem following gastric bypass surgery?

31

PELVIC ORGAN PROLAPSE

William H. Staples, PT, DHSc, DPT, GCS, CEEAA

You have been referred a 63-year-old woman who has undergone surgery to repair a first-degree uterine prolapse with a bladder prolapse. She had surgery 4 weeks ago following several years of urinary incontinence and more recently (previous 6 months) chronic low back pain. Prior to surgery, she had been using a pessary. Her primary care physician had prescribed Tofranil-PM (imipramine pamoate), which she tried for 3 months, but she stopped taking it because she disliked the side effects. She has no other medical problem and would like to get back on a regular exercise program, which she quit because she would "leak" in the gym. She was very embarrassed of this problem. She has had vaginal delivery of three children. Vital signs are HR 74 beats per minute regular, RR 16 breaths per minute regular, BP 132/84, temperature 98.7°F, SpO$_2$ 97%, and denies any pain. Her BMI is 28.

■ CASE STUDY QUESTIONS

1. What occurs with a pelvic organ prolapse?

2. What is the most common organ to prolapse?

3. How common is pelvic organ prolapse?

4. What causes pelvic organ prolapse?

5. What can make the pelvic organ prolapse worse?

6. What are the symptoms of pelvic organ prolapse?

7. What medical tests and examinations would the patient have to aid in diagnosis?

8. What is a pessary?

9. What is the nonsurgical treatment for pelvic organ prolapse?

10. What type of incontinence was this patient having prior to surgery?

11. What is the surgery for a pelvic organ prolapse?

12. Is physical therapy helpful after surgery?

13. What is Tofranil-PM (imipramine pamoate), and what are some of the possible side effects?

32

OSTEOARTHRITIS?

William H. Staples, PT, DHSc, DPT, GCS, CEEAA

A 71-year-old patient comes to you after seeing his primary care physician due to pain in his hips and shoulders and has a medical diagnosis of osteoarthritis. He had radiographs taken of both hips and shoulders, but they were normal. A lab report lists blood cell counts normal, the serum erythrocyte sedimentation rate (ESR) as 65 mm/h, slightly elevated CRP 5 mg/dL (C-reactive protein), and negative results for antinuclear antibody, rheumatoid factor, and anticyclic citrullinated antibody.

He has had pain and limitation in both shoulders for the last 3 to 4 weeks that has been getting progressively worse. He is taking two 220-mg Aleve (naproxen sodium) twice a day for pain. He denies any trauma and states, "They keep getting worse and I'm having trouble driving." "I guess I'm just getting old."

Vital signs are HR 74 regular, RR 16 regular, BP 130/78, SpO$_2$ 97%, temperature 99.8°F. A musculoskeletal examination reveals decreased active range of motion in bilateral shoulders in flexion (145°-150°), abduction (140°-145°), and external rotation (60°-65°) due to pain (6/10) throughout the range. Passive range is only lacking 5° in range in all motions and less painful (2/10). The patient's hip range of motion is decreased bilaterally in all motions due to pain (3/10), and due to the pain he has difficulty standing up from a chair. Palpation and observation of the joints and muscles reveal no tenderness, crepitus, heat, or redness, except both hands that appear swollen. Strength of all four extremities is 5/5. Gait is slightly antalgic due to the hip pain. The patient states that the pain decreases (2/10) as the day goes on unless he sits for a long time, then the stiffness returns.

Functional tests performed include the Timed Up and Go (10.2 seconds), and Five-Time Sit to Stand (19 seconds). You decide to see the patient three times a week for therapeutic exercise and to instruct in a home exercise program to decrease pain and increase active range of motion to prevent further loss of function.

■ CASE STUDY QUESTIONS

1. Although these symptoms may be osteoarthritis, is there something with the patient history that sounds strange?

2. What does the sedimentation rate tell you?

3. What are the normal ranges for sedimentation rate?

4. Is there another disease that may have been overlooked?

PART 2

After 2 weeks, the patient has not improved and you refer the patient to rheumatologist as you suspect something else is occurring with this patient. The patient comes back in 2 weeks with a diagnosis of polymyalgia rheumatica, and is now taking 15 mg of prednisone per day and has much less joint pain (1/10) in the shoulders.

■ CASE STUDY QUESTIONS: PART 2

1. What is polymyalgia rheumatica?

2. Should this person continue with the physical therapy program of exercise?

3. Are there any precautions now that the person is taking steroids?

4. About 2 weeks later, the patient comes to therapy complaining of a headache and blurred vision. Is this related to the polymyalgia rheumatica?

5. Are these new symptoms potentially harmful?

6. How is diagnosis of giant cell arteritis made?

33

IDIOPATHIC PULMONARY FIBROSIS: PART 1

William H. Staples, PT, DHSc, DPT, GCS, CEEAA

A 78-year-old male retired truck driver resident of a senior living community reported symptoms of increasing dyspnea over the last 3 days with thick, purulent sputum present, increased difficulty with ambulation, and confusion. The patient's daughter brought him to his physician, and he was subsequently admitted to the hospital. Upon admission to the hospital, radiographs were taken, which revealed a left lower lobe infiltrate. Oxygen saturation (SpO_2) was noted at 78% room air in readings before the patient was placed on 3 L nasal oxygen.

He was diagnosed with community-acquired pneumonia and started on Solu-Medrol, Levaquin (an antibiotic), DuoNeb, Mucomyst, Mucinex, to improve breathing. Additionally, he did have a course of IV antibiotics during the hospital stay. His physician suggested a brief stay in a skilled nursing facility following hospitalization, but the patient adamantly refused, returned home, and was referred to a home health care agency.

He was seen the day after hospital discharge by a physical therapist to admit for home health care. His previous medical history included idiopathic pulmonary fibrosis diagnosed 12 months ago, pulmonary embolism, type 2 diabetes mellitus, hypertension (HTN), congestive heart failure (CHF), prostate carcinoma, coronary artery disease (CAD), multiple episodes and locations of skin carcinoma, open wound on the right great toe, hyperlipidemia, and a transluminal angioplasty 2 years ago. He has an allergy to penicillin. Although he quit 4 years ago, the patient had a 52-year one-pack-per-day smoking history.

The patient is a widower who was previously quite active in the senior community. A daughter who lives 10 miles away is now the primary caregiver. She takes care of finances, medication setup, and shopping. Meals are provided to residents of this senior community, but the patient must make it down to the dining hall or there is a $25 room service charge per meal. The patient is in a room that is 400 ft from the dining hall. There is also an availability of in-house nurse, which also costs $25 to walk in the room for a scheduled visit, and $35 if the call button is used for an unscheduled visit. The patient is concerned about his finances due to these extra costs.

The medications he was taking upon home health admission were the same as hospital admission except for the two marked "NEW."

Glipizide XL 2.5 mg PO q 24 hours (for diabetes)

DuoNeb nebulizer qid (to aid in loosening mucosal secretions)

Warfarin (Coumadin) 2.5 mg PO M, W, F, Sa, Su (anticoagulant) and 5.0 mg PO Tu, Th

Bacitracin ointment (R) great toe, wrap with sterile gauze bid

Bisacodyl 5 mg PO bid (laxative-stimulant)

Zocor 20 mg PO Daily (for cholesterol)

Paroxetine (Paxil) 20 mg PO qh6 (antidepressant)—NEW

Docusate 100 mg PO bid (Colace-lubricant)

Prednisone 50 mg PO Daily (steroid)—NEW patient was on 20 mg prior to hospitalization

Mucinex 1200 mg PO bid (expectorant)

Furosemide (Lasix) 80 mg PO tid (diuretic)

K-Dur 20 mEq PO tid (potassium supplement due to use of Lasix)

3.0 L/min nasal oxygen

His lab values

Test	Patient	Normal Range
Blood urea nitrogen (BUN)	43.8 mg/dL (H)	10.0-20.0
Creatinine	1.5 mg/dL (H)	0.6-1.2
Glucose	69 mg/dL	70-110
Glycosylated hemoglobin (HbA1c)	9% (H)	4%-6%
Potassium	3.0 mEq/L (L)	3.5-5.5
Sodium	139 mEq/L	135-145
Chloride	85 mEq/L (L)	95-105
Carbon dioxide	41.7 mEq/L (H)	20.0-29.0
Calcium	9.6 mg/dL	9-11.0
Prothrombin	18.9 s (L)[a]	20.5-29.5[a]
INR (international normalized ratio)	1.9 (L)	2.0-3.0

[a]Protime range is in the therapeutic range. Normal range for patients not on anticoagulant medication is 11.0 to 13.0 seconds.

The standardized OASIS evaluation was performed per Medicare Part A requirements. The evaluation found that the patient used a lounge chair for sleeping, as he was unable to lie flat. The lounge chair has an electric motor lift that enables the patient to come to standing, and assist for transfers. His vital signs were a heart rate (HR) of 96 and regular; a respiratory rate (RR) of 36 and regular; and a blood pressure (B/P) of 104/66 while sitting. Oral temperature was 98.0°F. No carotid bruits present. He was on 3 L/minute nasal oxygen with a saturation of 94% at rest. This sat level dropped rapidly with accompanying shortness of breath with any activity, even minimal such as using a urinal, indicating severe debility. His vision was adequate and he wears glasses for reading. He was hard of hearing in both ears, but communication can be made by raising the volume of speech. He was only able to speak with short phrases between breaths. He denied any pain. Assessment of the integument system revealed an open circularly shaped wound that measured 0.5 cm in diameter and 0.25 cm in depth on the medial nail bed border of the left great toe. The wound had been covered with gauze but had fallen off. It was redressed with sterile gauze following the assessment. Both lower extremities had absent hair growth. There were many areas of ecchymosis on the upper extremities, which the patient stated were from the IV and repeated blood draws in the hospital. Sensation to light touch was diminished in a stocking-type distribution in both legs.

The patient reported a height of 5 ft 6 in and a weight of 205 lb. He has episodes of urinary incontinence, urinal present at side of chair. The urine was dark yellow in color and clear. His abdomen was soft. Cognition was normal and he scored a 30/30 on the Mini Mental State Examination. There were no outward signs of depression, and he was taking an antidepressant. He has a daily bowel movement and has bedside commode next to chair at 45° and a standard wheelchair on the opposite side of the lounge chair at 45°. There was a rolling walker with a seat and hand brakes in the center that the patient uses to transfer between the lounge chair, commode, and wheelchair.

The durable medical equipment (DME) that was present was an oxygen concentrator that he was currently using, a portable tank for travel that can be filled from a liquid oxygen container, and 50 ft of cannula tubing. Additional equipment included a tub seat and a long-reacher. He had one needed piece of equipment, a basket for the walker, in order to carry the portable oxygen tank. Medicare does not pay for this, so the daughter was contacted to purchase this item as it is necessary for patient independence.

A home environmental assessment shows an apartment that can be negotiated with a walker, but is not truly wheelchair accessible to small doorways and tight corners. It was not possible to get the wheelchair into the bathroom without taking the door off the hinges, which was done. No fall hazards were present including a pet, wires, area rugs, or general clutter.

EXAMINATION

His functional abilities were quite limited. He needed assistance for all activities of daily living (dressing, grooming, and bathing). His meals were being brought by staff to the room. His transfers required maximal assist to stand from a chair, but independent to pivot from chair to the commode. With the use of the lift chair, he can come to standing independently. Bed mobility was not tested due to his inability to lie flat. Gait used a two-wheeled rolling walker to ambulate up to 8 ft with moderate assist before tiring. During that brief period of gait his oxygen saturation (sat) dropped to 82%, the heart rate increased to 112, the respiratory rate increased to 40, and the blood pressure remained stable at 112/66. No irregular heart rate noted with activity. His gait pattern consisted of bilateral short strides, approximately 5 to 6 in with forward flexed posture. The feet barely cleared the floor surface and had no discernable "push-off" or heel strike. A Gait Assessment Rating Score (GARS) and the modified functional ambulation tool were not able to be performed. His strength was measured grossly at 4+/5 all four limbs. Sitting balance was normal, and standing balance was limited as he had to use the upper extremities for support to prevent a fall. He was unable to perform any of the standardized screens/tests for balance (POMA, Berg Balance Scale) due to the fatigue status. Functional reach was 0 in.

Throughout the examination, the patient had shortness of breath, particularly with exertion and a chronic dry, hacking cough. He complained of fatigue and weakness, discomfort in the chest, loss of appetite, and states that he has lost almost 10 lb in the last month.

His functional abilities have recently shown significant deterioration because 3 months ago he was independently ambulating with a rolling walker approximately 500 ft independently to get to meals in the communal dining area. He was also independent in all transfers and ADLs and was able to use the bathroom. He did not previously use oxygen, but had had several episodes of "panic attacks." These might be linked to periods of low oxygen saturation (sats) that were not previously detected.

The significance of all these findings is that this patient needs a lot of time and work. He is very dependent for activities due to poor ventilation and is a high risk for rehospitalization. Rehospitalization is one of the quality measures used in home care. One of the primary goals of home health care is to prevent rehospitalization because of the extensive costs involved.

Following completion of the evaluation, the physician was contacted to get an order to titrate oxygen with activity to maintain oxygen saturation at or above 90%. An additional order for occupational therapy was obtained to assist this patient with ADLs, energy conservation, and donning TED hose. The patient has TED hose but is unable to don them independently.

■ CASE STUDY QUESTIONS

1. What are the normal changes with the aging pulmonary system?
2. What is idiopathic pulmonary fibrosis?
3. What is the cause of idiopathic pulmonary fibrosis?
4. What are the signs and symptoms of idiopathic pulmonary fibrosis?
5. What is a typical course of idiopathic pulmonary fibrosis?
6. Is there an effective treatment for idiopathic pulmonary fibrosis?
7. Can a person diagnosed with idiopathic pulmonary fibrosis exercise?
8. Are there other names for idiopathic pulmonary fibrosis?
9. Why was the physician contacted about titrating the oxygen?
10. What is the prevalence of this disease?
11. How would a therapist determine the risk for pulmonary embolus?
12. How would a therapist measure dyspnea?
13. What do you know about the BUN lab value?
14. Is this a medically complex patient? Why?
15. What is an OASIS?
16. What are TED hose?
17. What are the top 10 reasons (diagnoses) older adults are admitted to the hospital?

34

IDIOPATHIC PULMONARY FIBROSIS: PART 2

William H. Staples, PT, DHSc, DPT, GCS, CEEAA

You do not need to read Part 1 before answering these questions.

This is Part 2 of a 78-year-old male retired truck driver living in a senior living community who reported symptoms of increasing dyspnea, thick, purulent sputum production, increased difficulty with ambulation, and confusion, and subsequently hospitalized. He was begun on home care and was seen three times per week for 1 week but was rehospitalized when he went into severe hyperglycemia with blood glucose of 290 mg/dL.

His previous medical history included idiopathic pulmonary fibrosis diagnosed 12 months ago, pulmonary embolism, type 2 diabetes mellitus, hypertension (HTN), congestive heart failure (CHF), prostate carcinoma, coronary artery disease (CAD), multiple episodes and locations skin carcinoma, hyperlipidemia, and a transluminal angioplasty 2 years ago. He has an allergy to penicillin. Although he quit 4 years ago, the patient had a 52-year one-pack-per-day smoking history.

His vital signs are heart rate (HR) of 96 and regular; a respiratory rate (RR) of 36 and regular; a blood pressure (B/P) of 104/66 while sitting, and oral temperature is 98.4°F. No carotid bruits are present. He is on 3 L/minute nasal oxygen with a saturation (SpO_2) of 94% at rest. He was also independent in all transfers and ADLs and was able to use the bathroom. He did not previously use oxygen, but had had several episodes of "panic attacks." These might be linked to periods of low oxygen sats that were not previously detected.

The medications he was taking upon original home health admission were the same as hospital discharge except for the two marked "NEW."

Sliding scale insulin NEW

Glipizide XL 2.5 mg PO q 24 hours (for diabetes)

DuoNeb nebulizer qid (to aid in loosening mucosal secretions)

Warfarin (Coumadin) 2.5 mg PO M, W, F, Sa, Su (anticoagulant) and 5.0 mg PO Tu, Th

Bacitracin ointment (R) great toe, wrap with sterile gauze bid

Bisacodyl 5 mg PO bid (laxative-stimulant)

Zocor 20 mg PO Daily (for cholesterol)

Paroxetine (Paxil) 20 mg PO qh6 (antidepressant)

Docusate 100 mg PO bid (Colace-lubricant)

Prednisone 50 mg PO qd (steroid) (the patient was on 20 mg prior to original hospital stay)

Mucinex 1200 mg PO bid (expectorant)

Furosemide (Lasix) 80 mg PO tid (diuretic)

K-Dur 20 mEq PO tid (potassium supplement due to use of Lasix)

3.0 L/min nasal oxygen

His new lab values:

Test	Patient	Normal Range
Blood urea nitrogen (BUN)	25.2 mg/dL (H)	10.0-20.0
Creatinine	1.5 mg/dL (H)	0.6-1.2
Glucose	153 mg/dL	70-110
Glycosylated hemoglobin (HbA1c)	9.5% (H)	4%-6%
Potassium	3.4 mEq/L (L)	3.5-5.5
Sodium	139 mEq/L	135-145
Chloride	95 mEq/L	95-105
Carbon dioxide	39.7 mEq/L (H)	20.0-29.0
Calcium	9.6 mg/dL	9-11.0
Prothrombin	18.9 s (L)[a]	20.5-29.5[a]
INR (international normalized ratio)	2.5 (L)	2.0-3.0

[a] Protime range is in the therapeutic range. Normal range for patients not on anticoagulant medication is 11.0 to 13.0 seconds.

The reevaluation again found that the patient still uses a lounge chair for sleeping, as he is unable to lie flat. The lounge chair has an electric motor lift that enables the patient to come to standing, and assist for transfers. His vital signs are heart rate (HR) of 96 and regular; a respiratory rate (RR) of 36 and regular; a blood pressure (B/P) of 104/66 while sitting, and oral temperature is 98.4°F. No carotid bruits are present. He is on 3 L/minute nasal oxygen with a saturation (SpO2) of 94% at rest. This oxygen sat level dropped rapidly to 86% with accompanying shortness of breath with any activity, even minimal such as using a urinal, indicating severe debility. His vision is adequate and he wears glasses for reading. He is hard of hearing in both ears, but communication can be made by raising the volume of speech. He was only able to speak with short phrases between breaths. He denies any pain.

Assessment of the integument system revealed an open circularly shaped wound that measured 0.5 cm in diameter and 0.25 cm in depth on the medial nail bed border of the left great toe. The wound had been covered with gauze but had fallen off. It was redressed with sterile gauze following the assessment. Both lower extremities had absent hair growth. There were many areas of ecchymosis on the upper extremities, which the patient stated were from the IV and repeated blood draws in the hospital. Sensation to light touch was diminished in a stocking-type distribution in both legs.

The patient reported a height of 5 ft 6 in and a weight of 205 lb. He has episodes of urinary incontinence, despite a urinal present at side of the chair. The urine was dark yellow in color and clear. His abdomen was soft. Cognition was normal and he scored a 30/30 on the Mini Mental State Examination.

A home environmental assessment shows an apartment that can be negotiated with a walker, but is not truly wheelchair accessible to small doorways and tight corners. It was not possible to get the wheelchair into the bathroom without taking the door off the hinges, which was done. No fall hazards were present including a pet, wires, area rugs, or general clutter. The bedside commode next to chair is at a 45° angle and a standard wheelchair on the opposite side of the lounge chair also at 45°. There was a rolling walker with a seat and hand brakes in the center that the patient uses to transfer between the lounge chair, commode, and wheelchair.

His functional abilities remain quite limited. He needed assistance for all activities of daily living (dressing, grooming, and bathing). His meals were being brought by staff to the room. His transfers required maximal assist to stand from a chair, but independent to pivot from chair to the commode. With the use of the lift chair, he can come to standing independently. Bed mobility was not tested due to his inability to lie flat.

Today, gait used a two-wheeled rolling walker to ambulate up to 80 ft with several rest periods before tiring. During that brief period of gait his oxygen saturation (sat) dropped to 82%, the heart rate increased to 112, the respiratory rate increased to 40, and the blood pressure remained stable at 112/66. No irregular rate noted with exercise. Gait pattern consisted of bilateral short strides, approximately 5 in with forward flexed posture. The feet barely cleared the floor surface and had no discernable "push-off" or heel strike. He was unable to perform any of the standardized screens/tests for balance (POMA, Berg, and Functional Gait Assessment [FGA]) due to the fatigue status. Functional reach was 0 in.

His strength was measured grossly at 4+/5 all four limbs. Sitting balance was normal, and standing balance was limited as he had to use the upper extremities for support to prevent a fall.

■ CASE STUDY QUESTIONS

1. What do you think caused this patient to be rehospitalized?
2. What are the normal changes with the aging cardiac system?
3. What is idiopathic pulmonary fibrosis?
4. Can a person diagnosed with idiopathic pulmonary fibrosis exercise?
5. What functional outcome measure would be the best way to measure endurance?
6. How would a therapist measure dyspnea?
7. What are prothrombin time and INR (International normalized ratio), and why are we concerned about them?
8. What is glycosylated hemoglobin (HbA1c), and what does it measure?
9. Why is assessing the wound important?
10. What is a sliding scale for insulin dosage?
11. Would you screen this patient for depression?
12. What are the top five reasons older adults are readmitted to the hospital? (Not diagnosis)
13. Why is preventing rehospitalization important?
14. Is decreased aerobic capacity a significant concern?
15. What type of exercise program would you set up for this patient?

35

SARCOPENIA*

Haniel J. Hernandez, PT, DPT

Michael O. Harris-Love, PT, MPT, DSc

Mr Jones is an 80-year-old Caucasian male who has been recently admitted to a community living center for generalized weakness and a history of falls. He was previously living alone in his home, and he typically had visits by his children once or twice per week. He recently fell 2 weeks ago trying to carry some groceries into the home. Mr Jones' house has five steps with a right side hand rail to enter from the outside.

His biggest complaint is his diminished ability to independently stand from the sitting position. He also reports that he used to be very active with cleaning chores and modest maintenance projects within the home, but decreasing strength and endurance has limited his ability to complete these tasks.

Upon reviewing his history, you find the following: hypertension, congestive heart failure (ejection fraction 50%), cardiomyopathy, and atrial fibrillation, with pacemaker placement in left upper chest. Echocardiogram does not indicate any thickening of the walls of the heart. The medical history was also significant for sensorineural hearing loss, obsessive compulsive disorder, depression, benign prostatic hyperplasia without urinary obstruction, and dysphagia that requires speech therapy intervention. Mr Jones' current medications are notable for his long-term use of anticoagulants. Anthropometric measures and vital signs include height 5 ft 9 in; body weight 179.1 lb; BP 135/78; HR 81 beats per minute. The physical examination is unremarkable except for 3−/5 hip abductor strength bilaterally with manual muscle testing (MMT). His balance scores with the Berg Balance Test revealed that he is at a medium risk for falls (score of 21). He is independent with bed mobility, but requires moderate assistance for sit-to-stand transfers from the bed side to standing with a rolling walker.

Given the patient's age, general complaints, and lack of clinical findings pointing to a systemic cause of his decreased strength, you opt to perform a brief screening examination for sarcopenia. Both the US and European sarcopenia consensus groups use customary gait speed to screen for sarcopenia. Therefore, you conduct a 10-Meter Walk Test and find that Mr Jones has a gait speed of 0.9 m/s. In addition, you perform objective strength assessment considering the observed strength limitations despite the minimal MMT findings. Given your limited time with the patient, and the resources available in your clinic, you decide to use a brief, pragmatic assessment via grip strength testing using a handheld dynamometer (HHD). The test results reveal that the average grip strength (based on three trials) was 75 lb on the dominant side, and 67 lb on the nondominant side.

At the subsequent patient care conference for the community living center unit, you summarize the status and evaluation findings for the new admission, Mr Jones. You inform the attending physician and the rest of the medical team that the patient's clinical presentation and low gait speed constitute positive screening findings for sarcopenia and may merit follow-up. The attending physician notes that Mr Jones would soon undergo a DXA examination to assess his bone mineral density (BMD) and help determine his fracture risk. Therefore, the medical order for the DXA scan was amended to include both BMD and body composition assessment. The subsequent report from the radiologist includes the following:

- Total mass (g) = 81,241
- Lean mass (g) = 53,549
- Lean mass – arms = 5635
- Lean mass – legs = 19,093
- Fat mass (g) = 27,693
- Bone mineral content (g) = 3088
- Android/gynoid ratio = 1.26

Determine how the imaging data and previous clinical findings augment your assessment of Mr Jones. Answer the questions below regarding the patient diagnosis, the utility and limitations of the imaging data, clinical body composition assessment, and the treatment approach for your patient.

■ CASE STUDY QUESTIONS

1. What are the clinical stages of sarcopenia?
2. Does this patient meet the clinical criteria for having the geriatric syndrome of sarcopenia?
3. Calculate the BMI for this patient.
4. Does the patient's calculated BMI place him at risk for sarcopenia?
5. How could you evaluate the effect of body size, as estimated via BMI, as a contributor to the sarcopenia diagnosis?
6. Name three common methods of assessing lean body mass in order of the most reliable to the least reliable.
7. What is the risk of DXA?
8. Can all forms of DXA assess both bone mass density (BMD) and lean body mass (LBM)?
9. Do the benefits of DXA justify its risks? Why or why not?
10. What does the ejection fraction mean?
11. Based on the information presented, what are you able to conclude about this patient's type of heart failure?
12. Based on the available information, is he a safe candidate for endurance exercise intervention?
13. Based on the available information, is he a safe candidate for resistive exercise intervention?

*Any opinions or recommendations expressed in this publication are those of the authors and do not necessarily reflect the view of the US Department of Veterans Affairs.

Funding for this project was provided by the VA Office of Academic Affiliations (OAA; 38 U.S.C 7406) and the VA Office of Research and Development.

36

SHOULDER PAIN

William H. Staples, PT, DHSc, DPT, GCS, CEEAA

The administrator of the nursing home in which you work asks you to check her 60-year-old husband, a retired police officer who has been complaining of diffuse "nagging" right shoulder pain for the last 2 months. On examination, the patient complains of pain that comes and goes even at night, making it difficult to get a full night's sleep. He denies any recent trauma. The pain is described as "achy" with an occasional increase in sharpness of the pain. The pain is a 4/10 on a verbal analog scale with the least (best) a 2/10 and most (worse) 6/10. He states that the shoulder pain has been making feel fatigued lately. Range of motion of the shoulder, elbow, and cervical spine in all planes is pain free and muscle strength is 5/5 throughout without any increase or decrease in the pain with testing. Sensory testing for light touch is intact and DTRs of the right arm are normal (2/4). No impingement or instability is noted in the shoulder. Cervical Distraction Test, Spurling Test, and Shoulder Depression Test are all negative. A Bakody sign is also negative. Palpation does not elicit or provoke any increase in the pain. Vital signs are a pulse of 74 beats per minute, respiration 14 per minute, blood pressure in the left arm of 138/84, and pulse oximetry of 98%. You decide to check the blood pressure in the right arm to compare and get a 136/82. He has been taking extra strength Tylenol three to four times per day, otherwise he only takes 81 mg of aspirin per day and is in otherwise good health. He has tried a heating pad on the shoulder with only slight temporary relief of pain. He denies any other pain including pain during urination.

■ CASE STUDY QUESTIONS

1. Why do you test strength and range of motion in the elbow and cervical spine?

2. What are the Cervical Distraction Test, Spurling Test, and Shoulder Depression Test, and why did you perform them?

3. Describe how to perform a Spurling Test.

4. What is a Bakody sign, and how do you test for this?

5. Why would you take blood pressure readings in both arms?

6. Does the patient's complaint of pain at night concern you?

7. What does the inability to ease or provoke pain in the shoulder make you suspect?

8. Can shoulder pain be caused by nonshoulder tissues?

9. What could cause pain during urination?

10. Are there any follow-up tests or question you would now ask the patient?

11. Would you schedule this patient for treatment?

12. What would you tell this patient?

13. What was the final outcome/diagnosis for this patient?

37

WHAT IS THE DIAGNOSIS?

William H. Staples, PT, DHSc, DPT, GCS, CEEAA

You are referred a 60-year-old female home health patient who has a new diagnosis of right foot cellulitis of unknown etiology and Sjögren syndrome. Until 4 years, she had no medical problems. She was diagnosed with Sjögren syndrome after a rheumatologist ruled out a previous diagnoses of rheumatoid arthritis and fibromyalgia, which had been previously made by different physicians over the past 4 years. Her current physician has ordered weight bearing as

tolerated (NWB) gait due to the pain and swelling but can progress weight bearing as tolerated (WBAT).

Upon examination, you see a fairly fit woman who had been an avid runner until 1 year ago and has been frustrated by her medical care and has been to multiple physicians looking for an answer to her medical problems. She has a current complaint of right ankle and heel pain of 4/10 throughout the day and night that increases to 6/10 with weight bearing, but is not tender to palpation at either malleoli, the midfoot, or over the navicular bone. The ankle is slightly warm to the touch. She also has a complaint of mild pain in her thoracic spine. Muscle strength and range of motion of the extremities were normal except for the right ankle with 0° of dorsiflexion and 27° of plantar flexion compared to 22° of dorsiflexion and 58° plantar flexion on the left. She is independent with crutches NWB right lower extremity on all surfaces. She does complain of generalized fatigue and malaise. Before she made NWB, she states that she tires rapidly when she attempts to do any housework.

Posture analysis revealed a slightly forward head. Ankle and foot size was measured by use of a figure 8 and at midfoot using the navicular bone as a reference point measuring cloth tape to determine edema. The edema was localized in the forefoot and the ankle joint and did not extend above the malleoli or into the toes. Edema measured 24 cm at midfoot and 50.5 cm with figure 8 compared to 20.5 and 42 cm, respectively on the left. Her vital signs were heart rate 66, respiratory rate 12, blood pressure 108/76, SpO_2 99%. Unable to palpate a pedal pulse in the right foot, but toes are warm and have normal color. Her vision was 20/20 and she did not complain of a dry mouth. She had just finished a course of general antibiotics and was taking Vicodin (acetaminophen and hydrocodone) 500 mg/5 mg four to five times per day for pain.

This patient was seen twice weekly over the course of 6 weeks where her ankle pain diminished to 1/10 and she resumed normal ambulation weight bearing as tolerated without crutches. The ankle swelling would diminish with manual therapy and drainage techniques but return by the next day. After week 2, an elastic bandage with closed heel was obtained to use following treatment. The bandage helped decrease the edema return but not completely and if she failed to wear the bandage the edema would fully return. The patient had been instructed in home exercise of ROM and positional drainage techniques to minimize the swelling. At week 4 following treatment, her right ankle had decreased to 22 cm midfoot and 46.5 cm figure of 8, but her generalized back pain had worsened to 3/10.

■ CASE STUDY QUESTIONS

1. What is Sjögren syndrome?

2. Is this patient taking the pain medication correctly?

3. What are the side effects of Vicodin?

   For the following questions: Are there any tests or measures that you could do or would recommend to help clarify a physical therapy diagnosis or rule in/out one of the following medical conditions? Do you think her current, previous, or new diagnosis may need to be made?

4. Could you rule in or out a deep vein thrombosis (DVT)?

5. Could you rule in or out fibromyalgia?

6. Could you rule in or out lymphedema?

7. Could you rule in or out rheumatoid arthritis?

8. Could you rule in or out an ankle fracture?

9. Could you rule in or out gout?

10. Could you rule in or out ankylosing spondylosis?

38

SYSTEMIC LUPUS ERYTHEMATOSUS

William H. Staples, PT, DHSc, DPT, GCS, CEEAA

A 65-year-old African American woman with a 15-year history of systemic lupus erythematosus (SLE) is now referred to physical therapy due to loss of endurance including inability to perform instrumental activities of daily living (IADLs). She frequently becomes short of breath during the day and has lost 5 lb in the last 6 weeks of which her physician is aware. She has been medically cleared by her physician to perform endurance activities. Medications include naproxen (Aleve) controlled-release 375 mg two tablets twice per day, azathioprine (Imuran) 100 mg per day, Zestril (lisinopril) 20 mg per day, Prilosec (omeprazole) 20 mg, clobetasol propionate (0.05%) a corticosteroid cream manually applied to her rash daily, and Plaquenil (hydroxychloroquine) 200 mg per day.

On examination, she presents with generalized weakness through the extremities and trunk, grossly 4/5 muscle strength. She complains of mild joint pain 2-4/10 on a verbal analog scale in her fingers, hands, wrists, and knees. She has a darkened (hyperpigmented) "butterfly" shaped are on both cheeks and across the bridge of her nose. Sensation to light touch is intact but she complains of numbness in her fingers and toes. She was unable to complete a 6MWT and had to stop after 3 minutes due to shortness of breath after walking 600 ft (183 m). At 2 minutes, she had ambulated 45 m without assistive device, but complains of pain in both of her knees of 2/10. Vital signs at rest were a blood pressure of 138/82, heart rate of 72, respiratory rate of 20, and a pulse oximetry of 95%, and temperature of 99.1°F. With ambulation, her blood pressure does not change but her heart rate increases to 104, respiratory rate is 32, and oxygen stat is 92%. Auscultation reveals no adventitious lung sounds and normal heart sounds. Using a Snellen eye chart, you determine her vision is 20/40 in both eyes. A Wells criteria scoring for pulmonary embolus and deep vein thrombosis are both 0.

■ CASE STUDY QUESTIONS

1. What is systemic lupus erythematosus (SLE)?
2. What epidemiological factors would be important to know for this patient?
3. What organs does SLE affect?
4. What are instrumental ADLs, and how might they be affected by this diagnosis?
5. How might these disease processes affect the rehabilitation process?
6. Why is the monitoring of vital signs especially important with this patient?
7. Are there any special precautions or monitoring that need to be taken for someone with SLE during therapy?
8. What abnormal breath or heart sounds might you hear in a patient with SLE?
9. Are there any possible neurological problems associated with SLE?
10. Is the knee pain consistent with the primary diagnosis of SLE, or most likely due to another problem?
11. Is the slight fever something to be concerned about? Why or why not?
12. What might be the cause of the weight loss?
13. How does walking 600 ft compare to the normative data for this person?
14. What other tests/measures would be useful?
15. What interventions would be useful for this patient?
16. What would you set for long-term and short-term goals?
17. Why is the patient taking each of the medications?
18. What are the side effects of each of the medications?
19. Are the Wells criteria for assessing for pulmonary embolism or deep vein thrombosis useful in people with SLE?
20. Why was it important to check the patient's vision?
21. What other advice would you give to this person?

39

THE OLDER ADULT WITH MULTIPLE COMORBIDITIES

Cathy H. Ciolek, PT, DPT, GCS, CEEAA

The patient, Mrs Ethel Hannigan, is a 78-year-old woman who sustained a comminuted intertrochanteric fracture of the left hip when she slipped and fell while getting up in the middle of the night to go to the bathroom, becoming incontinent and slipping on the wet floor. Her past medical history included a fall on an icy sidewalk 10 years previously that resulted in a right intertrochanteric fracture, which was reduced with a compression screw. Other past medical history includes hypertension, hypercholesteremia, osteoporosis, lung cancer (CA) (now 2 years postlobectomy), and irritable bowel syndrome (IBS).

She reported taking medications including metoprolol, simvastatin, lubiprostone, and alendronate sodium with addition of cefazolin and ketorolac (while in hospital). Prior to injury, she needed no assistance in any basic activities of daily living (ADLs) and instrumental activities of daily living (IADLs). The patient lived alone in an apartment. She did volunteer work for her church. Before the most recent hip fracture, the patient was active; she enjoyed walking and assisted in the care of her young grandchildren.

The second hip fracture was surgically repaired with open reduction and internal fixation (ORIF) using an intramedullary rod and a gamma nail. Physical therapy interventions included 2 days of physical therapy in the acute care setting, 20 days of inpatient rehabilitation at a skilled nursing facility, and six home care visits over 3 weeks. After a follow-up visit with her orthopedic surgeon, she has been progressed to full weight bearing, and she now presents to outpatient physical therapy at with the following:

Strength:

	Hip Flexion	Hip Ext	Hip Abd	Knee Ext	Knee Flexion	Ankle PF	Ankle DF
Left	4/5	3/5	3/5	4/5	3/5	4/5	4/5
Right	5/5	4/5	4/5	5/5	4/5	5/5	5/5

The patient's average free gait speed was 0.94 m/s with the cane and 0.56 m/s without the cane.

6-Minute Walk Test: 1046 ft with straight cane, with 2- to 20-second standing rest breaks

Timed Up and Go (TUG): 21.3 seconds with straight cane

Five times sit to stand: 20 seconds

Pain at evaluation was 3/10 along incision and generally 2/10 in lower extremity

Single leg stance: 15 seconds right, 2 seconds left

BP 142/88, HR 68, RR 16, SpO$_2$ 98%, temp 98.6°F

Her goals are to return to previously independent ambulation, to be able to get down to the floor and up again to care for her grandchildren, and resume her walking program and church work.

■ CASE STUDY QUESTIONS

1. What do the outcome measures tell you about this individual at this moment?
   a. Aerobic capacity
   b. Balance
   c. Muscle strength
   d. Safe/efficient walking
2. What would be a reasonable exercise prescription to address her musculoskeletal weakness?
3. What precautions do you need to be aware of with her medical history before initiating an aerobic exercise program?
4. What would be a reasonable exercise prescription to address her aerobic/endurance limitations?
5. Is this patient a fall risk?
6. What would be a reasonable exercise program in the clinic to address her balance impairments?
7. Why is urinary incontinence a concern for older adults?
8. What types of urinary incontinence are more common in older women?
9. How might her issues with urinary incontinence be assessed?
10. How might her urinary incontinence be treated?
11. What is lubiprostone, and what are the possible side effects of this medication?

40

URINARY INCONTINENCE—FOUR OF A KIND

Lucy H. Jones, PT, DPT, MHA, GCS, CEEAA

A 63-year-old patient comes to your outpatient clinic with a complaint of incontinence that has recently worsened. She had read in a magazine that physical therapy might help her with this problem. She has three adult children and a new 2-year-old grandchild that she cares for while her daughter is working. She has noticed that chasing after her grandchild has led to more episodes of incontinence. She states that she had some leakage episodically prior to this, but she managed that with an absorbent pad. She is embarrassed with this increase in fluid loss. She has no other medical conditions and takes Tylenol for occasional joint pain.

Continence is defined as "a state in which a person possesses and exercises the ability to store urine and micturate at a socially acceptable place and time."[1] Incontinence is defined as "the involuntary leakage of urine."[1] There is gross undertreatment of this disabling condition, and serious consequences for the older adult. Regrettably, the tendency is for symptoms to become worse with age. There may be embarrassment, a restriction of activity away from home, and/or concerns about odor. Physical therapy management of the patient with incontinence may be an important alternative to surgical interventions and medication.[2] There are several considerations in the study of this impairment. First being that the individual must realize that everyone needs to urinate, second realizing the need to locate the appropriate place to urinate, third to get to that place in the appropriate time needed, fourth to retain the urine until the proper place is reached, and last be able to urinate once that place is reached. Many of us may take all these steps for granted, but if any of these steps fail, incontinence may occur.[3]

■ CASE STUDY QUESTIONS

1. What is the prevalence of urinary incontinence among those over 65?
2. What is the incidence of men versus women with urinary incontinence?
3. What is the process of micturition?
4. What are the four types of urinary incontinence?
5. What are the gender-specific causes of urinary incontinence in women?
6. How is urinary incontinence evaluated and diagnosed?
7. What are examples of self-assessment tests for urinary incontinence?
8. What are the reversible causes of incontinence?
9. What is the relationship between urinary incontinence and quality of life?
10. What is the association between urinary incontinence and falls?
11. How does the physiology of aging impact urinary incontinence?
12. What are the medications used for continence management?
13. What are various physical therapy treatment options for urinary incontinence?

REFERENCES

1. Incontinence. MediLexicon Web site. www.medilexicon.com/medical dictionary.php?t=20067. Accessed June 20, 2015.
2. Borello-France D. Management of urinary incontinence in women and men. In: Guccione A, Wong R, Avers D, eds. *Geriatric Physical Therapy.* 3rd ed. St Louis, MO: Elsevier; 2012:382-398.
3. Prevalence of incontinence among older Americans. Centers for Disease Control and Prevention Web site. http://www.cdc.gov/nchs/data/series/sr_03/sr03_036.pdf. Accessed June 20, 2015.

INTRODUCTION

OTHER IMPORTANT ISSUES FOR THE AGING ADULT

William H. Staples, PT, DHSc, DPT, GCS, CEEAA

There are a few other issues that the geriatric physical therapist needs to understand. An important factor is understanding how the payment system works, in order to get paid for what you do. Writing a case study about Medicare payment is a risk because the laws, rules, and payment schedules change often. I have done the best under the current guidelines but some of the answers may be altered by subsequent health care regulation changes. Payment for providing services is essential to being considered a professional. All entry-level physical therapy programs in the United States provide a doctoral education and therapists should expect to be paid appropriately. But it is also essential to understand how payment for services works in order to justify that payment.

Elder abuse is another important factor to understand when treating older adults. Elder abuse can affect people of all ethnic backgrounds and social status and can affect both men and women. Elder abuse is an umbrella term referring to six areas of any knowing, intentional, or negligent act by a caregiver or any other person that causes harm or a serious risk of harm to a vulnerable adult. The specificity of laws may vary from state to state, but can be classified as physical, emotional, sexual, financial, neglect, and abandonment. The types of abuse may be briefly defined in the following paragraphs.[1-4]

Physical abuse, the most obviously recognized form of abuse can be defined as inflicting, or threatening to inflict, physical pain or injury on a vulnerable elder, or depriving them of a basic need. Physical abuse may include, but is not limited to, such acts of violence as striking (with or without an object), hitting, beating, pushing, shoving, shaking, slapping, kicking, pinching, and burning. In addition, inappropriate use of drugs and physical restraints, force-feeding, and physical punishment of any kind also are examples of physical abuse.[1-4]

Emotional abuse is the inflicting mental pain, anguish, or distress on an elder person through verbal or nonverbal acts. Emotional/psychological abuse includes, but is not limited, to verbal assaults, insults, threats, intimidation, humiliation, and harassment. In addition, treating an older person like an infant; isolating an elderly person from his/her family, friends, or regular activities; giving an older person the "silent treatment"; and enforced social isolation are all examples of emotional/psychological abuse.[1,3,4]

Sexual abuse is the nonconsensual sexual contact of any kind. Sexual contact with any person incapable of giving consent is also considered sexual abuse. It includes, but is not limited to, unwanted touching, all types of sexual assault or battery, such as rape, sodomy, coerced nudity, and sexually explicit photographing.[1,3,4]

Financial abuse or exploitation is the illegal taking, misuse, or concealment of funds, property, or assets of a vulnerable elder. Examples include, but are not limited to, cashing an elderly person's checks without authorization or permission; forging an older person's signature; misusing or stealing an older person's money or possessions; coercing or deceiving an older person into signing any document (eg, contracts or will); and the improper use of conservatorship, health care representative, guardianship, or power of attorney.[1,3,4]

Neglect is the refusal or failure by those responsible to provide food, shelter, health care, or protection for a vulnerable elder. Neglect may also include failure of a person who has fiduciary responsibilities to provide care for an elder (eg, pay for necessary home care services) or the failure on the part of an in-home service provider to provide necessary care.

Neglect typically means the refusal or failure to provide an elderly person with such life necessities as food, water, clothing, shelter, personal hygiene, medicine, comfort, personal safety, and other essentials included in an implied or agreed-upon responsibility to an elder. This is the most difficult to enforce as legal obligations differ from what many would consider societal norms of caring for family members and these can be different across different cultures.[1,3,4]

Abandonment is the desertion of a vulnerable elder by anyone who has assumed the responsibility for care or custody of that person. Abandonment may include the desertion of an elder at a hospital, a nursing facility, or other similar institution; the desertion of an elder at a shopping center or other public location; or a person's own report of being abandoned.[1,3]

Lastly, there is self-neglect. Self-neglect is characterized as the behavior of an older person that threatens his/her own health or safety. Self-neglect generally manifests itself in an older person as a refusal or failure to provide himself/herself with adequate food, water, clothing, shelter, personal hygiene, medication (when indicated), and safety precautions. The definition of self-neglect excludes a situation in which a mentally competent older person, who understands the consequences of his/her decisions, makes a conscious and voluntary decision to engage in acts that threaten his/her health or safety as a matter of personal choice.[1,3,4]

Another issue deals with the end-of-life decisions that can vary between personal, family, cultural, societal, and religious differences. The difficult position that health professionals are placed can differ from their own thoughts and feelings, and can be a very emotional journey. Some individuals chose to end their lives prematurely for a variety of reasons, so therapists working with older adults must be able to recognize the signs of suicide.

Lastly, nutrition is a factor in overall health of individuals and especially so with people as they age. A geriatric therapist should be aware of nutritional factors so that they can respond appropriately if clients bring up issues related to nutrition. There are two major problems with the nutrition for older adults. The first is overnutrition or obesity and the second is undernutrition or malnourishment. The medical complex chapter had a three-part case study on obesity. This chapter will have a case of malnourishment.

REFERENCES

1. Drench ME, Noonan AC, Sharby N, Ventura SH. *Psychological Aspects of Health Care*. 3rd ed. Upper Saddle River, NJ; 2012:321-335, chap 15.
2. Robnett RH, Chop W. *Gerontology for the Health Care Professional*. 3rd ed. Burlington, MA: Jones & Bartlett; 2015:315-316.
3. Ferrini RL, Ferrini AF. *Health in the Later Years*. 5th ed. McGraw-Hill; New York, 2012:453-456.
4. Administration on Aging. What is elder abuse? US Department of Health and Human Services. http://www.aoa.gov/AoA_programs/Elder_Rights/EA_Prevention/whatIsEA.aspx. Accessed March 29, 2015.

1

DRIVING

William H. Staples, PT, DHSc, DPT, GCS, CEEAA

Betty is an 86-year-old retired teacher who was widowed 5 years ago. She has hypertension, osteoarthritis in both knees, and a slight thoracic kyphosis due to osteoporosis. Following a recent car accident, she was sent to physical therapy due to continued mild cervical pain and stiffness. Cervical mobility was limited in rotation to the left. The comprehensive evaluation by the physical therapist also included the St Louis University Mental Status Examination (SLUMS),[1] and she scored 20 out of 30. Her eyesight was reported to be 20/60 and upward gaze was limited secondary to the kyphosis and deep set eyes. Her 10-Meter Walk Test was 1.1 m/s, and the Toe-Tap Test was 16 in 10 seconds. Her grip strength was 8.5 kg force bilaterally. After reading the literature, you also perform a 20-Foot Walk Test where the patient walks 10 ft, turns, and returns to the start. The patient is able to perform this in 10 seconds. Medications that she is taking include metoprolol (Lopressor) for the hypertension, risedronate (Actonel) for osteoporosis, and Tylenol for arthritis pain. Her physician added Flexeril (cyclobenzaprine) to relax the cervical muscle spasms for the next 2 weeks. You notice she has great difficulty parking in a lined space, and departing in her car from your clinic you have witnessed a couple of near misses with both parked and moving cars. The pain subsided in 2 weeks of moist heat application and soft tissue mobilization but should you be concerned about her ability to drive safely?

■ CASE STUDY QUESTIONS

1. What are the demographics of older drivers?
2. Why was each of the functional tests important?
3. How is the Toe-Tap Test performed, and where does this patient fit compared to the age-related norms?

4. Functionally, for driving, how do the test results affect the ability to drive? (Consider vision, cognition, and motor function.)
5. Why is it so important to check Betty's vision?
6. What are the possible side effects of the prescribed medications that could affect driving?
7. What physical therapy interventions would you initiate to assist with her driving?
8. What would you suggest for this patient regarding driving safety?
9. Would this patient benefit from a formal driving assessment?
10. How might you suggest to the family the best way to discuss the unsafe driving issue?
11. Does your state/province/country require health professionals to report possible unsafe drivers?
12. What are the most common moving violations for older adults?

REFERENCE

1. Older adult drivers. Centers for Disease Control & Prevention Web site. http://www.cdc.gov/Motorvehiclesafety/Older_Adult_Drivers/. Accessed July 7, 2013.

2

ELDER ABUSE: CASE 1

William H. Staples, PT, DHSc, DPT, GCS, CEEAA

Mr Roberts is an 82-year-old man. He is thin and somewhat frail, but, except for blood pressure medication and a diagnosis made last year of early stage of Alzheimer disease, is in generally good health. Up until the last several weeks, he has been independent with his ADLs and ambulated independently in the home and community. His wife has been deceased for 5 years, and for the last 2 years, he has been splitting his time among his three children with 4-month rotations at each of their homes. The children all live in different parts of the country.

Mr Roberts is currently residing with his 44-year-old daughter, Rose, in Indianapolis. She is a single mom (had a messy divorce approximately 2 years ago) with two teenage children. Although Rose has a professional position at a large pharmaceutical company with good benefits, money has been a constant concern since the divorce. She is currently back in court with her ex-husband, trying to increase his child support payments. She desperately wants to keep the home and lifestyle to which she and the children have been accustomed. Her husband is remarried and lives out of state and rarely gets his child support payments to Rose in a timely basis.

The children are good students, but recently, the 14-year-old girl has had lots of extracurricular expenses, including an expensive computer program for her advanced math class, a new color guard uniform, and another round of orthodonture. The 16-year-old son has just gotten pretty hot and heavy with his girlfriend, and although "house rules" state that there should be no friends around when mom is not home, 2 weeks ago, Rose caught her son and girlfriend entwined and partially undressed on the couch when she came home early from work. Rose was angry with her father for not supervising them. She also called the girl's parents and her son has not spoken to his mother since that time.

Mr Roberts has been living with Rose for 6 weeks. He has typically been safe spending the days at home alone. In the last few weeks, however, he has left the stove on twice and has locked himself out of the house, and been doing some wandering around the neighborhood. Against Rose's wishes, he took out the car last week, got confused about how to get home, had an accident, and had to be brought home by the police. He has been stiff and sore since the accident. Mr Roberts repeats himself constantly and is very demanding of Rose's time when she is home. In the last 2 weeks, she has had to call him at home two to three times a day to check on him.

Rose admitted her father to a full-time program (8 hours/day, 5 days/week) at the local adult day care center where you, a physical therapist, work two mornings a week. Typically with a new guest, you do a complete physical therapy examination to document admission status and prepare a plan of care for the activities director regarding safety, gait status, transfers, and ability to use the restroom. This morning when Rose arrived with her father, you spent a brief time with her prior to the examination. She looked haggard and was very short with you about the questions you were asking until you discovered that you had a mutual friend. She then became more talkative and states she "had a late night, last night" and described that she was pleased to be able to bring her dad to the center in spite of the fact that her siblings had forbidden her to do so because of the cost which they are unwilling to share. She reported that she found herself unable to cope with caring for him at home because of stress.

During your examination, you noticed that whenever you made a sudden move, Mr Roberts flinched. You also noted that he had several burns on his hands and arms. You note limited neck ROM and when asked, Mr Roberts reported that he injured his neck when Rose pushed him onto the floor during an angry outburst 3 to 4 days ago. He also states that his daughter is always yelling at him.

■ CASE STUDY QUESTIONS

1. What is elder abuse?
2. How would you define physical abuse?
3. What are the signs and symptoms of physical abuse?
4. How would you define emotional abuse?
5. What are the signs and symptoms of emotional abuse?
6. How would you define sexual abuse?
7. What are the signs and symptoms of sexual abuse?
8. How would you define exploitation?
9. What are the signs and symptoms of exploitation?
10. How would you define neglect?
11. What are the signs and symptoms of neglect?
12. How would you define abandonment?
13. What are the signs and symptoms of abandonment?
14. What makes an older adult vulnerable to abuse?
15. Who are the abusers of older people?
16. Are there criminal penalties for the abusers?
17. How many people are suffering from elder abuse?
18. Who do I call if I suspect elder abuse?
19. What should I expect if I call someone for help?
20. How can elder abuse be prevented?
21. Does elder abuse occur in nursing homes? If so, what might be the cause?
22. How can abuse be prevented in long-term care facilities?

ELDER ABUSE: CASE 2

William H. Staples, PT, DHSc, DPT, GCS, CEEAA

The home health agency was referred a patient from a physician's office whose family member (niece) called concerned about his health. The police department had made a visit upon the daughter's request earlier in the week, but the patient refused to let them in. The police reported that the home had a foul smell, but they have no reason to follow up as the person is alive as no crime has been reported. The patient is an 86-year-old male who the family reports has always been something of a "hermit" since his wife left him almost 20 years ago after retiring as a plumber. Over the last year, the niece would occasionally drop off food for her uncle, but he would never let her in the home, telling her "all you want is my money."

The patient does not have a phone as service was turned off last year due to nonpayment of his bill, so all appointments are made through the niece. A registered nurse made the initial visit and was able to gain entrance to the house. The house was foul smelling, and the nurse noted that the patient had at least three cats that were not well fed. The description of the patient was that he appeared confused, malnourished, dehydrated, had matted hair, and wore dirty clothes including two coats. Upon questioning, the patient appeared evasive.

The nursing assessment includes patient's vital signs which were HR 102 with an occasional irregularity, RR 20, BP 86/62, SpO_2 94%, temp 99.8°F. The patient had poor skin turgor. His medical history consists of angina, a myocardial infarction 10 years ago, and type 2 diabetes. He is 6-ft tall and weighs 121 lb. His blood sugar was 178. Lungs are clear and the patient reports no open wounds but would not let the nurse perform a complete body inspection. The house smells like urine, but the patient denies urinary incontinence, and he cannot recall the last time he had a bowel movement. He has prescriptions for metformin (Glucophage), nifedipine (Procardia), nitroglycerin, but it does not appear that he has been taking the metformin as the prescription is old. The bottle of nitroglycerin is 2 years old and has been opened. The patient reports he has not had any chest pain in 2 years. The nurse finds the refrigerator essentially empty except a stale loaf of bread, a small bottle of ketchup, and a couple of beers. There are two microwavable dinners in the freezer.

The patient is able to negotiate inside the home holding onto furniture, but stumbles occasionally. The patient refuses to demonstrate any ADL skills.

The nurse tries to convince the patient to go to the hospital for a thorough medical checkup, but the patient adamantly refuses. She does convince the patient to have a physical therapist come to assess his mobility and function as he appears to be a fall risk. The nurse also contacts the patient's physician about medications, but the physician wants to see him in his office before changing any medications. The nurse encourages the patient to drink lots of water and take his current medications as prescribed. She reorders all his medications. The nurse also contacts a social worker to help obtain meals on wheels and/or food stamps.

The physical therapy evaluation is performed 2 days later. You follow the patient to the kitchen and observe a slow, shuffling gait pattern with forward leaning posture. You continue your evaluation sitting at the kitchen table. Besides the pungent odor of urine, you notice that the patient has a sickly sweet, fruity breath odor. Vital signs are HR 106 with irregularity, RR 28, BP 86/60, SpO_2 94%, temp 99.9°F. The patient states he has not taken his blood sugar today and does not plan to despite your request to do so. The patient appears confused and complains of a headache. You attempt to perform some physical tests but the patient is quite lethargic. A skin turgor test strongly suggests severe dehydration.

■ CASE STUDY QUESTIONS

1. How would you define self-neglect?
2. What are the signs and symptoms of self-neglect?
3. How common is self-neglect?
4. What signs and symptoms of self-neglect are similar to those seen in dementia or depression?
5. Why is self-neglect of importance?
6. Does the patient have the right to remain in his home under these conditions?
7. What would have to happen to get him out of his home?
8. What are the rules for developing a conservatory in your state?
9. What is a power of attorney?
10. What are the reasons he has been prescribed the medications he is taking?
11. What are the signs of dehydration?
12. How would a therapist check skin turgor?
13. What is diabetic ketoacidosis?
14. What are the symptoms of diabetic ketoacidosis?
15. What should you as a therapist do next?
16. What happens if the patient were to refuse your choice of what to do next?

ELDER ORPHANS

William H. Staples, PT, DHSc, DPT, GCS, CEEAA

An 83-year-old male is admitted to your long-term care facility after a 5-day hospitalization before which the patient attempted to take his own life by overdosing with pain killers. Luckily, he was found conscious the following day when a neighbor saw 2 days of newspapers on the front porch, which was unusual as the patient was unable to leave his home without assistance. The medical team decided that the patient would not be able to go back to living by himself because of his condition and complications while in the hospital. He has no local support mechanism. He is widowed and his only son lives across the country. He also has no social support in the area except for his neighbor who is 86 years old and just able to care for himself. The patient was placed, possibly permanently, in a nursing home.

■ CASE STUDY QUESTIONS

1. What is an elder orphan?
2. What percent of older adults are elder orphans?
3. Will this affect the health care system?
4. What is the current population in nursing homes?

5. What causes someone to become an elder orphan?
6. What percentage of nursing home residents do not have regular visitors?
7. What are the risk factors for admission to a nursing home?
8. How much will the nursing home population grow in the next few years?
9. Who pays for most nursing home care?
10. How many nursing homes are in the United States?
11. Is there a way society could help older adults age in place and cost the system (tax payers) less money?

END-OF-LIFE DECISIONS: CASE 1

Lucy H. Jones, PT, DPT, MHA, GCS, CEEAA

Living wills, advanced directive, and do not resuscitate (DNR) orders can all be confusing as we prepare our elders for end-of-life decisions.[1] Many people may think they have already addressed this earlier in their lives, but questions to ask are: Is the language current, and is the statement of their wishes succinct enough to be understood?[2] What health professionals are finding, nationwide, is there is a lack of communication of a person's wishes as they go to the final stages of their lives.[3] Either the language is not clear enough as to what services they do or do not want, or presented with so much legalese that there is no time to decipher it when needed.[4] Therefore, in the process of an emergency there is little time to listen to precisely what the family is saying.[5]

Case Study: An 86-year-old man, Stan, thought that he and his wife, Louise, had dealt with the end-of-life issue years ago. Their "living will" from the state of Missouri stated, "No extreme measures were to be used to keep alive either party should there be no chance of recovery or quality of life to preserve." His wife was failing from pneumonia, and had end-stage Alzheimer disease. She was admitted from their home of 47 years to an assisted living facility after she had become essentially nonverbal and nonambulatory without assistance 5 months previously. She was transferred to the nursing facility 2 months ago. Stan moved into an independent senior living apartment that was part of the same continuing care community, so he could remain near to her. Her nighttime restlessness was all that could reveal discomfort and her shallow breaths signified to him and the caregivers that she was in distress. She had a scheduled visit with the facility's medical director, who never addressed end-of-life wishes at any previous or at this current visit, took one look at her and said in a panic, "She needs to go the hospital right now!" This raised everyone's emotions and 911 was called.

To the credit of the ambulance attendant, he asked, "What would you like us to do?" Seeing his wife in distress, Stan said, "Could you just give her a little oxygen to make her breathe more easily?" He did not realize that the word "oxygen" meant initiate bagging and establishing an airway, thus a full code. Once at the hospital, because bagging was initiated in the ambulance, the resuscitation would continue as protocol.[6] Stan had a copy of his wife's "living will," which he showed to the doctor. It was dated February 1990, and was three pages of legal terms with no clear-cut distinction of a desire not to resuscitate.[5] Here was an educated man who sought the advice of his lawyers, but never had the document reviewed, thinking once was enough.[7] Upon entering her room, Stan found that she was intubated with several tubes, indicating multiple systems' failure. Her husband of 56 years began to cry and said, "Couldn't they just let her go; she wouldn't want to be this way."

Family members began to gather and asked three times to talk to the doctor, who never came out to see them.[8] Finally, as most of the family arrived, they were all shocked at the lack of communication at every turn concerning a "do not resuscitate (DNR)" wish. When the family finally got someone to listen 3 hours later, a quality assurance person had to interview Stan and get his signature to approve the removal of the breathing tube by the respiratory therapist, which occurred 2 hours after he signed their document.[9] Louise lived four more days with labored breathing, in a coma, with just enough antibiotics and oxygenated blood to linger.

■ CASE STUDY QUESTIONS

1. How could Louise and her family's suffering been alleviated?

2. Why was it so hard to have someone listen to the family's wishes?

3. Why and how could this circumstance happen?

4. Would things have been different if the facility had a copy of the living will for all residents?

5. Why are end-of-life documents not standardized nationally?

6. Where might physical therapists assist with this issue?

7. What is a durable power of attorney for health care?

8. What is an advanced medical directive, also known as a living will?

9. How are advanced medical directives implemented?

10. When do you use living will or a durable power of attorney, and what is the difference?

11. Can you have both a living will and a health care power of attorney?

12. What are the disadvantages in not having a power of attorney?

13. How can we help our older adults navigate the process and establish their wishes, and how should they be honored in their last days?

REFERENCES

1. Miles SH, Koepp R. Advance end-of-life treatment planning: research review. *Arch Inter Med*. 1996;156(10):1062-1068.

2. Teno JM, Licks S. Do advance directives provide instruction that direct care? *J Am Geriatr Soc*. April 1997;45(4):508-512.

3. Ashby M, Wakefield M. General practitioners' knowledge and use of living wills. *Brit Med J*. January 1995;310:230.

4. Schonwetter R, Walker R. Life values, resuscitation preferences, and the applicability of living wills in an older population. *J Am Geriatr Soc*. August 1996;44(8):954-958.

5. Gordon M, Levitt D. Acting on a living will: a physician's dilemma. *Can Med Assoc J*. 1996;155(7):893-895.

6. Morrison S, Olson E. The inaccessibility of advance directives on transfer from ambulatory to acute care settings. *JAMA*. 1995;274(6):478-482.

7. Ashby M, Wakefield M. General practitioners' knowledge and use of living wills. *Brit Med J*. 1995;310(6974):230.

8. Hanson L, Danis M. What is wrong with end-of-life care? Opinions of bereaved family members. *J Am Geriatr Soc*. 1997;45(11):1339-1344.

9. Terry M, Steven Z. Prevalence of advance directives and do-not-resuscitate orders in community nursing facilities. *Arch Fam Med*. 1994;3(2):141-145.

END-OF-LIFE DECISIONS: CASE 2

William H. Staples, PT, DHSc, DPT, GCS, CEEAA

A couple that has been married for 60 years determines that is time to plan for the end of their lives. End-of-life decisions can be very difficult and they realize they need to find an attorney who will understand their wishes when the time comes. They have limited funds but want to ensure that they can be comfortable in their last years. They discuss several topics between themselves and their attorney.

■ CASE STUDY QUESTIONS

1. Are there attorneys who specialize in older adults?

2. What are advanced care directives?

3. What is a DNR?

4. What is a living will?

5. What is a physician orders for scope of treatment (POST), or physician orders for life-saving treatment (POLST)?

6. Do many people have or use an advanced care directive?

7. Who usually makes the decision to implement a DNR?

8. Where do people die, and what does it cost?

9. Do nursing home residents often get transferred to a hospital before they die?

10. What do people in the United States die from?

11. What is euthanasia?

12. What is assisted suicide?

13. What is hospice care?

14. What do terminally ill people want?

RESTRAINT ASSESSMENT

Cathy H. Ciolek, PT, DPT, GCS, CEEAA

James is an 84-year-old retired architect who never married and lives alone in an apartment with elevator access. He has a medical history of hypertension, hyperlipidemia, and type 2 diabetes currently, and a history of ankle fracture in his teens and humerus fracture as a child. He has intermittently used a rolling walker for the last 2 years when walking outside, but did not need one in the apartment. He was admitted to the hospital 1 week ago with abdominal pain and vomiting blood. The hospital workup determined that he had a peptic ulcer and he underwent an upper endoscopy 2 days later. During his recovery, it was noted that he had developed a fever, changes in mental status, and cloudy urine. He was diagnosed with a urinary tract infection (UTI) and was started on antibiotics 2 days ago. He was discharged to your skilled nursing facility last night and nursing has consulted physical therapy. The nurses note that he started having loose bowels during the previous night and was trying to get up and go to the bathroom without assistance.

Your evaluation shows an alert male who knows his name, date of birth, and state. He does not know the name of the facility. He is concerned with where the therapy bathroom is located. His medication list includes metoprolol for the hypertension, simvastatin for hyperlipidemia, Glucophage for the diabetes, and Cipro (ciprofloxacin) for the UTI.

On evaluation, you note he is able to tolerate resistance to manual muscle test in most major muscle groups against gravity. However, he fatigues easily and gets confused with directions of two steps or more. He tells you he has intermittently used a rolling walker for the last 2 years when walking outside, but did not need one in the apartment. Resting BP 134/90, HR 88, RR 13, SpO$_2$ 98%.

He requires three attempts to stand from the wheelchair when asked. The Berg Balance Score is 40/56. He does complete the TUG with close supervision with a rolling walker in 20 seconds. His 6-Minute Walk Test with the walker is 250 ft before he asks to stop and rest, at that point he notes a difficulty level of 7 on the 1-10 Borg (RPE) scale. Post 6-minute walk vitals: BP 142/92, HR 92, RR 16, SpO$_2$ 96%.

Nursing has requested that he have a bed with four side rails elevated and a seat belt on his wheelchair since he was trying to get up to go to the bathroom.

■ CASE STUDY QUESTIONS

1. Are restraints commonly used in health care facilities?

2. How is a physical restraint defined?

3. What are some examples of physical restraints?

4. What are some alternatives to restraints?

5. What are the primary negative sequelae of restraint use?

6. What is the APTA's position on restraints?

7. What is the position of other health professions regarding restraints?

8. What, if any, devices or restraint interventions are appropriate in this case?

9. What are the considerations needed in making this decision with the care team?

10. What do the outcome measures tell you about this individual at this moment?

11. What else should the physical therapist be concerned about?

NUTRITION AND AGING: MALNUTRITION

William H. Staples, PT, DHSc, DPT, GCS, CEEAA

A referral to your home health agency is an 85-year-old male who lives alone and has a diagnosis of "failure to thrive." He lives in a small apartment and lives on his Social Security check of $450 per month. He is 70 in tall and weighs 122 lb. His vital signs are HR 78 beats per minute, RR 16 breaths per minute, BP 118/72, SpO$_2$ 96%. The home health OASIS evaluation contains the Nutrition Checklist, which when completed scores an 8/21. Grossly his strength is 4/5, and ROM has no functional limitations. He ambulates independently in the home without an assistive device, although he occasionally grabs furniture for support as he walks. He tires easily and needs to rest after 2 minutes of active exercise. He is taking ibuprofen for

osteoarthritic knee pain, and an over-the-counter laxative as he has occasional constipation. He states that he sometimes has two to three beers at dinner time. He also states that he usually only has a bowel movement every 3 days or so. His last bowel movement was 2 days ago. His abdomen is not swollen or painful to palpation.

■ CASE STUDY QUESTIONS

1. What is the patient's BMI?

2. What are some of the physical barriers to adequate nutrition in aging adults?

3. What are some of the social and/or economic problems that could interfere with adequate nutrition in aging adults?

4. What did the Key Indicators of Well-Being (Older Americans 2012) state about nutrition in older adults?

5. What are the consequences of poor nutrition?

6. Certain components of diet and nutrition are more critical to healthy aging. Why is vitamin B$_6$ important?

7. Certain components of diet and nutrition are more critical to healthy aging. Why is vitamin B$_{12}$ important?

8. Certain components of diet and nutrition are more critical to healthy aging. Why is folic acid important?

9. Certain components of diet and nutrition are more critical to healthy aging. Why is vitamin D important?

10. What is MyPlate for Older Adults?

11. What is the Nutrition Checklist, and how can it be used?

12. Is this patient in need of outside nutritional help?

13. What major categories do the questions of the nutritional checklist cover?

14. What is protein-energy malnutrition (PEM)?

15. What do infrequent bowel movements have to do with poor nutrition?

16. You determine that the patient needs additional nutrition, what can you do?

17. Would vigorous exercise be important for this patient?

PAYMENT CASE STUDY: PART 1

Acute Care Hospital

William H. Staples, PT, DHSc, DPT, GCS, CEEAA

Writing a case study about Medicare payment is a risk because the laws, rules, and payment schedules change often. I have done the best under the current guidelines, but some of the answers may be altered by subsequent health care regulation changes.

Mrs Smith is an 82-year-old woman (retired secretary) living alone (widowed for 2 years) in a two-story, one-bedroom walk-up apartment on the east side of Indianapolis. The closest market and pharmacy are more than a mile from her home. She receives $690.00 from social security (before any government fees—hint Part B) every month. Her rent is $500.00/month; medications (after insurance—Medicare Part D) cost her $110.00/month. Her daughter, who lives in Chicago with her husband and three children, sends her mom $300.00 per month. She has Medicare Parts A and B. She has a supplemental insurance from AARP that costs $800.00 per year. She has meager savings of only $1500.00, because she spent a lot of money caring for her husband in the last 2 years of his life after he suffered a severe CVA.

Mrs Smith has a medical history of osteoporosis, osteoarthritis, congestive heart failure (CHF), non-insulin-dependent diabetes mellitus (NIDDM), depression, and atherosclerotic heart disease (ASHD). She received six sessions of outpatient physical therapy (Medicare paid $600) 2 months ago (this calendar year) for adhesive capsulitis in her right shoulder.

She fell in her apartment this morning, with a resultant closed femoral neck fracture. A neighbor called 911 this afternoon when she returned home from work, hearing Mrs Smith's screams for help.

The Medicare payment for the DRG for a fractured hip is $20,000. The cost of the hospital is $3500/day to care for Mrs Smith. She underwent an open reduction internal fixation (ORIF) for the left femoral neck fracture with a compression screw and plate the night of admission. The referral to physical therapy is to evaluate and treat NWB left lower extremity.

■ CASE STUDY QUESTIONS

1. How do you qualify for Medicare Part A?
2. What type of care is covered under Part A?
3. How much do Medicare Part A cost her per year?
4. What is a DRG?
5. How is therapy reimbursed? Be specific.
6. How much will Mrs Smith have to pay out of pocket?
7. Are there funds she could obtain to assist her?
8. Are there any requirements for reimbursement?
9. What is the ICD-10 code for this diagnosis?
10. What would be the physical therapy diagnosis?
11. What is the episode of care?
12. What are CPT codes, and what proposed interventions with appropriate CPT/HCPCS codes will be used?
13. What assistive devices or equipment are needed?
14. What is your proposed frequency, number of visits? Why?
15. What is the proposed length of stay? Why?
16. What impairments and functional limitations are present?
17. When should discharge occur? Where will she go?
18. What cost containment methods will be used by facility? By you?
19. Does the patient have other needs (outside the scope of direct interventions) that need to be addressed?
20. Do you see any ethical questions or dilemmas?
21. Would you recommend referral to another professional? Why?

10

PAYMENT CASE STUDY: PART 2

Inpatient Rehabilitation Facility

William H. Staples, PT, DHSc, DPT, GCS, CEEAA

Writing a case study about Medicare payment is a risk because the laws, rules, and payment schedules change often. I have done the best under the current guidelines, but some of the answers may be altered by subsequent health care regulation changes.

Mrs Smith is an 82-year-old woman (retired secretary) living alone (widowed for 2 years) in a two-story, one-bedroom walk-up apartment on the east side of Indianapolis. The closest market and pharmacy are more than a mile from her home. She receives $690.00 from social security (before any government fees—hint Part B) every month. Her rent is $500.00/month; medications (after insurance—Medicare Part D) cost her $110.00/month. Her daughter, who lives in Chicago with her husband and three children, sends her mom $300.00 per month. She has Medicare Parts A and B. She has a supplemental insurance from AARP that costs $800.00 per year. She has meager savings of only $1500.00, because she spent a lot of money caring for her husband in the last 2 years of his life after he suffered a severe CVA.

Mrs Smith has a medical history of osteoporosis, osteoarthritis, congestive heart failure (CHF), non-insulin-dependent diabetes mellitus (NIDDM), depression, and atherosclerotic heart disease (ASHD). She received six sessions of outpatient physical therapy (Medicare paid $600) 2 months ago (this calendar year) for adhesive capsulitis in her right shoulder.

She fell in her apartment this morning, with a resultant closed femoral neck fracture. A neighbor called 911 this afternoon when she returned home from work, hearing Mrs Smith's screams for help.

The Medicare hospital inpatient payment for the DRG for a fractured hip is $20,000. The cost of the hospital is $3500/day to care for Mrs Smith. She underwent an open reduction internal fixation (ORIF) for the left femoral neck fracture with a compression screw and plate the night of admission. The referral to physical therapy is to evaluate and treat NWB left lower extremity.

An inpatient rehabilitation facility/hospital (IRF) at first denies admission secondary to inability to tolerate enough hours of therapy per day but relents with pressure from social worker (MSW) and the physician to a 1-week trial (ramp-up) program.

She now has orders for toe-touch weight bearing (TTWB) left lower extremity (LLE). The IRF will receive $12,000 to care for Mrs Smith and it will cost the facility $750 per day to care for her.

■ CASE STUDY QUESTIONS

1. Who would pay for the stay at the inpatient rehabilitation hospital?
2. What is the 75% rule, and does she qualify under those guidelines?
3. Are there any exceptions to the 75% rule?
4. How are inpatient rehabilitation facilities paid under Medicare?
5. How is therapy reimbursed? Be specific.
6. How much will Mrs Smith have to pay out of pocket?
7. Are there funds she could obtain to assist her?
8. How many hours of therapy must a patient participate in to qualify?
9. Are there any other requirements for reimbursement?
10. What is a ramp-up program?
11. What is the ICD-10 code for this diagnosis?
12. What would be the physical therapy diagnosis?
13. What is the episode of care?
14. What are CPT codes, and what proposed interventions with appropriate CPT/HCPCS codes will be used?
15. What assistive devices or equipment are needed?
16. What is your proposed frequency, number of visits? Why?
17. What is the proposed length of stay? Why?
18. What impairments and functional limitations are present?

19. What cost containment methods will be used by facility? By you?

20. Does the patient have other needs (outside the scope of direct interventions) that need to be addressed?

21. Do you see any ethical questions or dilemmas?

22. Would you recommend referral to another professional? Why?

23. She develops thrombophlebitis in left lower extremity in the first week and is rehospitalized for 6 days. What happens to reimbursement at the hospital?

24. After the rehospitalization, she discharged to a skilled nursing facility, what happens to reimbursement at the rehabilitation hospital?

11

PAYMENT CASE STUDY: PART 3

Skilled Nursing Facility

William H. Staples, PT, DHSc, DPT, GCS, CEEAA

Writing a case study about Medicare payment is a risk because the laws, rules, and payment schedules change often. I have done the best under the current guidelines, but some of the answers may be altered by subsequent health care regulation changes.

Mrs Smith is an 82-year-old woman (retired secretary) living alone (widowed for 2 years) in a two-story, one-bedroom walk-up apartment on the east side of Indianapolis. The closest market and pharmacy are more than a mile from her home. She receives $690.00 from social security (before any government fees—hint Part B) every month. Her rent is $500.00/month; medications (after insurance—Medicare Part D) cost her $110.00/month. Her daughter, who lives in Chicago with her husband and three children, sends her mom $300.00 per month. She has Medicare Parts A and B. She has a supplemental insurance from AARP that costs $800.00 per year. She has meager savings of only $1500.00, because she spent a lot of money caring for her husband in the last 2 years of his life after he suffered a severe CVA.

Mrs Smith has a medical history of osteoporosis, osteoarthritis, congestive heart failure (CHF), non-insulin-dependent diabetes mellitus (NIDDM), depression, and atherosclerotic heart disease (ASHD). She received six sessions of outpatient physical therapy (Medicare paid $600) 2 months ago (this calendar year) for adhesive capsulitis in her right shoulder.

She fell in her apartment this morning, with a resultant closed femoral neck fracture. A neighbor called 911 this afternoon when she returned home from work, hearing Mrs Smith's screams for help.

She underwent an open reduction internal fixation (ORIF) for the left femoral neck fracture with a compression screw and plate the night of admission. She was treated in an inpatient hospital for 5 days.

She is admitted to a skilled nursing facility (SNF), the new referral to physical therapy is to evaluate and treat NWB left lower extremity. The patient can progress to WBAT at 8 weeks post-op. The evaluating therapist scheduled the patient to receive 500 minutes of therapy per week under RUGS pattern RVB (very high).

■ CASE STUDY QUESTIONS

1. Who would pay for the stay at skilled nursing facility?

2. What qualifies someone for a Medicare Part A stay in an SNF?

3. How is therapy reimbursed? Be specific.

4. What is an MDS?

5. What is an RUGs classification?

6. What are the major classifications of RUGs?

7. How are the rehabilitation RUGs groups further subclassified?

8. How much will Mrs Smith have to pay out of pocket?

9. Are there funds she could obtain to assist her?

10. Are there any requirements for reimbursement?

11. What is the ICD-10 code for this diagnosis?

12. What would be the physical therapy diagnosis?

13. What is the episode of care?

14. What are CPT codes, and what proposed interventions with appropriate CPT/HCPCS codes will be used?

15. What assistive devices or equipment are needed?

16. What is your proposed frequency, number of visits? Why?

17. What is the proposed length of stay? Why?

18. What impairments and functional limitations are present?

19. When should discharge occur? Where will she go?

20. What cost containment methods will be used by facility? By you?

21. Does the patient have other needs (outside the scope of direct interventions) that need to be addressed?

22. Do you see any ethical questions or dilemmas?

23. Would you recommend referral to another professional? Why?

12

PAYMENT CASE STUDY: PART 4

Home Health Care

William H. Staples, PT, DHSc, DPT, GCS, CEEAA

Writing a case study about Medicare payment is a risk because the laws, rules, and payment schedules change often. I have done the best under the current guidelines, but some of the answers may be altered by subsequent health care regulation changes.

Mrs Smith is an 82-year-old woman (retired secretary) living alone (widowed for 2 years) in a two-story, one-bedroom walk-up apartment on the east side of Indianapolis. The closest market and pharmacy are more than a mile from her home. She receives $690.00 from social security (before any government fees—hint Part B) every month. Her rent is $500.00/month; medications (after insurance—Medicare Part D) cost her $110.00/month. Her daughter, who lives in Chicago with her husband and three children, sends her mom $300.00 per month. She has Medicare Parts A and B. She has a supplemental insurance from AARP that costs $800.00 per year. She has meager savings of only $1500.00, because she spent a lot of money caring for her husband in the last 2 years of his life after he suffered a severe CVA.

Mrs Smith has a medical history of osteoporosis, osteoarthritis, congestive heart failure (CHF), non-insulin-dependent diabetes mellitus (NIDDM), depression, and atherosclerotic heart disease (ASHD). She received six sessions of outpatient physical therapy (Medicare paid $600) 2 months ago (this calendar year) for adhesive capsulitis in her right shoulder.

She fell in her apartment this morning, with a resultant closed femoral neck fracture. A neighbor called 911 this afternoon when she returned home from work, hearing Mrs Smith's screams for help.

Mrs Smith underwent an open reduction internal fixation (ORIF) for the left femoral neck fracture with a compression screw and plate 8 weeks ago. She spent 1 week in an acute care hospital followed by 8 weeks in a skilled nursing facility. She now has a referral to home health physical therapy is to evaluate and treat with new orders for weight bearing as tolerated (WBAT) for the left lower extremity.

You are the case manager and are sent to open the case and complete the OASIS. She is now full weight bearing on the left lower extremity.

■ CASE STUDY QUESTIONS

1. Who would pay for the home health care?

2. How much does Medicare Part A cost her per year?

3. How are home health agencies paid under Medicare?

4. What is the OASIS?

5. Who can be a case manager and open a Medicare Part A home care patient?

6. What are the responsibilities of the case manager?

7. How is therapy reimbursed? Be specific.

8. How much will Mrs Smith have to pay out of pocket?

9. Are there funds she could obtain to assist her?

10. Are there any requirements for reimbursement?

11. How does Medicare define "homebound?"

12. What is the ICD-10 code for this diagnosis?

13. What would be the physical therapy diagnosis?

14. What is the episode of care?

15. What are CPT codes, and what proposed interventions with appropriate CPT/HCPCS codes will be used?

16. What would be a very important factor in your evaluation?

17. What assistive devices or equipment are needed?

18. What is your proposed frequency, number of visits? Why?

19. What impairments and functional limitations are present?

20. When should discharge occur? Where will she go?

21. What cost containment methods will be used by facility? By you?

22. Does the patient have other needs (outside the scope of direct interventions) that need to be addressed?

23. Do you see any ethical questions or dilemmas?

24. Would you recommend referral to another professional? Why?

13

PAYMENT CASE STUDY: PART 5

Outpatient Therapy

William H. Staples, PT, DHSc, DPT, GCS, CEEAA

Writing a case study about Medicare payment is a risk because the laws, rules, and payment schedules change often. I have done the

best under the current guidelines, but some of the answers may be altered by subsequent health care regulation changes.

Mrs Smith is an 82-year-old woman (retired secretary) living alone (widowed for 2 years) in a two-story, one-bedroom walk-up apartment on the east side of Indianapolis. The closest market and pharmacy are more than a mile from her home. She receives $690.00 from social security (before any government fees—hint Part B) every month. Her rent is $500.00/month; medications (after insurance—Medicare Part D) cost her $110.00/month. Her daughter, who lives in Chicago with her husband and three children, sends her mom $300.00 per month. She has Medicare Parts A and B. She has a supplemental insurance from AARP that costs $800.00 per year. She has meager savings of only $1500.00, because she spent a lot of money caring for her husband in the last 2 years of his life after he suffered a severe CVA.

Mrs Smith has a medical history of osteoporosis, osteoarthritis, congestive heart failure (CHF), non-insulin-dependent diabetes mellitus (NIDDM), depression, and atherosclerotic heart disease (ASHD). She received six sessions of outpatient physical therapy (Medicare paid $600) 2 months ago (this calendar year) for adhesive capsulitis in her right shoulder.

She fell in her apartment this morning, with a resultant closed femoral neck fracture. A neighbor called 911 this afternoon when she returned home from work, hearing Mrs Smith's screams for help.

She underwent an open reduction internal fixation (ORIF) for the left femoral neck fracture with a compression screw and plate. She has been through rehabilitation at a skilled SNF for 8 weeks, followed by two to three times/week for 4 weeks home health physical therapy. She is full weight bearing and ambulates independently with a cane. She wants to continue therapy as an outpatient to continue to strengthen her lower extremities and reduce the risk for future falls.

■ CASE STUDY QUESTIONS

1. How do you qualify for Medicare Part B?

2. What type of care is covered under Part B?

3. How much does Medicare Part B cost her per year?

4. How are outpatient rehabilitation facilities/clinics paid under Medicare Part B?

5. How much will Mrs Smith have to pay out of pocket?

6. Are there funds she could obtain to assist her?

7. Are there any requirements for reimbursement?

8. What is the ICD-10 code for this diagnosis?

9. What would be the physical therapy diagnosis?

10. What is the episode of care?

11. What are CPT codes, and what proposed interventions with appropriate CPT/HCPCS codes will be used?

12. What is the "rule of 8s?"

13. What are G-codes?

14. What is your proposed frequency, number of visits? Why?

15. What impairments and functional limitations are present?

16. What functional tests would you perform?

17. When should discharge occur?

18. What are some examples of durable medical equipment that are paid for by Medicare Part B?

19. What cost containment methods will be used by facility? By you?

20. Does the patient have other needs (outside the scope of direct interventions) that need to be addressed?

21. Do you see any ethical questions or dilemmas?

22. Would you recommend referral to another professional? Why?

14

SUICIDE

William H. Staples, PT, DHSc, DPT, GCS, CEEAA

A home health referral is made for a 78-year-old white male with worsening Parkinson disease that has been decreasing his functional abilities. He is married and lives with his wife of 42 years. His physician has just increased his Sinemet (carbidopa levodopa) due to increased rigidity and bradykinesia. He has also been taking Requip (ropinirole) since his diagnosis 10 years ago. He was also just started on Paxil (paroxetine).

On evaluation, the patient has a flat affect, is slow to respond, but answers all questions except for a few where he cannot remember some of his medical and social history. He has slight cogwheel-type rigidity and his bilateral ROM limitations are as follows:

	Passive ROM	Active ROM
Shoulder flexion	0°-135°	0°-110°
Shoulder abduction	0°-120°	0°-105°
Hip extension	0°	0°
Ankle plantar flexion	20°	14°
Ankle dorsiflexion	12°	5°

The limitations in shoulder flexion and abduction are affected by a moderately severe kyphosis and forward head posture. A wall to occiput measure is 5.5 cm. Manual muscle test is 5/5 in all four extremities except for hip extensors and quadriceps, which are 4−/5.

There is a slight tremor in the right hand and reflexes are 3+ in the upper extremities and 2+ in the lower extremities. Sensation to light touch is intact. A Timed Up and Go Test takes 19.3 seconds, but the patient takes several attempts to get up from the chair accounting for half of the time. Once standing, the gait is safe and the steps are short and wide-based, and he does not require an assistive device. Single leg stance time is 3 seconds on the right and 2 seconds on the left. He also states that he feels "tired all the time."

The patient first states that his goals would be able to do yard work "since I feel pretty useless around the house." When asked about something he thought would be more reasonable to start with he says, "I want to be able to get my cereal box out of the kitchen cabinet." When asked why he does not just leave them on the kitchen counter, the wife interjects strongly stating, "The cereal boxes belong in the cupboard not the counter!"

You finish the evaluation; give the patient a few exercises to help with single leg stance, hip extension, and posture (wall standing). You suggest the purchase of a three-step step-stool that has a bar for balance that you saw at a home store, and will work on the cereal issue on the next visit.

You return 2 days later and the patient's wife has purchased the three-step step-stool that has a bar to hold onto for balance. The patient is not overly enthused about learning how to use the step stool. Several trials using moderate assist and verbal were used to get up and down two steps. You also begin to realize that the relationship between the husband and wife is strained as she complains about everything she has to do for the patient.

On your third visit, the patient remains very passive and somewhat unmotivated. Then the conversation leads to a common interest of coin collecting and the patient's attitude changes for the positive and he makes progress in using the step stool. On your fourth visit, the patient has much of his coin collection spread out on the table and you spend several minutes looking through the collection and discussing some rare coins. The collection is obviously worth thousands of dollars. The patient says that this used to be his pride and joy but has lost interest in it lately due to his disability. Eventually, you work on the balance and strengthening exercises and the patient continues to make progress.

After 3 weeks, the patient is almost safe and independent with using the step stool you ask the patient what else he would like to accomplish and he says that he wants to play catch. As a therapist, you think this would be great for standing balance, rotational movements, and coordination. Luckily you have a light-weight ball and play catch with him able to toss a ball underhand for almost 10 ft. Before leaving, the patient states that he knows that you really enjoyed his coin collection and asked if you would want it. At first, you go wow in your head, but then realize that it would be highly unethical to take a gift from a current patient, and while graciously thanking him you explain why you could not possibly take the gift.

You get a call from the home health agency the next day telling you that the patient took the step-stool out to the garage and thrown a rope over the beam and hung himself to death. You are very upset with this turn of events and decide to investigate suicide.

■ CASE STUDY QUESTIONS

1. What is Paxil?
2. How common is depression in the elderly?
3. What are the signs and symptoms of depression?
4. What is a good way to screen for depression?
5. Can patients with depression take Paxil with their Parkinson medications?
6. What are the side effects of SSRI antidepressants?
7. How well do SSRI antidepressants work to cure depression?
8. How long does it take before an SSRI antidepressant starts to work?
9. Is suicide common in older adults?
10. Who commits suicide?
11. Are suicide rates for older adults underestimated?
12. Are there any clues or signs that a person may be considering suicide?
13. Are older adults more likely to succeed in suicide than younger people?
14. Will talking about suicide increase the risk for it?
15. What should you do if you expect that someone is considering suicide?
16. Do people residing in nursing homes have depression?

15

TELEHEALTH—THE FUTURE?

William H. Staples, PT, DHSc, DPT, GCS, CEEAA

A nurse has opened a new home health patient and believes that the person would benefit from physical therapy. The patient lives on a rural farm almost 50 miles from the agency's office.

The patient is a 63-year-old woman with diagnoses of diabetes mellitus, obesity, congestive heart failure, and osteoarthritis in both knees. The home health agency has installed home monitoring equipment for vital signs and weight via a phone line, and the patient has a laptop computer, which she knows how to operate. Besides daily monitoring of the vital signs, the agency will do a "televisit" once weekly. Her current vital signs are HR 78, RR 20, BP 148/90, SpO_2 95%, her weight 247 is lb, and blood sugar is 120 mg/dL. The patient is 5 ft 6 in tall and is taking the following medications: Novolin (insulin) injection 70/30 bid, Cardizem (diltiazem) 180 mg bid, and Aleve (naproxen) 375 mg bid. The pain in her knees at rest is 2/10 but increases to 5/10 when ambulating and 7/10 while attempting stairs. She ambulates in her home independently with a cane but struggles going up and down the stairs due to pain and weakness, even with handrails and the cane. Although she might benefit from bilateral total knee replacements, her physician will not operate until she loses 30 lb. Her insurance company will not pay for a power-operated vehicle.

The agency would like you to make "televisits" as well to cut the cost of drive time and mileage, and improve your productivity. At the time of writing this question, telehealth for nursing and physical therapy has become a reality and may be a much bigger part of the future of health care. The following questions will help guide you through the process.

■ CASE STUDY QUESTIONS

1. Is it possible to perform physical therapy by way of the Internet?

2. Are all patients appropriate for telehealth physical therapy?

3. What are some of the operational/technological needs to utilize telehealth?

4. What are some of the legal requirements for setting up a patient for telehealth visits?

5. What needs to be in your documentation?

6. Do insurances/Medicare pay for telehealth?

7. Why would a therapist/clinic/agency consider utilizing telehealth to provide services?

8. If your home health agency is in one state, can you treat a patient through telehealth who resides in a different state?

9. What is an interstate compact agreement? What does this have to do with health care?

10. What items would you include in a problem list for this patient?

11. What is the patient's body mass index (BMI)?

12. What interventions could you utilize to improve her problem list?

13. Are there any guidelines regarding telehealth?

14. Are any organizations currently using telehealth?

15. What is the risk for liability using telehealth?

INDEX